AF429427

SERIES

Student's Companion

Medicinal Chemistry - III

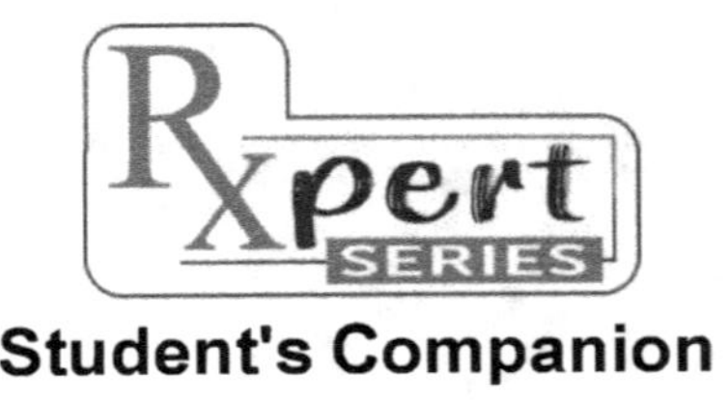

Student's Companion

Medicinal Chemistry - III

Manoj Kumar Dalai

Biswaranjan Behara

Biswakanth Kar

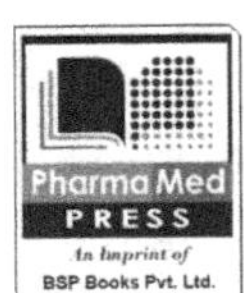

PharmaMed Press

An imprint of BSP Books Pvt. Ltd.

4-4-309/316, Giriraj Lane,

Sultan Bazar, Hyderabad - 500 095.

Medicinal Chemistry - III

by Manoj Kumar Dalai, Biswaranjan Behara and Biswakanth Kar

© 2024, *by Publisher*

Disclaimer: The authors and the publishers have taken due care to provide the authentic, reliable and up to date information related to the subject. However, neither the authors nor the publisher shall be responsible for any liability for any damage caused as a result of use of this book. The respective user must check the accuracy from other sources too.

Published by

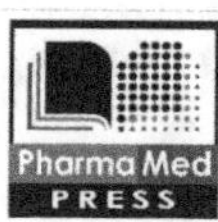

PharmaMed Press

An imprint of BSP Books Pvt. Ltd.

4-4-309/316, Giriraj Lane, Sultan Bazar, Hyderabad - 500 095.

Phone: 040-23445688; Fax: 91+40-23445611

E-mail: info@pharmamedpress.net

www.bspbooks.net/www.pharmamedpress.net

ISBN: 978-93-95039-61-1 (Hardback)

Preface

Medicinal chemistry is a branch of science that combines chemistry and pharmacy to study the design and development of medicinal drugs. Medicinal chemistry encompasses the discovery, synthesis, and development of novel chemical substances with therapeutic potential. It also includes researching existing drugs, their biological features, and drug structure-activity correlations. This book aims to simplify medicinal chemistry so that aspiring graduates can understand the importance of drug design. The enormous scientific effort in the field of drug design that has been performed recently has altered the entire notion of medicinal chemistry.

- Authors

Contents

CHAPTER 1

Antibiotics-I

CHAPTER 2

Antibiotics-II

CHAPTER 3

Anti-Tubercular Agents, Urinary Tract Anti-Infective Agents, Antiviral Agents

CHAPTER 4

Antifungal Agents Anti-protozoal Agents Anthelmintics Sulphonamides and Sulfones

CHAPTER 5

INTRODUCTION TO DRUG DESIGN AND COMBINATORIAL CHEMISTRY

CHAPTER 1

ANTIBIOTICS - I

1.1 β-Lactam Antibiotics

Definition

Medicinal Chemistry: It deals with the discovery, design, development and both pharmacological and analytical characterization of drug substances.

Drug: A chemical substance used in the treatment, cure, prevention or diagnosis of disease.

Antibiotic: These are chemical substances produced by various species of microorganisms that, in small concentrations, destroy or inhibit the growth of other species of microorganisms.

- ✓ Antibiotics; the term is extended to synthetic antibacterial agents such as sulphonamides and quinolones.
- ✓ Bacteria, fungi, and actinomycetes are the various species from which antibiotics are produced.

Historical Background

- ✓ Chinese people (500-600 BC) used molded curd to treat boils and carbuncles (a red, swollen, and painful cluster of boils that appeared under the skin).
- ✓ In the meantime, the **science of bacteriology** (the study of bacteria and their relation to medicine) was developed. During studies, it has been observed that microorganisms are capable of producing some therapeutic (relating to the healing of disease) agents.
- ✓ In the year 1877 - **Louis Pasteur & Joubert** found that an injection of *anthrax bacillus* into lab animals did not produce any harmful effect and did not have the deadly effect if common bacteria were injected along with it.
- ✓ After 1929 - the modern history of antibiotics was started.
- ✓ **Sir Alexander flaming** (Fig. 1.1), a British bacteriologist, detected a chemical substance from *Penicillium notatum* (a species of fungus in the genus *Penicillium*) which have bacteriostatic in nature. Later, another researcher developed the preparation and structure of the active compound that produced from the mould.

- ✓ 1941 - The **Penicillin** was first used clinically as an antibacterial agent.

- ✓ 1944 - **Selman A Waksman** (Fig. 1. 8) isolated streptomycin from *Streptomyces griseus* (*Actinomycete* species). After that large number of antibiotics were discovered by other scientist. These includes natural origin and semisynthetic (structural analogues of natural origin) antibiotics. While a very small proportion of antibiotics have shown therapeutic value.

- ✓ The efficacy, toxicity, stability, economics of production, and rendering into suitable formulation are the parameters that should meet the acceptance of new antibiotics products. After successful evaluation, the new antibiotics are included in different pharmacoapeias as monograph.

Nature of antibiotics: Either, it has shown as **bactericidal** and **bacteriostatic** in nature.

Bacteriostatic: An antibiotic reversibly inhibits the growth of susceptible microorganisms.

Bactericidal: Antibiotics shall kill or destroy the microbes in *in vitro*.

Antibacterial property of antibiotic in concentration label: At low concentration antibiotic produces **bacteriostatic** action. While, at certain or higher concentration antibiotic produces **bactericidal** action.

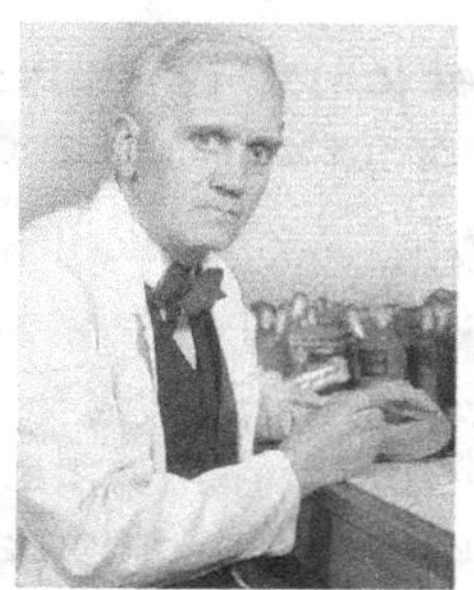

Fig. **1.1** Sir Alexander Fleming at St Mary's, Hospital, London (1943).

Drawbacks of frequent use of antibiotics: Microbial resistance may develop during prolonged use of antibiotics. Microbes could develop resistance to one antibiotic and another antibiotic, termed "cross-resistance". The resistance develops due to a stable genetic change that passes from generation to generation.

Classification

1. **On the basis of antimicrobial properties:**

   (a) **Narrow spectrum antibiotics:** These types of antibiotics are effective against a few species of bacteria, gram-positive or gram-negative, fungi, or protozoa.

   (b) **Broad-spectrum antibiotics:** These types of antibiotics are effective against a variety of microorganisms, including both gram-positive and gram-negative bacteria, rickettsia, and even protozoa.

2. **On the basis of chemical classification:**

   (a) Amino acid derivatives: Ex. cycloserine and chloramphenicol

   (b) β-lactam ring containing antibiotic (Natural): Ex. benzylpenicillin, procaine penicillin

   (c) Semisynthetic penicillin: Ex. ampicillin, amoxycillin, cloxacillin

   (d) Cephalosporin group antibiotic: Ex. cephalosporin group also called as "C family"

(i) First generation: Ex. cephaloridine, cefatrizine

(ii) Second generation: Ex. cefoxitin

(iii) Third generation: Ex. cefotaxime

(iv) Fourth generation: Ex. cefepime

(e) Non-β-lactam ring containing antibiotic: Ex. imipenem

(f) β-lactamase inhibitor: Ex. clavulanic acid

(g) Polypeptide antibiotic: Ex. bacitracin A, polymyxin B

(h) Aminoglycoside antibiotic- derived from sugars: Ex. gentamicin, amikacin, tobramycin, neomycin, and streptomycin

(i) Derived from acetate or propionate unit: Ex. tetracycline, oxytetracycline, chlortetracycline

(j) Fusidic acid containing antibiotic: Ex. clindamycin, vancomycin

(k) Macrolide ring containing antibiotic: Ex. Erythromycin, azithromycin, clarithromycin

(l) Miscellaneous: chloramphenicol

1.1.1 Penicillin

Historical Background

- ✓ **Penicillin** was the first & most important group of antibiotics.

- ✓ In 1928- **Sir Alexander Fleming** (worked at Saint Mary's Hospital. London (Fig. 1.1) of Scotland observed that a mould (*Penicillium notatum*) contaminated culture medium (*Penicillium notatum*) prevented the growth of *staphylococcal* bacterial in the culture media. Later, he identified that the mould has antibacterial properties. Thereafter, the chemical substance is named Penicillin, Penicillin II, or Penicillin G.

- ✓ In 1938 - **Howard Walter Flory** (an Australian pharmacologist and pathologist), **Ernest Boris Chain** (German refugee & a German-British biochemist), and **Edward Abraham** (an English biochemist) found that the crude material of the mould had antibacterial properties against *streptococcal* infected mice. They won a Nobel Prize in 1945 with Fleming.

- ✓ In 1941 - Penicillin has undergone a clinical trial. The first dose of penicillin was administered to a policeman at Oxford, who suffered from mixed *staphylococcal* and *streptococcal* infection.

- ✓ Same year, penicillin was produced by the deep fermentation process at the Northern Regional Research Laboratory, USA, and a clinical trial was held at Yale University and the Mayo Clinic in 1942. The penicillin was named as **Penicillin I** or **Penicillin F**.

- ✓ The yield of penicillin from *Penicillium notatum* was low, and it was replaced by *P. chrysogenum*

- ✓ 1943 - The chemical structure of penicillin was determined by **Sir Robert Robinson** of Oxford and **Karl Folkers** of Merck.
- ✓ 1957 - Penicillin was synthesized by **John Sheehan** and **K R Henery-Logan** of MIT, USA.

Nomenclature: Basic Chemical Structure of Penicillin ring

The basic structure of penicillin consists of a thiazolidine ring which is fused with a β-lactam ring, and there is a side chain at the C-6 position (Fig.1. 2).

Structure-Activity Relationship of Penicillin group (Fig.1.2)

1. Substitution at R = $C_6H_5CH_2$ group obtained as a **Benzyl Penicillin** or **Penicillin G** which occurs from *P. notatum*. It is a narrow spectrum of antibiotic and only natural occurring penicillin and used as clinically.

2. By substituting R = $C_6H_5OCH_2$ (2-Phenoxymethyl) group at C-6; forms a new antibiotic product known as Penicillin V, and the resultant compound shows antimicrobial activity.

3. A wide range of penicillin has been prepared by changing substitutions in the 6-amino group of penicillin.

Example of Penicillin compound	Chemical Name	R = Substitution group
Benzyl Penicillin	6-(2-Phenylacetamido) penicillinic acid	$C_6H_5CH_2$--
Phenoxy methyl Penicillin or Penicillin - V	6-(2-Phenoxyacelamido) penicillinic acid	$C_6H_5OCH_2$--
Ampicillin	6-(α-D-Phenylglycylamino) Penicillic acid	NH_2 ...CH—
Amoxycillin	6-(α-D-P-hydroxy Phenyl glycylamino) Penicillic acid	HO— ...NH_2 ...C H
Cloxacillin	6-(3-(2-chlorophenyl)5-methylisoxazol-4-carboxamido)penicillinic acid	Cl ...N O ...CH_3

Fig. 1.2 General Structure of Penicillin and their derivatives.

4. The acylated product of penicillin is termed semisynthetic penicillin. The nature of the acyl group (C=OR) has a significant effect on properties of the penicillin. The derived product has greater acid stability and resistance against penicillinase-producing bacteria. Hence, they are termed as a broader spectrum of antibiotics.

5. Methicillin was the first product of the penicillin group which shows resistance against penicillinase-producing *staphylococcal* bacteria. There are several aromatic (ampicillin) and heteroaromatic (oxacillin, carbenicillin, amoxycillin, etc.) substitutions in the C6-amino group that are more active than benzylpenicillin. However, they are not resistant to penicillinase enzyme-producing bacteria.

6. D--amino phenyl acetamido side chain of ampicillin has shown acid stability and is effective against gram-ve bacteria. While *P*-hydroxyl of benzene nucleus of amoxycillin shows better absorption in GIT.

7. S-atom at position 1 & N at 5 positions of the penicillin is essential for antibacterial activity.

8. Dimethyl group at C-2 of penicillin possesses antibacterial activity.

Chemical Degradation of Penicillin (Fig.1.3)

1. Penicillin is a strong monobasic acid. The free acid in penicillin is unstable.

2. The dry form of penicillin salt (either with an alkali metal or organic acid) is stable. The breakdown of the chemical structure of penicillin occurs under different conditions, such as biochemical and chemical processes.

3. The enzyme penicillinase or in the presence of an alkali, brake up the β-lactam system. Penicillin forms penicilloic acid, which on further heating, undergoes decarboxylate to form penilloic acid. This acid was then reacted with $HgCl_2$ to produce penilloaldehyde.

4. In a dilute acid solution (pH 5.0), intermolecular rearrangement occurs which forms penilic acids. This acid was then reacted with $HgCl_2$ to produce penillamine.

5. In the presence of strong mineral acids or mercuric chloride break up the thiazolidine ring. Thus, penicillin forms penicillamine and penaldic acid (unstable state). The unstable state of penaldic acid on further reaction with penilloaldehyde to form the desired product.

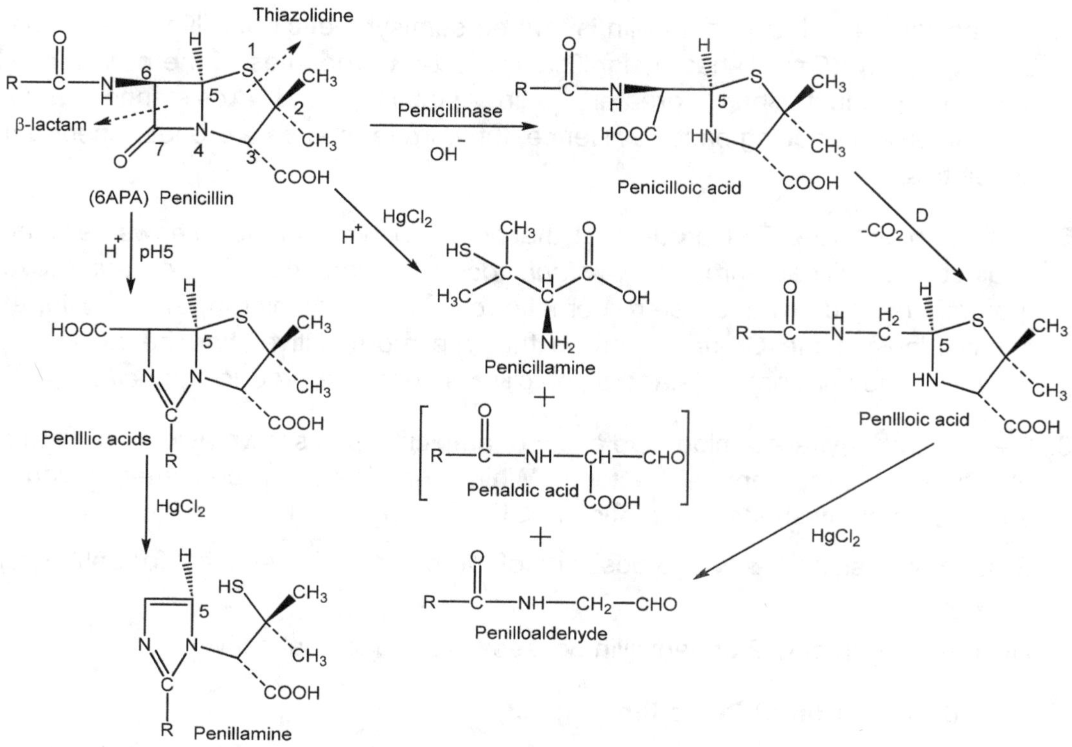

Fig. 1.3 Break down product of Penicillin.

Mechanism of Action of Antibiotic

Each class of antibiotic has a different type of mechanism of action. Some may have disorganized cell walls that cause loss of viability, which leads to cell death. Others may act on the cell membrane of the microorganism. Certain types of antibiotics affect the function of ribosomes and cause reversible inhibition of protein synthesis. Some antibiotics affect the function of the 30S or 50S subunits of the ribosome and change protein synthesis. Another type of antibiotic may affect nucleic acid metabolism.

Mechanism of Action of Penicillin

The term penicillin is used generically for the entire group of penicillins (prepared from biosynthetic or semisynthetic sources). They are usually bactericidal. They have inhibitory effects on the synthesis of the bacterial cell wall. The biological half-life is 30-60 minutes (a short period). They are well absorbed and widely distributed throughout the body. They are rapidly eliminated through glomerular filtration and renal tubular secretion.

Benzylpenicillin could be considered the parent compound of the penicillin family. It is active against gram-+ve bacteria, gram-ve *cocci*, *actinomycetes*, and *spirochetes*. In the presence of gastric acid, it becomes unstable and inactivated by bacteria that produce penicillinase-producing bacteria. **Penicillin V** is acid stable.

β-lactam Antibiotics inhibit peptidoglycan synthesis. Peptidoglycan is a heteropolymeric component of the cell wall. It is essential for the normal growth and development of bacteria. This provides mechanical stability for a highly cross-linked structure. It inhibits the enzyme transpeptidase and makes it inactive. So the synthesis of peptidoglycan is inhibited.

Uses:

- ✓ Treatment of *streptococcal* infection & rheumatic fever.
- ✓ Used in less sever types of microbial infection & UTI.

1.1.2 Cephalosporins

Historical Background

- ✓ Cephalosporins were discovered from *Cephalosporium acremonium* by **G. Brotzn** in the year 1945. He collected the fungus from seawater near a sewage outlet on the coast of Sardinia (a large Italian island). He found that the fungus has shown therapeutic activity against *staphylococcal* infections and typhoid fever.

- ✓ Many workers have shown interest in *Cephaosporium* species. Seven different antibiotic products were isolated from the species. Among them, five are fat soluble (one is steroidal - **Cephalosporin P**) and two (**Cephalosporin N & C**) are water-soluble.

- ✓ During the study, it was proved that **Cephalosporin N** is a penicillin-type. Later, it was marketed as **Penicillin N**. **Cephalosporin C** type is studied here due to its therapeutic value and the number of antibiotics generated by this group, and many of them possess its therapeutic value.

General Structure of Cephalosporin

- ✓ Official cephalosporin group is resembling the cepham general structure. But the chemical name for the official drug refers to the two general structures.

- ✓ Structure of cephalosporins corresponds to cepham (Structure - I) or 5-thia-1-azabicyclo [4.2.0] octane (Structure-II) (Fig.1.4).

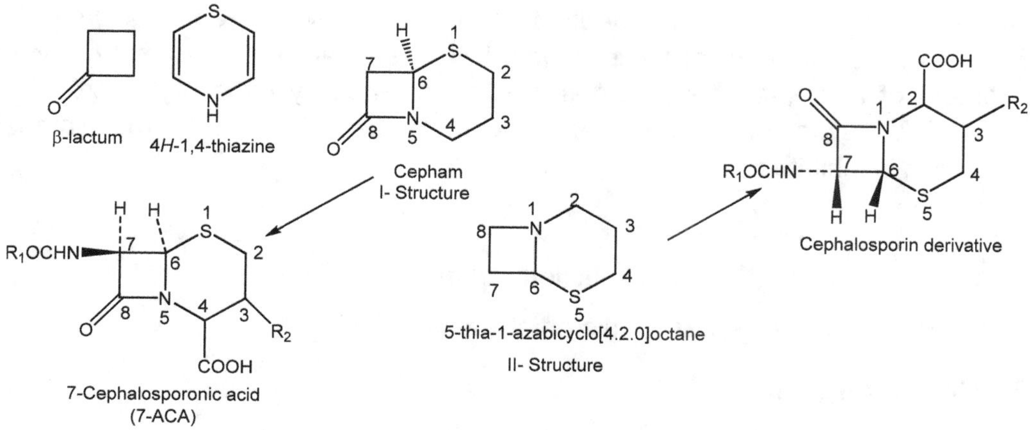

Fig.1.4 General structure of Cephalosporin.

- ✓ The β-lactam ring is fused with the 1,3 dihydro thiazine ring in place of the thiazolidine ring of penicillin. The fusion of the thiazine ring with β-lactam produces a stable antibiotic product. But, it is unable to resist acid and penicillinase-producing microbes.

- ✓ 7-amino acylation (acyl (R-C=O) group) at C-7 of the cephalosporin (Fig.1.4) structure produces a number of semisynthetic compounds.

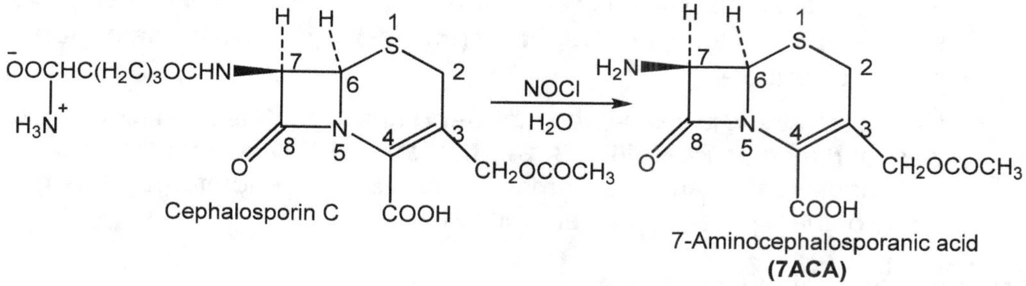

Fig.1.5 Chemical degradation of Cephalosporin C.

Chemical Degradation of Cephalosporin (Fig.1.5)

- ✓ **6-aminopenicillinic acid (6-APA)** is used for the preparation of semisynthetic penicillin. While **7-aminocephalosporanic acid (7-ACA)** is used for the preparation of semisynthetic cephalosporin compounds. There are a number of cephalosporin compounds generated by modification or substitution at the C-3 & C-7 positions.

- ✓ The breakdown of cephalosporin C with nitrosyl chloride (NOCl) in the presence of formic acid and followed by hydrolysis gives a new compound known as 7-aminocephalosporanic acid (Fig.1.5).

- ✓ Any suitable substitution at C-7 affects the antibacterial activity, and substitution at C-3 changes the pharmacokinetic properties of the compound.

Classification of Cephalosporin C (Fig. 1.6).

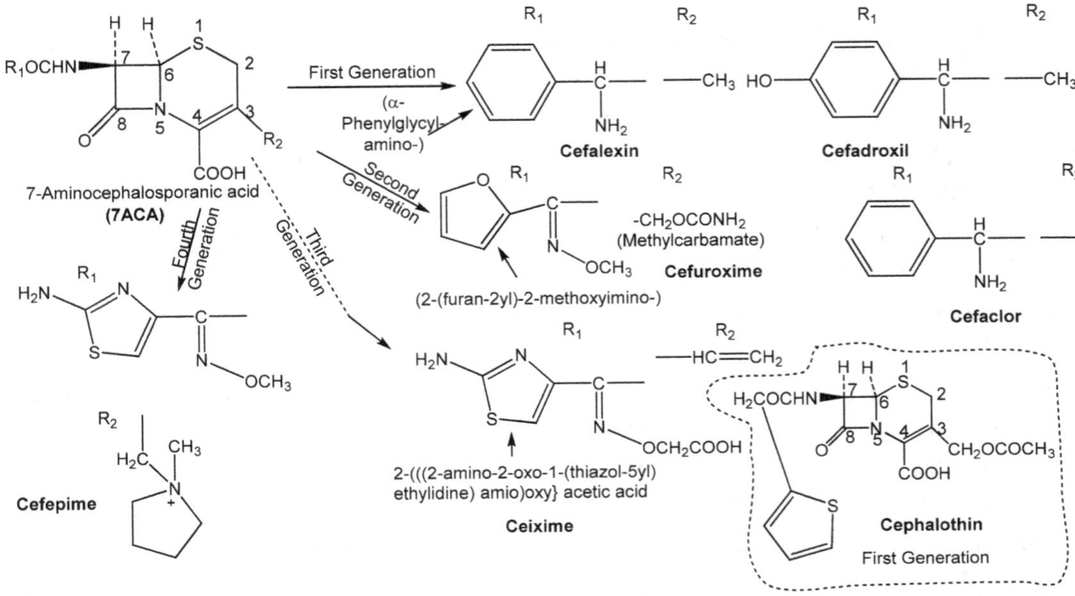

Fig. 1.6 Different classified generation of cephalosporin compounds.

1. **First generation Cephalosporins:** Ex. **Cephalothin** was first introduced and **Cephaloridine, Cephalexin, Cefadroxil, Cefradine, and Cefatriazine** were included in this group. These compounds are active against both gram-+ve and gram-ve bacteria and administered through the parental route due to their poor absorption character.

2. **Second generation:** Ex. **Cefamandole** was the first drug available in this group. Later, **Cefaclor, Cefoxitin, and Cefuroxime** are included in this group. These compounds are less active against gram+ve bacteria and more stable against β-lactamase-producing gram-ve bacteria.

3. **Third generation:** Ex. **Cefotaxime, Ceftriaxone, Cefixime,** and **Ceftazidine** are the compounds of this group. They are more active against gram-ve bacteria.

4. **Fourth generation:** Ex. **Cefepime.** It is active against a wide range of gram+ve and gram-ve bacteria.

Structure-Activity Relationship (Fig.1.6)

Any substitution at C-7 affects the antibacterial activity, and substitution at C-3 changes the pharmacokinetic properties of the compound.

1. Substitution at C-7 position of Cephalosporin ring.
   (a) Acylation (R-C=O) of the amino group, increases therapeutic potency against gram +ve bacteria.
   (b) Substitution of the aromatic ring increases its antibacterial property and lipophilic character.

(c) A heteroaromatic ring such as a thiophene, furan, or pyridine ring as a side chain improves its spectrum of activity.

(d) α-methoxy substitution improves the resistance to hydrolysis of β-lactamase-producing bacteria.

2. Substitution at C-3 position of Cephalosporin ring.

(a) Substitution of a suitable group at C-3 affects its pharmacokinetic and antibacterial activity.

(b) Substitution of the benzoyl ester group improves its gram +ve activity and lowers its gram -ve activity.

(c) Substitution of a heterocyclic ring such as pyridine or pyrimidine improves its antibacterial property.

(d) Substitution of aromatic thiol groups improves the antibacterial activity against gram -ve and pharmacokinetic properties.

(e) Substitution of the $-CH_3$ & $-Cl$ groups in place of the acetoxy ($-CH_3COO$) group improves its oral absorption property.

3. Oxidation of 'S' to sulfoxide (SO), decreases its antibacterial property.

4. The replacement of 'S' with 'O' retains its antibacterial properties. Similarly, replacing the -S group with the methylene group enhances chemical stability and has a longer biological half-life.

5. Carboxyl (C(=O)OH) group at C-4 has been converted to ester, shows increasing the bioavailability of the compound.

6. A double bond at the 2,3 position loses its antibacterial character.

Mechanism of Action

Cephalosporins have a similar mechanism of action as penicillin. Cephalosporins are bactericidal in nature. They inhibit bacterial cell wall synthesis. **First-generation** cephalosporin groups have effective antibacterial activity against gram +ve & moderate activity against some gram-ve bacteria. They are effective against *staphylococci* bacteria. **Second-generation** cephalosporins are less active against gram +ve but are stable to hydrolysis by gram-ve bacteria. They are active against Enterobacteriaceae and the influenza virus. **Third-generation** cephalosporins are more active against β-lactamase-producing gram-ve and less active against gram+ve bacteria. The **fourth generation** is effective against both gram+ve and β-lactamase-producing gram-ve bacteria.

Uses

✓ Used in the treatment of *staphylococci*, *enterobacteriaceae*, and influenza virus infections.

✓ Cephalosporin is active against both gram+ve and gram-ve bacteria.

1.1.3 β-Lactamase Inhibitors

There have been certain agents developed that are structurally similar to β-lactams but they are not actually penicillin or cephalosporin compounds. Examples: Clavulanic acid and sulbactam are two such β-lactamase inhibitors.

Clavulanic Acid

It is isolated from *Streptomyces clavuligerus*. It consists of β-lactam ring with an oxazolidine heterocycle ring. Potassium clavulanate is an official product. It is well absorbed orally. It is given in combination with amoxicillin for oral and ticarcillin for parenteral use.

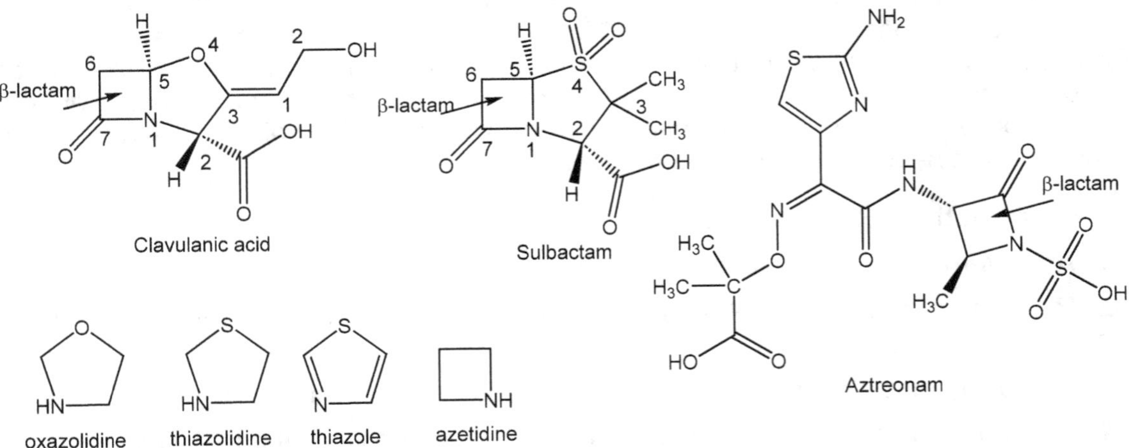

Fig. 1.7 Structure of Lactamase inhibitors and Monobactams.

Chemical Structure: see Fig.1.7

Chemical Naming:

(2R,5R,Z-)-3-(2-hydroxyethylidene)-7-oxo-4-oxa-1-azabicyclo [3.2.0] heptane-2-carboxylic acid

Uses

- ✓ Given combination with amoxicillin as first-line treatment of different types of infections, including sinus and urinary tract infections.
- ✓ Given combination with penicillins and cephalosporins to treat infections caused by β-lactamase-producing microbes.

Mechanism of action: Clavulanic acid is a semisynthetic β-lactamase inhibitor antibiotic, isolated from *Streptomyces* spp. It binds strongly to β-lactamase at or near its active site. This protects other β-lactam antibiotics from β-lactamase catalysis, thereby increasing their antibacterial effects.

Sulbactam: It is a semi-synthetic β-lactamase inhibitor. Structurally, it is penicillanic acid 1, 1-dioxide.

Chemical Structure: see Fig. 1.7

Chemical Naming:

(2S,5R)-3,3-dimethyl-7-oxo-4-thia-1-azabicyclo[3.2.0]heptane-2-carboxylic acid 4,4-dioxide.

Uses

- ✓ Combining with β-lactamase susceptible antibiotic, such as penicillins or cephalosporins, to treat infections caused by β-lactamase-producing microbes.

Mechanism of Action

The β-lactam ring of sulbactam irreversibly binds to β-lactamase at or near its active site, thereby blocking enzyme activity. Many β-lactam-containing antibiotics act as substrates for β-lactamase enzyme-producing bacteria. β-lactamase inhibitors type of antibiotics are bound to the active site of β-lactamase enzyme-producing bacteria and prevent the destruction of β-lactam inhibitor antibiotics. It has poor antimicrobial properties but is active against β-lactamase enzyme-producing bacteria.

Structure-Activity Relationship

1. Any alteration of β-ring loses its potency.

2. Removal of the hetero 'N' atom by any other heteroatom results in an inactive compound.

3. Removal of the C=O group from the ring reduces or loses its activity.

4. Sulfone group of sulbactam is essential and increases its antibacterial activity.

Monobactams: Ex. Aztreonam

Aztreonam, a β-lactam ring, is not condensed with another ring. It is a monocyclic-lactam compound and is also called a monobactam compound. It was isolated from *Chromobacterium violaceum*. It can be synthesized from threonine (an amino acid).

Chemical Structure: see Fig. 1.7

Chemical Naming:

2-((((Z)-1-(2-aminothiazol-4-yl)-2-(((2S,3S)-2-methyl-4-oxo-1-sulfoazetidin-3-yl)amino)-2-oxoethylidene) amino)oxy)-2-methylpropanoic acid

Uses

- ✓ Infections caused by gram-ve bacteria such as *Pseudomonas aeruginosa*.

- ✓ Used in the treatment of bone infections, pneumonia, and urinary tract infections.

- ✓ It is administered parenterally in the treatment of gram-ve aerobic infections, including *Pseudomonas aeruginosa*.

Mechanism of Action

It inhibits the synthesis of the bacterial cell wall, by blocking peptidoglycan cross-linking. It is bactericidal, but less active than cephalosporin compounds. It is resistant to β-lactamase-producing bacteria. It has a narrow spectrum of antibacterial activity.

Structure Activity Relationship

1. The sulphate (SO_3-) group does not distort (alter) the β-lactam ring but is sufficiently electronegative to activate it.

2. Carboxyl group increases its antibacterial activity.

3. Aminothiazole oxime group of the structure imparts effective against gram-ve bacteria.

4. α-methyl group increases resistance to β-lactamase-producing bacteria.

1.2 Aminoglycosides

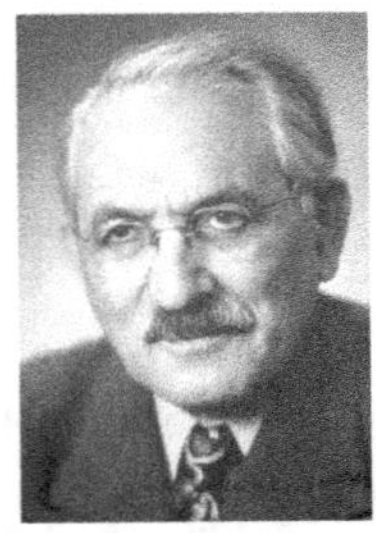

Fig. 1.8 Selman A. Waksman. N. Kresge, et al., 2004

✓ Aminoglycoside antibiotics are produced by (*Streptomyces* spp. Ex. **streptomycin, neomycin, framycetin, kanamycin** and **tobramycin** and *Micromonospora* spp. (Ex. **gentamicin** and **sisomicin**).

✓ Structurally, they are closely related to each other.

✓ They contain aminocyclitol (2-deoxystreptamine) with aminosugars linked glycosidically. Hence, they are called aminoglycosidic aminocyclitiols.

Mechanism of Action

Aminoglycoside antibiotics are bactericidal in nature. They are interfering with bacterial protein synthesis. They are most active against gram-ve rods (the shape of the bacteria). Gram+ve and anaerobic bacteria are resistant to aminoglycoside antibiotics. *Staphylococcus aureus* is resistant to aminoglycoside antibiotics. They have delayed absorption in GIT. Hence, it is preferred over the parental route. They are excreted through urine in unchanged form. Some of the members are useful as anti-tubercular drugs.

Toxicity: ototoxicity, nephrotoxicity, allergy, and neuromuscular blocking activity limit the use of aminoglycosides.

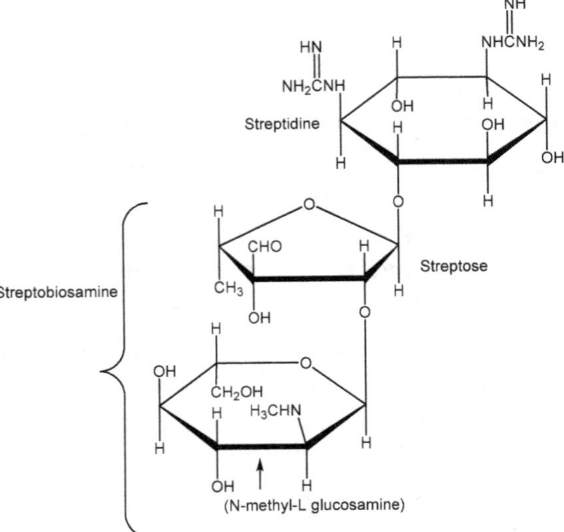

Fig. 1.9 Chemical structure of Streptomycin.

1.2.1 Streptomycin

Historical Background

1944 - **Selman A. Waksman** & his associates discovered streptomycin from *Streptomyces griseus*. It was the first aminoglycoside antibiotic and the first effective drug in the treatment of tuberculosis. He was considered the "Father of Antibiotics" (Fig. 1.8). Streptomycin sulphate is an official drug.

Chemical Structure

Streptomycin (Fig.1.9) is a triacidic base (capable of combining with three molecules of a monobasic acid) compound. The structure belongs to an aldehydic carbonyl group. It consists of three structural units of aminoglycoside **streptidine** (diguanidinyl compound corresponding to streptamine), **streptose,** and **N-methyl-L-glucosamine**. Each structure is connected through glycosidic linkages.

Chemical Breakdown of Streptomycin

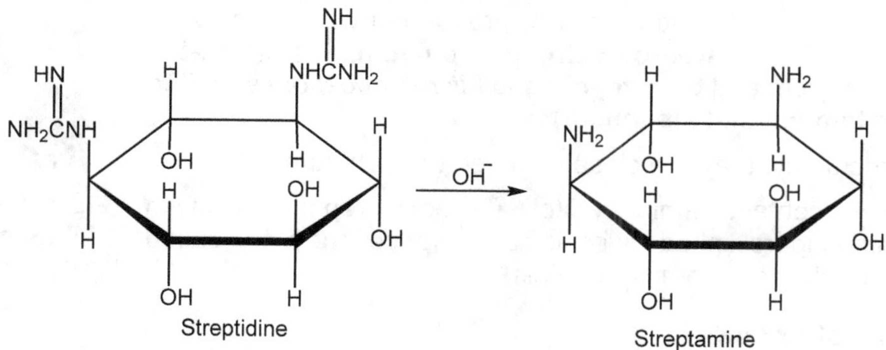

Fig.1.10 Chemical degradation of streptomycin.

1. Streptomycin on hydrolysis under acidic conditions gives diacidic base streptidine.
2. Streptidine on alkaline hydrolysis is converted to urea derivative and then diamine streptamine. It is a meso compound. (A meso compound or meso isomer is a non-optically active member of a set of stereoisomers, at least two of which are optically active. This means that despite containing two or more stereogenic centers, the molecule is not chiral.)
3. Mild hydrolysis with CH_3OH/HCl gives streptidine (Fig.1.10) and methyl streptobiosaminide dimethyl acetal.
4. Streptomycin on reduction gives dihydrostreptomycin, which is a semisynthetic antibiotic. During the conversion process, the aldehyde group of streptomycin is changed to a primary alcohol ($-CH_2OH$).
5. *Streptomyces humidus* fermentation has successfully isolated dihydrostreptomycin, which is also naturally occurring. However, dihydrostreptomycin is more ototoxicity than streptomycin. Therefore, it is used only for veterinary purposes and not for human use.

Uses

- ✓ It has particular activity against *Mycobacterium tuberculosis*. Therefore, its main use is in the treatment of tuberculosis, along with other antimycobacterial agents.

- ✓ It acts as an alternative to gentamycin. Hence, it has been given in combination with penicillin for the treatment of endocarditis (this is an infection of the endocardium, which is the inner lining of your heart chambers and heart valves)

- ✓ Used in the treatment of **plague** and **tularemia** (a severe infectious bacterial disease of animals transmissible to humans, characterized by ulcers at the site of infection, fever, and loss of weight)

1.2.2 Neomycin

Historical Background
1949 - **S. A. Waksman & H. A. Lechevalier** discovered neomycin, which is produced from *Streptomyces fradiae*. Neomycin sulphate is an official drug.

Chemical structure: Neomycins (Fig.1.11) is a mixture of three compounds such as neomycins A, B & C. The separation of the compound could be possible.

Chemical Breakdown of Neomycins

1. On methanolysis (alcoholysis using methanol) neomycins B & C gave methyl neobiosaminides B & C.

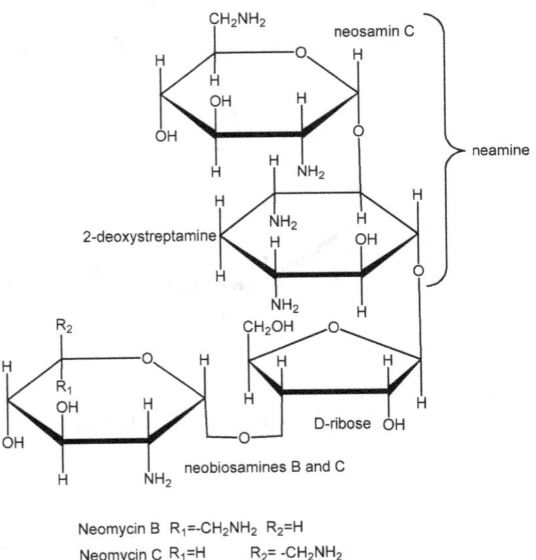

Fig.1.11 Chemical structure of Neomycin.

2. The difference between neobiosamines B & C can be distinguishing with stereochemistry at position 5 in the components neosamines B and C.

3. This is sole difference in between neobiosamines B & C and neomycins B and C.

Uses

- ✓ It is active against gram-ve bacteria and *Staphylococcus aureus*.
- ✓ It is applied topically in the treatment of ear, eye, and skin infections.
- ✓ It is given in combination with corticosteroids for topical application.
- ✓ It has been used as bowel preparation (cleansing the colon) before surgery and treatment of GIT.
- ✓ It possesses toxicity; which limits its use in systemic infections.

1.2.3 Kanamycin

Historical Background

1957 - **H. Umezawa** isolated the compound from cultures of *Streptomyces kanamyceticus*, the organism obtained from the soil of the Nagarov district of Japan.

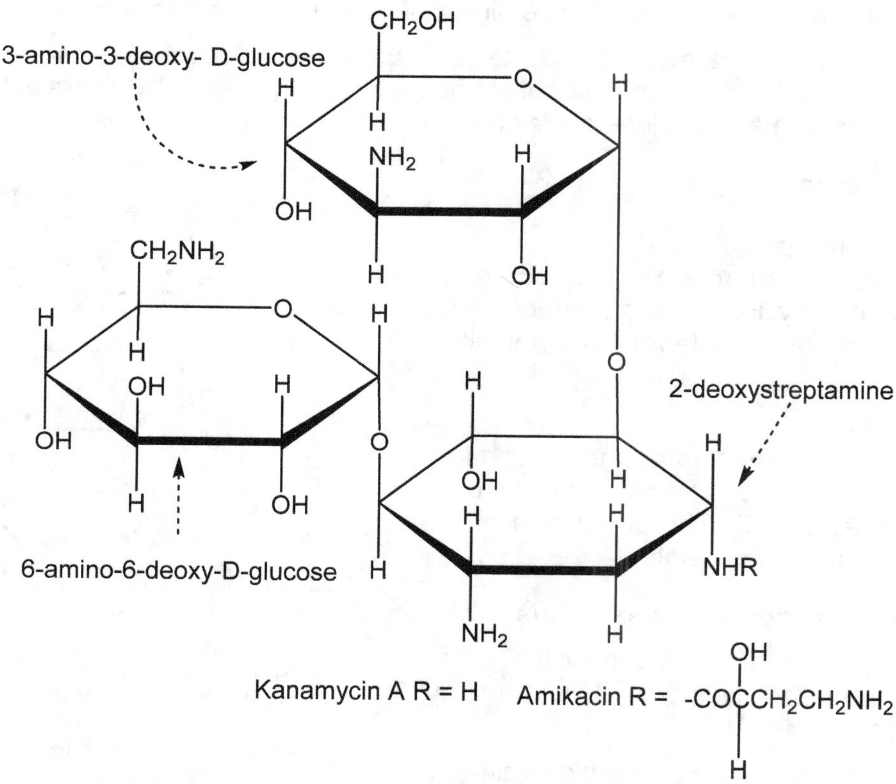

Fig.1.12 Chemical structure of Kanamycin.

Chemical Structure of Kanamycin

1. **Kanamycin A** (Fig.1.12) is the major and **kanamycins B & C** are the minor components.

2. The aminocyclitol 2-deoxystreptamine and 3-deoxy- 3-amino-D-glucose are present in all three components.

3. The difference is with regard to the second amino sugar, which is linked glyosidically to the 4-position of the central 2-deoxystreptamine. It is 6-amino- 6-deoxy-D-glucose in kanamycin A.

4. **Amikacin** is a semisynthetic derivative, The compound is prepared by acylation of the 1-amino group of 2-deoxystreptamine moiety with L-4-amino-2-hydroxybutyric acid of kanamycin A.

Uses

- ✓ Treatment of severe infections caused by microorganism resistance to gentamicin and tobramycin.
- ✓ Given in treatment of tuberculosis with other drugs. However, the toxicity of the drug limits its use.
- ✓ Treatment of intestinal infections and other infections caused by microorganisms.

1.3 Tetracyclines

Tetracycline (Fig.1.13) antibiotics are organic compounds. These group antibiotics are derived from acetic acid (CH_3COOH) & propionic acid (CH_3CH_2COOH) derivative compounds. Such derived antibioics as **tetracyclines, fusidic acid,** and **erythromycin** possess antibacterial properties. While, **griseofulvin, amphotericin.** and **nystatin** act as antifungal agents, **daunorubicin** and **doxorubicin** are antineoplastic agents.

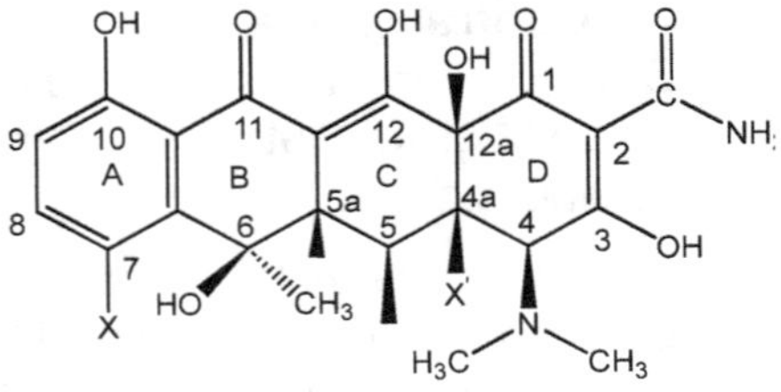

Fig.1.13 Chemical structure of tetracycline group.

Historical Background

- ✓ Tetracyclines are a group of antibiotics originally derived from *Streptomyces* spp.
- ✓ **Chlorotetracycline** was discovered as the first antibiotic of the series.
- ✓ 1948 - **B. M. Duggar** isolated chlorotetracycline from *Streptomyces aureofaciens.*
- ✓ **Oxytetracycline** was the next member of this group. It is isolated from *Streptomyces rimosus* species.
- ✓ **Tetracycline** was the third member of this group and was first obtained by catalytic hydrogenolysis of Chlorotetracycline and thereafter by fermentation in low-chloride media.

Classification of Tetracyclines: On the basis of duration of action (biological half-life):

- ✓ **Short acting tetracyclines** - Ex. Chlorotetracycline (6hr), Oxytetracycline (8hr), Tetracycline (9hr)
- ✓ **Intermediate acting (12-14hr):** Ex. Demeclocycline and Methycycline
- ✓ **Long acting (16-18hr):** Ex. Minocycline and Doxycycline

Chemical name of tetracycline: 4-(dimethylamino)-3,6,10,12,12a-pentahydroxy-6-methyl-1,11-dioxo-1,4, 4a,5,5a,6,11,12aoctahydrotetracene- 2-carboxamide OR 4-Dimethylamino-1,4,4a,5,5a,6,11,12a-octahydro-3,6,10,12,12a-pentahydroxy-6-meth-1, 11-dioxo-naphthacene-2-carboxamide.

Structural Elucidation

1. Structurally, tetracyclines have a common tetracyclic ring known as the **octahydronaphthacene** nucleus.

2. Each structure of this group has close chemical similarities. The difference in between the two antibiotics is that Chlorotetracycline has a chloro group(-Cl)group at the C-7 position and in **Oxytetracycline** has a hydroxyl (-OH) at position C-5.

3. **Chlortetracycline, oxytetracycline** and **tetracycline** are natural occurring product. Structurally, tetracycline has differ from chlortetracycline only by the absence of the methyl group at C-6. While doxycycline and minocycline are semisynthetic compounds.

4. In **Tetracycline** there are five chiral centers, and each of these centers has an S configuration. Tetracycline HCl is an official product. Eye ointment and drops of the product are used to treat ocular infections.

Structure-Activity Relationship

1. Keto-enol system of the ring A for antibacterial activity. If changes the functional group in this ring changes its character or loses its activity.

2. Carbamoyl group at C-2 is essential for antimicrobial activity. Unsubstitution or monosubstitution is acceptable. The large alkyl group in replacement of this position loses its antibacterial activity.

3. Keto-enol system at C-3 is suitable for antibacterial activity.

4. Dimethyl amino at C-4, which favorably contributes to the keto-enol system of the ring A. replacement of this group causes the loss of its activity.

5. α-hydrogen atom at C-4a & 5a is necessary for their antibacterial activity.

6. Substitution of hydroxyl group at C-5 (in the case of oxytetracycline) shows the more potent antimicrobial or broad spectrum of activity.

7. The antimicrobial activity is related to the substitution of the CH_3 group at C-6 and the -OH group. Replacement of the -OH group in this position forms a novel product known as doxycycline which also possesses a broad spectrum of activity.

8. Cl group at C-7 (Chlortetracycline) has produced potent antibiotics. Replace the group with NO_2 to produce a toxic effect against the host.

9. Hydroxyl group at C-10 is necessary for a broad spectrum of activity.

10. Keto-enol system at C-11 is required for antibacterial activity and at C-11a for binding of bacterial cell walls.

11. Hydroxyl group at 12a improves its lipophilicity character and is essential for antibacterial activity.

Mechanism of Action

At therapeutic concentrations, tetracyclines act as bacteriostatic agents. They interfere with protein synthesis, such as aminoglycoside antibiotics. The main site of action of tetracyclines is the bacterial ribosomes. They bind to the 30S bacterial ribosomes and prevent the access of aminoacyl tRNA to the acceptor (A) site on the mRNA -ribosome complex.

It possesses a wide spectrum of microbial activity, which includes gram+ve, gram-ve bacteria, chlamydiae, rickettsia, mycoplasma, spirochaetes, mycobacteria, and protozoa.

1.3.1 Oxytetracycline

Oxytetracycline dihydrate, oxytetracycline calcium, and HCl are the official products. Tablets, capsules, and injections are used in topical applications.

Chemical Name:

4-(dimethylamino)-3,5,6,10,12,12a-hexahydroxy-6-methyl-1,11-dioxo-1,4,4a,5,5a,6, 11, 12a-octahydronaphthacene-2-carboxamide

Structural Elucidation

1. Oxytetracycline (Fig.1.13) carries one additional chiral center at the C-5 position of S-configuration.
2. The configuration at positions 4a & 5a is the same as tetracycline.

1.3.2 Chlorotetracycline

Chlorotetracycline (Fig.1.13) HCl is the official product. The product is applied topically as an ointment to the eye or as a cream or ointment to the skin.

Chemical Name

(4S,4aS,5aS,6S,12aS)-7-chloro-4-(dimethylamino)-3,6,10,12,12a-pentahydroxy-6- methyl-1,11-dioxo-1,4,4a,5,5a,6,11,12a-octahydrotetracene (or naphthacene)-2-carboxamide.

Octahydronaphthacene

Minocycline

Doxycycline

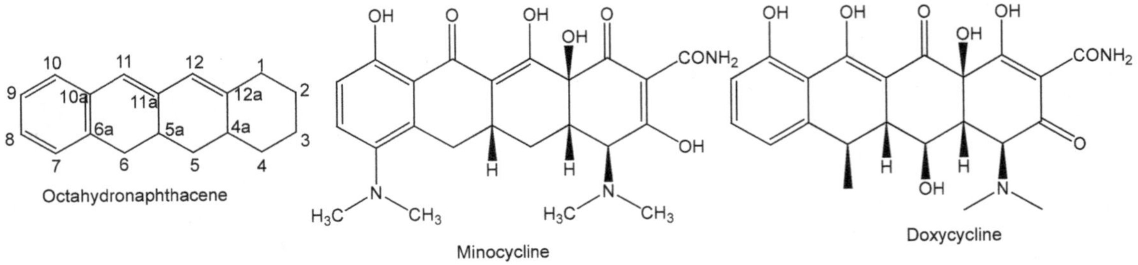

Fig. 1.14   Chemical structure of Doxycycline and Minocycline.

1.3.3 Doxycycline

Doxycycline (Fig.1.14) HCl, IP, and Doxycycline hyclate, BP are the official product. it is given in the oral route and occasionally given in the parental route.

Chemical Name

(4S,4aR,5S,5aR,6R,12aR)-4-(dimethylamino)-1,5,10,11,12a-pentahydroxy-6-methyl-3, 12-dioxo-4a,5,5a,6-tetrahydro-4H-tetracene-2-carboxamide

Structural Elucidation

1. Chemical naming of Doxycycline is similar to chemical naming of oxytetracycline.

2. Methyl group at C-6 are similar in both but Hydroxyl group at C-6 is absent.

3. The absolute configuration at the position has R-configuration in Doxycycline. While, it is S-configuration in oxytetracycline.

1.3.4 Minocycline

Minocycline (Fig.1.14) HCl, BP is the official product. Preferable, it is given in oral route.

Chemical Name

(4S,4aS,5aR,12aS)-4,7-bis(dimethylamino)-3,10,12,12a-tetrahydroxy-1,11-dioxo-1,4,4 a,5,5a,6,11,12a-octahydrotetracene-2-carboxamide

Uses

- ✓ Used in the treatment of *Rickettsia,* Mycoplasma, and Chlamydia infections and pelvic inflammatory disease. Tetracyclines are not suitable for the treatment of gram+ve and gram-ve infections.

- ✓ Treatment of cholera, severe acne, and amoebic dysentery.

- ✓ Given in combination with streptomycin or rifampicin in treatment of plague. In cases of malaria (*P. falciparum*), given in combination with quinine.

- ✓ Preferred route of administration is the oral route, but most cases are given via the IV route and are rarely chosen as IM. Except for use in the eye, topical application shall be avoided, because it poses a high risk of toxic effects.

CHAPTER 2

ANTIBIOTICS - II

2.1 Macrolide

Definition of Macrolide: The macrolides are a group of antibiotics produced by various strains of *Streptomyces* (spore forming bacteria that grow slowly in soil or water as a branching filamentous mycelium similar to that of fungi) and have a complex chemical (macrocyclic) structure.

✓ Certain antibiotics have a common structural feature. They consist of a large non-planar (not lying or able to be confined within a single plane: having a three-dimensional quality, sp^3 hybridize) strainless lactone ring (an internal cyclic mono ester formed by gamma or delta hydroxy acids spontaneously), hence, they are called macrolide antibiotics. There are more than three dozen such classes of compounds.

✓ Macrolide antibiotics are derived from *Streptomyces Spp.*

✓ Structurally, it consists of a large macrocyclic lactone ring to which one or more deoxy sugars, usually cladinose (neutral sugar) and/or desosamine (basic sugar), may be attached. The amino sugars are linked glycosidically to the lactone ring, and a neutral sugar is linked to the lactone ring or the basic sugar.

✓ This class of antibiotics consists of weak bases. Hence, they are only slightly soluble in water.

✓ They are **bacteriostatic** or **bactericidal**, depending upon the concentration and type of microbe desired to be used.

✓ All macrolide classes of antibiotics have similar properties to erythromycin. While the pharmacokinetic properties differ from each other.

✓ The lactone rings are usually 14-, 15-, or 16-membered. Macrolides belong to the polyketide (polyketides are a large group of metabolites which either contain alternating carbonyl groups (-CO-) and methylene groups ($-CH_2-$) class of natural products. Some macrolides have antibiotic or antifungal activity.

Classification

A. Natural or Prominent Macrolide antibiotic: Ex. erythromycin

B. Biosynthetic origin: Ex. spiramycin, oleanlomycin

C. Semi-synthetic derivative of erythromycin/ and more recent macrolide antibiotics: azithromycin, clarithromycin, dirithromycin, and roxithromycin

2.1.1 Erythromycin

Historical Background

1949 - **Abelardo B. Aguilar**, a Filipino scientist, sent some soil samples from the Philippine Archipelago (an island group) to his employer, **J. M. McGuire**, who worked at Eli Lilly, USA. **J. M. McGuire** and his associate managed to isolate erythromycin from the metabolic products of a strain of *Streptomyces erythreus*.

Chemical Structure & Elucidation

1. During the fermentation process, there are three i.e. A, B & C types of erythromycin (**Fig. 2.1**) produced. A is the major and most important component.

2. Erythromycin A has a lactone ring (erythronnolide A) attached to the basic sugar desosamine and neutral sugar cladinose (3-O-methylmycarose) glycosidically.

3. Erythromycin A & B have the same sugar moieties.

4. A hydroxyl (-OH) group at C-12 is the only difference between erythromycin A & B.

5. Erythromycin C contains lactone ring, desosamine, and mycarose instead of cladinose. They are linked glycosidically.

6. The tertiary amine of desosamine moiety conforms its basic character to erythromycin.

7. It readily forms salts with inorganic and organic acids and also forms esters.

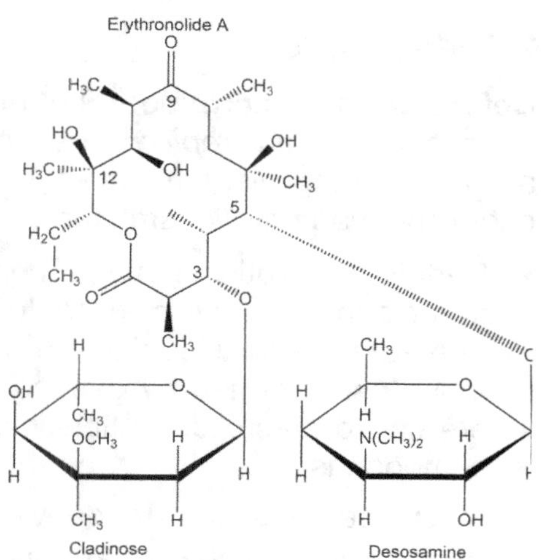

Fig. 2.1 Chemical structure of Erythromycin A.

Uses

✓ Treatment of diphtheria, pertussis (whooping cough), and respiratory infections.

✓ It is given as an alternative to penicillin-allergic patients and tetracycline in Chlamydia infections.

✓ Given topically in the treatment of neonatal conjunctivitis and in acne.

✓ It is unstable in gastric acid; therefore, it is given as an enteric coated formulation or stable salts or esters such as stearate or ethyl succinate.

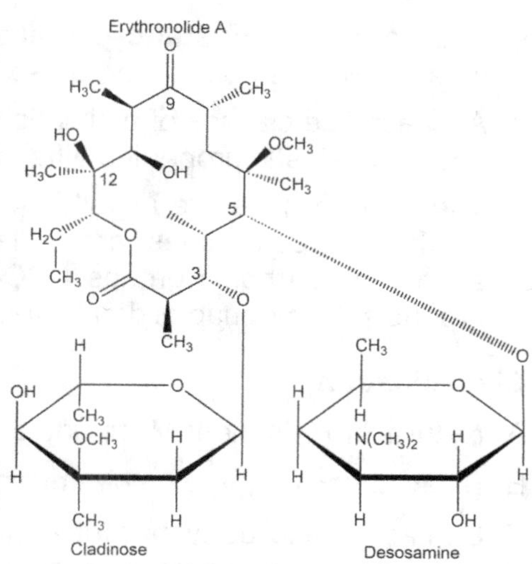

Fig. 2.2 Chemical structure of Clarithromycin.

2.1.2 Clarithromycin

1. Structural difference to erythromycin only by methylation of the -OH group at C-6 position.

2. The metabolite 14 (*R*) - hydroxy clarithromycin is more active than clarithromycin (Fig. 2.2).

3. Hydroxylation (Chemical process) is stereospecific. *R* and *S* - epimers occurs *in vitro*, *R*-epimer is present in a higher concentration and shows an increase in biological activity.

4. Stability and oral bioavailability are improved than erythromycin. It is well absorbed in GIT.

5. It is effective against *Haemophilus influenzae, Chlamydia,* and *mycobacterium.*

2.1.3 Azithromycin

1. It is very stable in acidic conditions (Fig. 2.3).

2. It is more active against respiratory infections caused by *Haemophilus influenzae, Moraxella trachomatis.* It is given in the treatment of urethritis (inflammation of the urethra) caused by *Chlamydia trachomatis* and is active against *Mycobacterium.* It is useful in the treatment of sexually transmitted diseases (STD).

3. It has unique pharmacokinetic properties and a prolonged biological half-life.

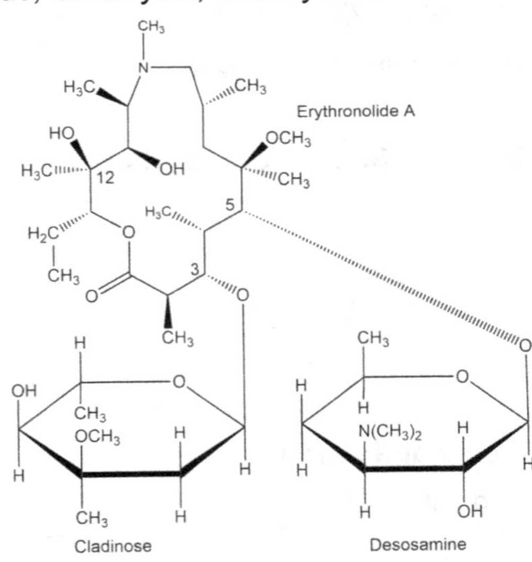

Fig. 2.3 Chemical structure of Azithromycin.

Mechanism of Action

The macrolide antibiotics are bacteriostatic or bactericidal in nature, and their activity depends upon their concentration and the types of microorganisms used. They inhibit protein synthesis by binding reversibly to the 50S ribosomal subunits of sensitive microorganisms. They have an antimicrobial spectrum which is similar to that of benzylpenicillin (active only gram+ve bacteria). Macrolide class antibiotics are active against gram-ve bacteria, including *Legionella pneumophila, Mycoplasma pneumonfae, rickettsia,* and *chlamydia.*

2.2 Miscellaneous

✓ Several antibiotics can also be obtained from amino acids. Some antibiotics are derived from single amino acids, two amino acids, or more than two amino acids, known as **polypeptide** antibiotics.

✓ **Cycloserine** (D-serine) & **chloramphenicol** (D-phenylserinol) are obtained from single amino acids.

✓ Amino acid-derived antibiotics are prepared from natural (*Streptomycetes. spp.*) and synthetic processes. However, the synthetic process is more economical than the fermentation process.

2.2.1 Chloramphenicol

Historical Background

✓ Chloramphenicol (also known as chloromycetin), was discovered in 1947. It was isolated from a mold *Streptomyces venezuelae* The mold was collected from a soil sample of Venezuela. Later, it was also produced by a number of different species of *Streptomyces*.

✓ It can be produced by a fermentation process.

✓ 1948 - **Q. R. Bartz** & his associate established the chemical compound.

✓ It was the first antibiotic produced synthetically and made available for clinical use.

Chemical Structure: Fig. 2.4

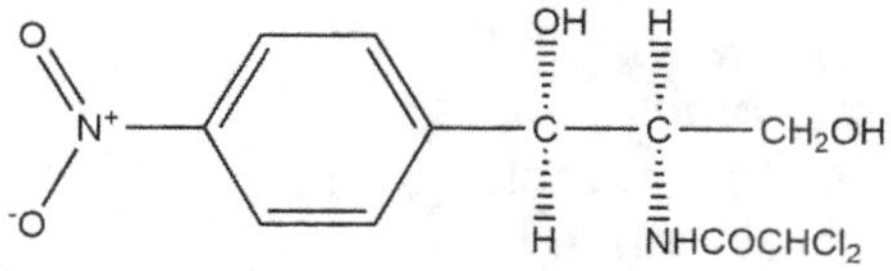

Fig. 2.4 Chemical structure of Chloramphenicol.

Chemical Naming

2,2-dichloro-N-((*1R,2R*)-1,3-dihydroxy-1-   4-nitrophenyl)   propan-2-yl)acetamide   or 2,2-dichloro-N-((*1R,2R*)-2-hydroxymethyl- 2-(4-nitrophenylethyl) acetamide.

Synthesis: (Fig. 2.5 & Fig. 2.6)

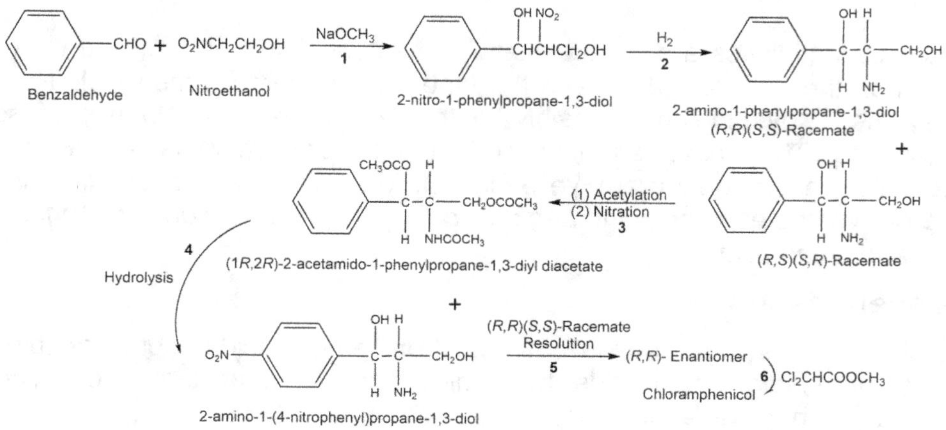

Fig. 2.5 Synthesis of chloramphenicol - First process.

Preparation of Chloramphenicol - First Process

1. Benzaldehyde on reaction with nitroethanol to form a new product, 2-nitro-1-phenylpropane-1,3-diol.

2. The obtained product on reduction gave a mixture of R,R- and S,S- and R,S- and S,R- stereoisomers compound.

3. With help of fractional crystallisation, the diastereomers were separated as (RR,SS & RS, SR) compound. The RS, SR stereoisomeric compound will be separated.

4. The remaining residue (RR,SS stereoisomer) compound under careful acetylation & nitration will obtain a crystallized diacetyl derivative compound.

5. The obtained product under hydrolysis process gave (R,R)-(S,S)-2-amino-1-(4-nitrophenyl)propane-1,3-diol.

6. The intermediate racemate was again separated by fractional crystallisation with (+)-camphorsulphonate salts. Thus, regenerate the free base with R,R- configuration.

7. The R,R- configured compound treated with dichloroacetate to afford purified form of chloramphenicol with right stereochemical structure.

Preparation of Chloramphenicol - Second Process (Fig. 2.6)

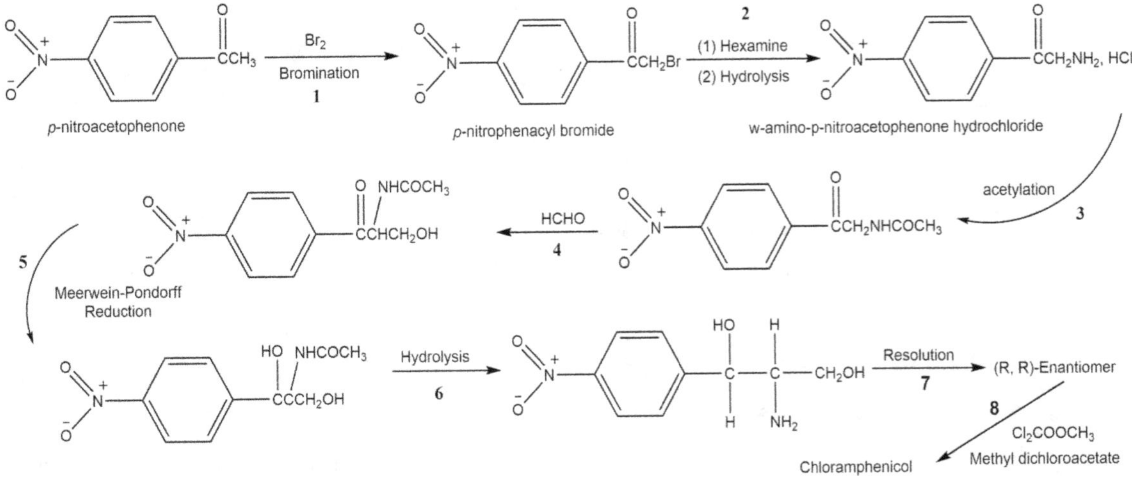

Fig.2.6 Synthesis of chloramphenicol - Second process.

1. p-nitroacetophenone treated with bromine under bromination process to obtain p-nitrophenacyl bromide.

2. The resultant product treat with heaxamine and hydrolysis to produce ω-amino-p-nitroacetophenone hydrochloride.

3. The resultant product of the acetylation process is an acetamide derivative compound.

4. The acetamide derivative compound is condensed with formaldehyde a hydroxymethylol derivative product will form.

5. The acetamide derivative is under the **Meerwein-Pondorff** reduction process to give *R,R-S,S* racemic mixture. There also obtain *R,S-S,R-* racemate as a minor product.

6. The racemic product under hydrolysis to gives a racemic base. The racemic base is under chemical treatment (resolved) to obtain the *R, R* -enantiomer.

7. The *R, R* -enantiomer product is treated with methyl dichloroacetate to afford chloramphenicol.

Stereochemistry

1. Chemically, chloramphenicol has two asymmetric centers and is able to form four isomers. They are D-(-)-*threo*, D-(+)-*threo*, D-(-)-*erythro*, & D-(+)-*errythro* isomeric compound or DL-*threo* & DL-(-)-*erythro* racemic pairs (Fig. 2.7).

2. Chloramphenicol has D-(-)-*threo* (*R,R*) confirmational structure & biological active compound. The remaining isomeric compounds are inactive.

3. Chloramphenicol has a stereochemical relationship with D-serine (amino acid) residue.

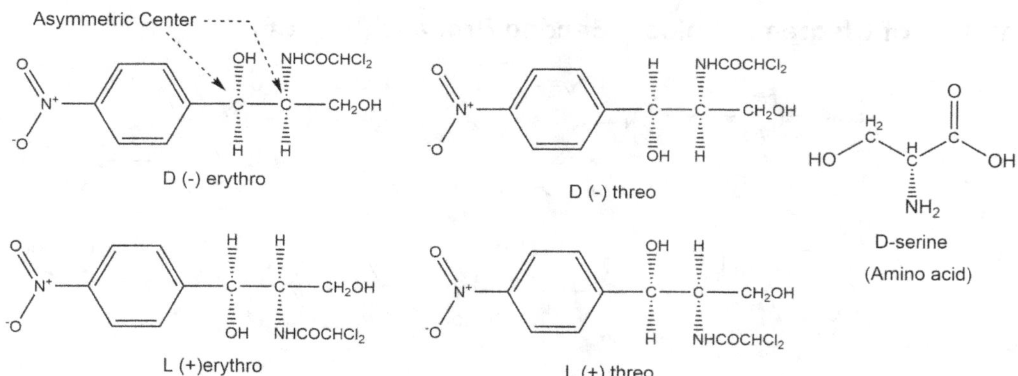

Fig.2.7 Stereochemistry of Chloramphenicol.

Structure-Activity Relationship

1. D-(-)-*threo* (*R,R*) structural arrangement is necessary for antimicrobial activity. L-*threo* (*S, S*) and D- and L- *erythro* isomeric form of chloramphenicol does not show the antibacterial property (Fig. 2.7).

2. Dichloroacetyl group at C-2 is essential for antibacterial activity.

3. The nitro group of the phenyl ring has been replaced by another radical group, i.e., methanesulfinate (CH_3O_2S-) from a new compound known as thiamphenicol. Thiamphenicol shows a broad spectrum of activity, like chloramphenicol. *p*-NO_2 group replaced by strong electron-withdrawn substituents like the acetyl (CH_3CO-) group has loses antibacterial activity.

4. The propanediol group of chloramphenicol should be present in threo configuration for antibacterial activity.

5. Biologically active compounds can also be obtained by removing or transferring chlorine atoms, shifting the p-NO$_2$ group to the ortho position, or esterifying the -OH group.

6. Replacement of the phenyl ring of chloramphenicol by other aromatic and heterocyclic rings has reduced biological activity.

Mechanism of Action

Chloramphenicol inhibits protein synthesis by binding to the 50S subunit of the 70S ribosome. It inhibits peptide bond formation by blocking peptidyl transferase. This mechanism prevents aminoacyl transfer RNA from binding to the peptidyl transferase active site as well. It prevents translation, resulting in nonfunctional proteins, and causes bacterial cell death.

Chloramphenicol shows bacteriostatic action at low concentrations by preventing the protein synthesis of bacteria. In higher concentration, it acts as a bactericidal against Haemophilus influenzae.

It is a broad spectrum antibiotic. It is active against gram+ve & gram-ve bacteria, rickettsiae, chlamydiae, and mycoplasms.

Uses

✓ Used in the treatment of typhoid, bacterial meningitis, and salmonella infections.

✓ Applied locally for the treatment of ear, eye, and skin infections.

✓ Given orally in the form of capsules or suspension of palmitate ester. Chloramphenicol sodium succinate is given by injection.

2.2.2 Clindamycin

Historical Background

✓ 1967- **B J Magerlein** and his associates synthesized the compound **Clindamycin**. This is a semisynthetic derivative of a naturally occurring antibiotic, lincomycin.

✓ 1962 - **D. J. Mason** and his associates discovered lincomycin from *Streptomyces lincolnensis*, an *actinomycete* species. The species was collected from a soil sample of Lincoln, Nebraska, USA. Therefore, the compound is named as **Lincomycin**.

✓ Clinically, Clindamycin is preferred to lincomycin as it is more active, and fewer side effects, and has better oral absorption.

✓ Clindamycin has little structural difference from lincomycin. In the structure, substitution 7(R)-chloro- of the clindamycin is in place of the 7(R)-hydroxyl group of lincomycin.

Chemical Structure: (Fig. 2.8)

Chemical Name:

(2S,4R)-N-[(1S,2S)-2-chloro-1-[(2R,3R,4S,5R,6R)-3,4,5-trihydroxy-6-methyl sulfanyloxan-2-yl]propyl]-1-methyl-4-propylpyrrolidine-2-carboxamide

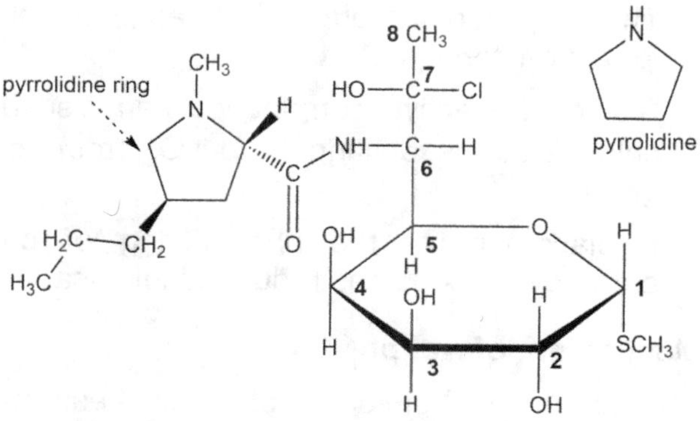

Mechanism of Action

Clindamycin is a semisynthetic broad spectrum antibiotic produced by chemical modification of the parent compound lincomycin.

Fig.2.8 Chemical structure of Clindamycin.

Clindamycin is more effective than lincomycin. Clindamycin has a primarily bacteriostatic effect (low concentration). At higher concentrations, it binds with the 50S ribosomal subunit of bacteria and inhibits protein synthesis. They also inhibit peptidyltransferase action.

Uses

- ✓ Clindamycin HCl capsule, Clindamycin palmitate HCl liquid preparation is given in oral route. Clindamycin phosphate is given by the parentral route.

- ✓ Used for the treatment of bone or joint infections, pelvic inflammatory disease, pneumonia, middle ear infections, and endocarditis.

- ✓ Given in the treatment of dental infections and respiratory tract, skin, and soft tissue infections. It can also be used to treat acne, and in some cases, it can be used against methicillin-resistant *Staphylococcus aureus* microbes.

- ✓ Combine with quinine, it can be used for the treatment of malaria. The cream is applied locally to the skin or vaginal infection.

2.3 Antimalarials

Historical Background

- ✓ Antimalarials are the drugs given in the treatment of "malaria".

- ✓ If the symptoms show periodic fevers, it means the disease is malaria. It is a infectious disease. Since ancient times, malaria cases have been reported in India, China, West Asia, and the Mediterranean region.

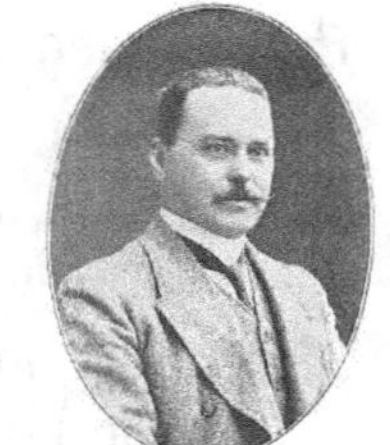

Fig. 2.9 Sir Ronald Ross / wiki.

- ✓ In the olden days, people believed that the disease was associated with swamps and marshlands (low land with flood) area. The harmful air in these areas caused malaria. This led to the coining of the word "malaria" ("mala" means bad & "aria" means air).

✓ **Case study:** There are 300-500 million malaria cases per year reported around the globe. The disease claimed mortality of 1.5-2.7 million per year. In the African region, more than a million children die every year. The country has nearly eradicated malaria, although there have been reports of cases. This is due to people of those countries traveling from or to the malaria region.

✓ 1880 - **Charles Louis Alphonse Laveran**, a French Army Physician, has identified *Plasmodium* protozoans as causative agents of malaria and trypanosomiasis diseases. He won a noble prize in medicine in 1907.

✓ **Sir Ronald Ross** (Fig. 2.9), a British Army surgeon in India, suggested that the Female *Anopheles* mosquito is the causative agent of malaria. He was awarded the Nobel Prize in medicine for his discovery in the year 1902.

2.3.1 Etiology of Malaria

✓ There are four types (*Plasmodium falciparum*, *P. vivax*, *P. malariae, and P. ovale*) of *Plasmodium* protozoa detected in infected humans.

✓ *Plasmodium falciparum* - Life threatening (dangerous) form of the malaria parasite. It causes a malignant (very virulent or infectious) tertian (symptom - fever that repeats every second day) type of malaria.

✓ *P. vivax* - the form of symptoms is milder than *Plasmodium falciparum.* It is the benign tertian type of malaria.

✓ *P. malariae* - an infection that occurs in localized areas of the tropics. It is a quartan (a mild form of malaria causing a fever that repeats every third day) malaria type.

✓ *P. ovale* - a rare form of malaria disease. The occurrence of symptoms is like that of *P. vivax*. It is a mild type of malaria, and the curing rate is rapid.

✓ Monkeys, rodents, birds, and apes are also infected with the protozoan *Plasmodium*.

2.3.1.1 Life Cycle of *Plasmodium*

A. Asexual Phase

1. All species of *Plasmodium* have two hosts i.e. vertebrate (an animal that has a backbone and a skeleton) and mosquito. Here, the role of the mosquito is both vector (by biting, it transmits a disease or parasite from one animal or plant to another) and a definite host.

2. During the biting of an infected mosquito (*Anopheles*) on a healthy human; it releases a *Sporozoites* [a motile spore (a minute, typically

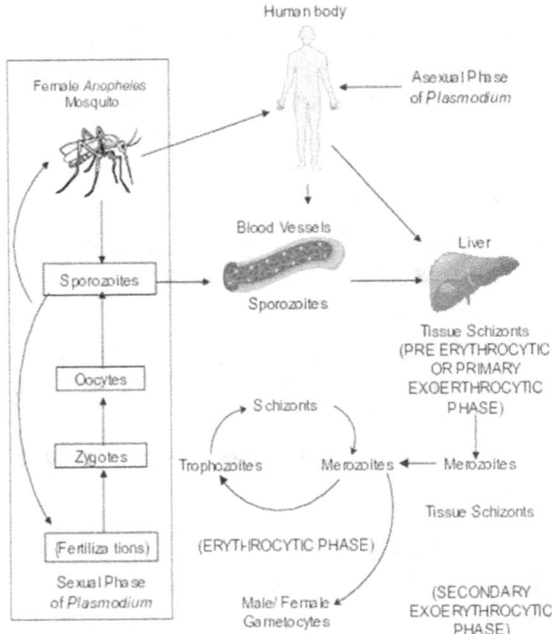

Fig. 2.10 Life cycle of plasmodium protozoa.

one-celled, reproductive unit capable of giving rise to a new individual without sexual fusion) stage] into the blood circulation (Fig. 2.10).

3. The sporozoites will travel to the parenchymal cells of the liver. Where it multiplies and develops into tissue *Schizonts*.

4. Till, this stage is called the **primary exoerythrocytic** or **pre-erythrocytic stage**. This stage remains for 5-16 days depending upon the nature or types of *plasmodium* species.

5. When tissue *schizonts* grow certain stage after that it ruptures, each releasing thousands of *merozoites*. The released *merozoites* enter into the blood circulation and get infected by erythrocytes. Here, is the start of **the erythrocytic phase** or **blood cycle**.

6. While some *merozoites* remain in the liver and get infect more cells of the liver. This stage is called the **secondary exoerythrocytic stage** and occurs only in *P. vivax* & *P. ovale* but not in *P. falciparum* & *P. malariae* types of parasites. Although, other dormant types of parasites remain for a long period (months or years) in an infected person.

7. The *merozoites* grow in the erythrocyte and change to *trophozoites* and finally mature into **schizonts** and is known as blood **schizonts**. This development stage is called as Asexual stage.

8. The mature blood **schizonts** then rupture **schizonts** containing erythrocytes. Each releasing 6-24 *merozoites*. Here, the patient feeling of chilled & a fever. The released *merozoites* again infect another erythrocyte and start the cycle anew.

9. The life cycle continues to the death of the infected patient or stops the cycle by a suitable drug or immunity (acquired) of the patient.

10. The period of fever in tertian or quartan malaria could be known on the timing of **schizonts** containing erythrocyte parasites.

11. The merozoites in humans are classified into two types i.e. male and female. They are also known as gametocytes. Here, is the start of the sexual phase. The sexual phase occurs in mosquitoes after biting an infected person.

B. Sexual Phase

1. After biting, it sucks the blood which consists of gametocytes. These gametocytes are passed to the stomach of a female mosquito and start the process of sporogony (sexual cycle).

2. In this cycle (fertilization), *Zygote* develops in the wall of the stomach as an *oocyst* and later, it develops as an infected *Sporozoite* and migrates to the salivary gland of a mosquito.

3. The infected mosquito again bit any healthy person to become infected. In this way, malaria is spread in a community or from person to person (Fig. 2.10).

2.4 Quinolines

Since 1948, - Mice with *P. berghei* has been used for screening of potential antimalarial drugs. Earlier, the screening of antimalarial drugs was attempted with *P. relictum* in birds (1926-35) and *P. gallinaceum* in chicks, ducks, etc.(1935-48).

Classification:

A. Chemical Classification

(i) Quinine derivatives: Ex. **quinine**, cinchonidine, quinidine, cinchonine, **mefloquine**

(ii) 4-aminoquinolines derivatives: Ex. **chloroquine, amodiaqulne,** cycloquine, Hydroxypiperaquine

(iii) 8-aminoquinolines derivatives: Ex. **pamaquine, primaquine,** quinocide

(iv) Amino alcohol derivatives: Ex. **halofantrine**

(v) 9-aminoacridines: Ex. **quinacrine**

(vi) Biguanides: Ex. **proguanil**

(vii) Triazines (metabolite products of proguanil) derivatives: Ex. **cycloguanil pamoate**

(viii) Aminopyrimidine: **pyrimethamine**, Trimethoprim

(ix) Artemisinin and its derivatives: Ex. artemisinin, dihydroartemisinin. **artemether,** arteeher, **sodium artesunate**

(x) Miscellaneous agents: Ex. **atovaquone**

B. Sites of the action at *Plasmodium* by drugs

(i) *Sporozoitocide*/pre-erythrocytic form - There is no such drug available to act on the parasite. However, some drugs are used as a casual prophylactic. Ex. **pyrimethamine** for *P. falciparum* malaria and **primaquine** (not recommended due to toxicity)

(ii) *Tissue schizontocides*/ secondary exo-erythrocytic form - (*P. vivax* and *P. ovale* in the liver) and drugs are used to prevent relapse of parasites. Drugs are used along with blood *schizontocides*) Ex. **primaquine** (anti-relapse drug), **pyrimethamine**

(iii) Blood *schizontocides*/asexual erythrocytic form - Drugs are for all types of *Plasmodium spp.*
a) Fast-acting *Schizontocides* - Ex. chloroquine, quinine, mefloquine
b) Slow-acting *Schizontocides* - Ex. pyrimethamine, sulphonamides, sulphones.

(iv) *Gametocytocides*/sexual erythrocytic form - drugs prevent transmission of the malarial parasite to the mosquito - Ex. primaquine (*P. falciparum*), & chloroquine, mepacrine, and quinine (*P.vivax* and *P. malariae*)

(v) *Sporontocides* - Drugs that prevent the formation of oocytes and sporozoites in infected mosquitoes Ex. proguanil and primaquine

Drugs used on the basis of Mechanism of Action

(a) Rapid *Schizontocidal* action: Ex. primaquine, quinine, chloroquine, and mefloquine (primaquine is less active in this group and also against erythrocytic stage than tissue stages of malaria parasites)

(b) Slow *Schizontocidal* action/antifolate properties: Ex. pyrimethamine and proguanil (dihydrofolate reductase inhibitor) and sulphones and sulphonamide (prevent folate synthesis)

Drawback: In 85% of malarial cases, it has been observed that *P. falciparum* has developed resistance against antimalarial drugs (chloroquine, pyrimethamine-sulphadoxine combination).

2.4.1 Quinine Sulphate

Historical Background

✓ Quinine is a prime alkaloid component found in cinchona bark and is extensively cultivated in South America, India & Indonesia. In European people in ancient times, preparation of bark part was used for the treatment of malaria.

✓ 1677 - The chemical compound was included in London Pharmacopoeia.

✓ 1820 - **E. Caventau and J. Pelletier** was isolated the compound & skeletal structure was established in the year 1908 by **P. Rabe** & **V. Prelong**, 1944.

✓ 2001 – The synthesis of quinine has been credited to **Gilbert stork** (Fig. 2.11), an organic chemist of Belgium.

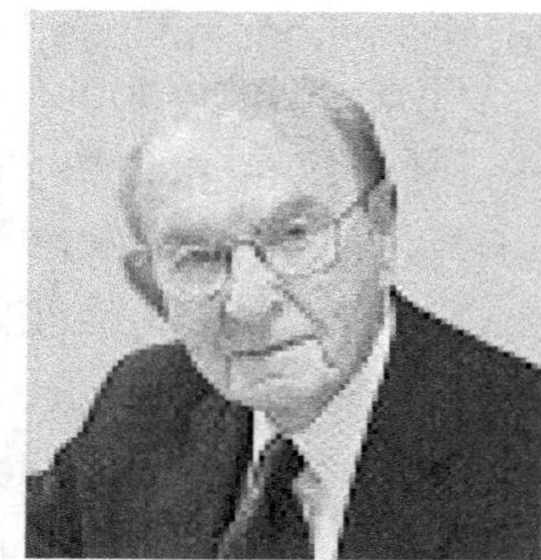

Fig. 2.11 Gilbert Stork.

Chemical Structure: (Fig. 2.12)

Chemical Name:

(*R*)-(6-methoxyquinolin-4-yl)((*1S,2S,4S,5R*)-5-vinylquinuclidin-2-yl)methanol sulfate OR (*8S, 9R*)- 6 methoxycinchonan-9-ol sulphate dihydrate

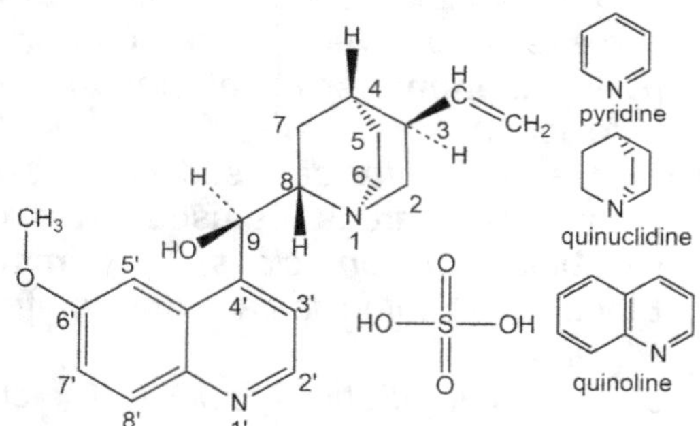

Fig. 2.12 Quinine sulphate.

Stereochemistry

1. Two pairs of optically isomeric alkaloid compounds (quinine, quinidine and cinchonine, cinchonidine) are found in the cinchona bark. Among them, quinine is the most important alkaloid compound.

2. Four chiral centers are located at positions C-3, C-4, C-8 & C-9. Quinine and cinchonidine possess an 8*S*, 9*R* conformation, and quinidine and cinchonine have 8*R*, 9*S* orientation.

3. All four isomers have antimalarial activity.

4. Quinine is a derivative of rubane (3-vinyl-6'-methoxyrubanol-9). Quinidine is a diastereoisomer of quinine. Cinchonidine and cinchonine are the desmethoxy (a methoxy group that has been removed) derivatives of quinine and quinidine, respectively. Quinine and cinchonidine are levorotatory, and their isomers quinidine and cinchonine are dextrorotatory (**Fig. 2.13).**

Structure-Activity Relationship

1. Quinoline (heterocyclic ring) is linked to quinuclidine moiety through a secondary alcohol in the structure of quinine (Fig. 2.14).

2. A vinyl group is directly attached to C-3 of quinuclidine. A methoxy group is positioned at C-6 of quinine and quinidine. The two groups(vinyl and methoxy) are not part of the antimalarial activity.

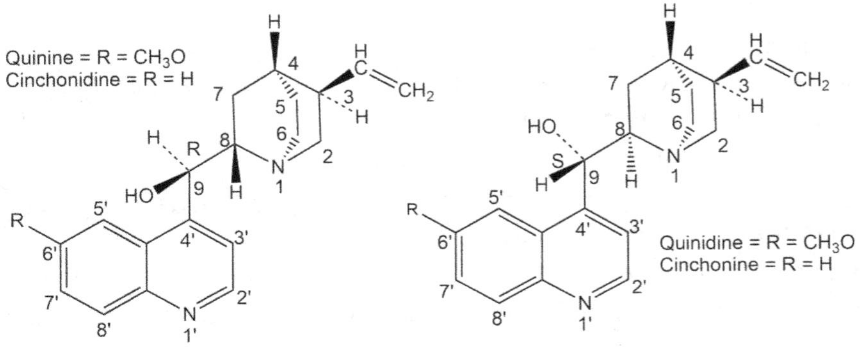

Fig. 2.13 Stereochemistry of quinine.

3. All four compounds have antimalarial properties. However, epimers at C-9 (8R,9R or 8S,9S configuration) have produced inactive compounds.

4. Any chemical changes such as esterification, oxidation, etc. in the secondary alcohol function at C-9 have reduced the antimalarial activity.

5. An alkyl tertiary amine in quinuclidine structure is necessary for antimalarial activity. Otherwise, quinuclidine part of quinine has not required for antimalarial activity.

6. This observation helps to study different amino alcohols with the following general structure (Fig. 2.14).

7. Quinine and related alkaloid compounds have this moiety in their structures. There are many compounds with this moiety that have been prepared and screened for antimalarial activity. 4-quinolyl, 1-naphthyl, or 9-phenanthryl substituted at aromatic ring position have resulted in the new antimalarial drug (mefloquine, halofantrine)

8. 1963- **Mefloquine** was developed by Walter Read Institute for Medical Research and had shown promising antimalarial activity against strains of *P. falciparum*.

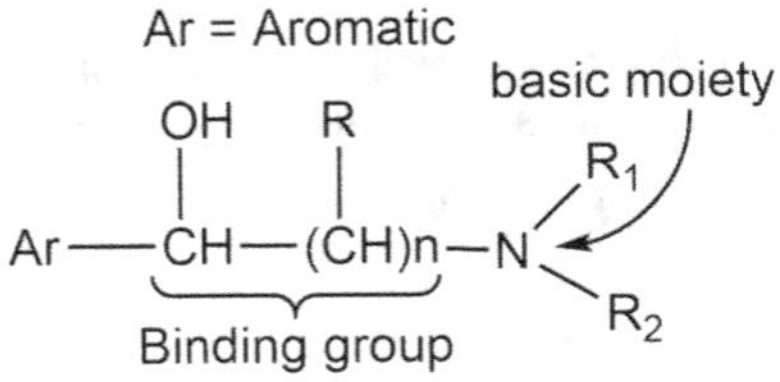

Fig.2.14 General structure of Anitmalarial drug.

Mechanism of Action

Primarily, quinine inhibits the parasite at the blood *schizontocide* label. It is less active against sporozoites or tissue forms of the malarial parasite. It is also act as gametocidal for *P. vivax* and *P. malariae,* but not for *P. falciparum*. It also functions as a DNA synthesizer.

The exact mechanism of action of quinine has not been fully understood, although in vitro studies indicate it inhibits nucleic acid and protein synthesis and inhibits glycolysis in P. falciparum. Quinine may target the purine nucleoside phosphorylase enzyme in malaria parasites.

Uses

- ✓ Sulphate, bisulphate, hydrochloride, and dihydrochloride are the official compound of quinine and are given the treatment of severe forms of chloroquine-resistant or multi-drug resistant *P. falciparum* of malaria.
- ✓ It is given by I.V. in the case of non-immune patients.
- ✓ Given combination with pyrimethamine, and a sulphonamide or with tetracycline to cure patients with multidrug resistant *P. falciparum* malaria.
- ✓ Quinine is given with primaquine for treatment of *P. vivax* or relapsing of malaria.
- ✓ It should not be given alone. Though, it produces less active or toxic effects on the host.

2.4.2 Chloroquine

Historical Background

- ✓ Chloroquine is a 4-aminoquinolines derivative compound. The chemical structure of the compound is similar to the 9-amino acridine derivative compound (quinacrine (mepacrine))
- ✓ Many 4-aminoquinolines derivative compounds were first studied in Germany. Which, Santoquine was studied for its antimalarial activity in the North African region people. This led to a study of the number of 4-aminoquinolines class compounds, among them chloroquine was found to be an effective antimalarial drug.

Chemical Structure: (Fig. 2.16)

Chemical Name:

N^4-(7-chloroquinolin-4-yl)-N^1,N^1-diethylpentane-1,4-diamine   or   (*RS*)-7-Chloro-4-(4-diethylamino-1-melhylbutylamino)-quinoline or (R S)-4- (7 -chloro- 4-quinolylamino) pentyldielhylamine.

Synthesis of Chloroquine

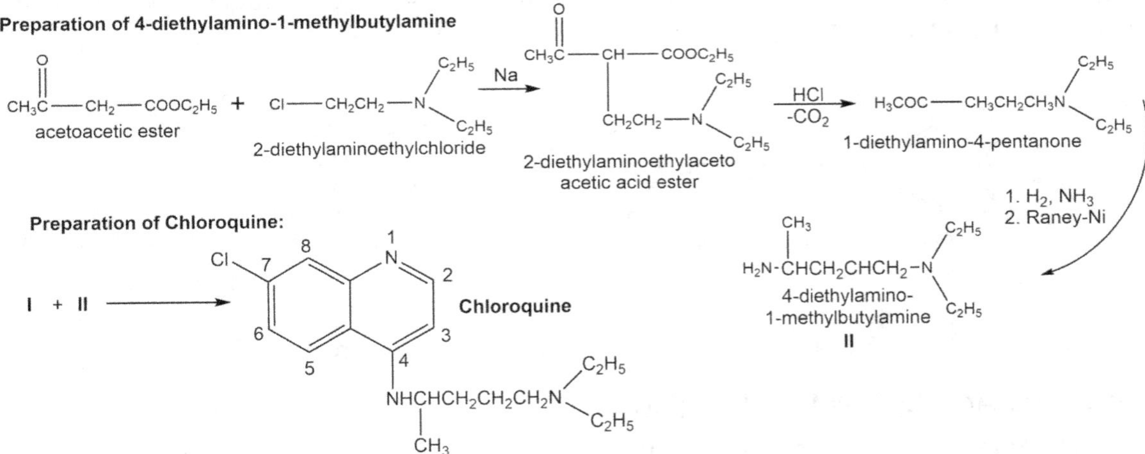

Fig. 2.15 Preparation of Quinoline ring.

Preparation of 4-diethylamino-1-methylbutylamine

Preparation of Chloroquine:

Fig. 2.16 Preparation of Chloroquine.

A. First Method

1. Preparation of 4,7-dichloroquinoline is attempted in several ways from 3-chloroaniline. One of these ways consists of reacting 3-chloroaniline with the diethyl ester of oxaloacetic acid in the presence of acetic acid to give the corresponding enamine.

2. Enamine, when heated to 250°C undergoes heterocyclization to form the ethyl ester of 7-chloro-4-hydroxyquinolin-2-carboxylic acid and a small amount of 5-chloro-4-hydroxyquinolin- 2-carboxylic acid.

3. The later product is separated from the main product by crystallization from acetic acid.

4. Alkaline hydrolysis of the ethyl ester of the 7-chloro-4-hydroxyquinolin-2- carboxylic acid and subsequent high-temperature decarboxylation of the resulting acid gives 7-chloro-hydroxyquin-4-ol.

5. The obtained product is reacting with phosphorus oxychloride (POCl₃) gives the product **4,7-dichloroquineoline** is the first step of reaction (Fig. 2.15).

6. The second component is necessary for synthesizing chloroquine. 4-diethylamino-1-methylbutylamine could be prepared in in various ways.

7. Acetoacetic ester is Alkylating (Na) with 2-diethylaminoethylchloride gives 2-diethylaminoethylacetoacetic acid ester.

8. The resultant product upon acidic hydrolysis (using hydrochloric acid) and simultaneous decarboxylation makes a compound 1-diethylamino-4-pentanone.

9. Subsequent reductive amination of this compound with hydrogen and ammonia using Raney nickel as a catalyst gives the second component **(4-diethylamino-1-methylbutylamine)** of Chloroquine (Fig. 2.16).

B. Second/Direct Method

Chloroquine is also prepared directly. In this method, 4,7-dichloroquinoline is reacting with 4-diethylamino-1-methylbutylamine at 180°C (Fig. 2.17)

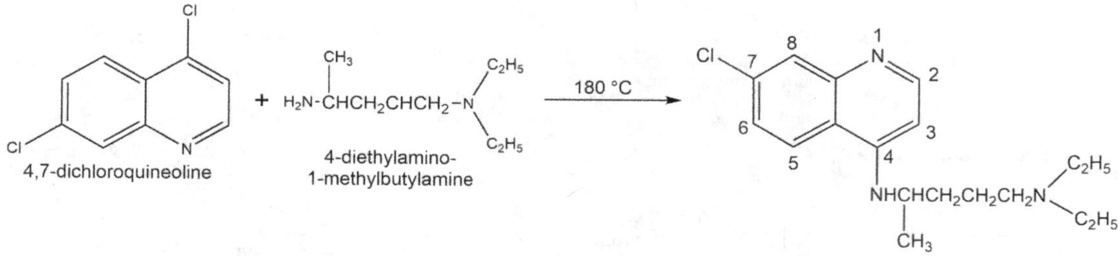

Fig. 2.17 Preparation of Chloroquine[Direct process].

Structure-Activity Relationship: (Fig. 2.16)

1. Dialkylaminoalkyl side chain - The length of the carbon chain (2-5) in between the nitrogen atom is optimal antimalarial activity as in chloroquine and quinacrine.

2. The amine group of chloroquine is responsible for the basic nature of the drug.

3. The tertiary amine in the aliphatic chain of chemical structure is important for activity.

4. Adding a double bond in the aliphatic chain of chemical structure is retain its activity.

5. The chlorine group at C-7 is required for antimalarial activity. Substitution of the CH₃ -group at C-3 reduces activity, and another substitution of the CH₃ group at C-8 completely abolishes the activity.

6. The substitution of the hydroxyl (-OH) group with any one of the ethyl groups on the tertiary amine of the aliphatic chain increases the antimalarial activity. The resultant product is one of the metabolites of chloroquine (hydroxychloroquine).

7. Replacement of the heterocyclic ring by an aromatic ring in the aliphatic chain gives a new compound, amodiaquine, which shows antimalarial activity similar to chloroquine.

8. The replacemant of the quinoline ring by three member acridine ring (mepacrine) in the aliphatic chain shows antimalarial activity but increases its toxicity properties.

9. The stereoisomer (d,l, and dl) forms of chloroquine have posses therapeutic effect against malaria in ducks. The d-form of chloroquine is more active and less toxic than L-form.

10. Secondary alkyl group attached to the carbon next to the amino group in the aliphatic chain have no major role in the antimalarial activity.

Mechanism of Action

It acts as a rapid *schizontocidal* effect and kills the erythrocytic forms of the malarial parasite at all stages of development without affecting human liver cells. It will inhibit *P. falciparum* but is not very effective against the relapse arising from the secondary exoerythrocytic phase of *P. vivax*, *P. ovale*, and *P. malariae*. Chloroquine and primaquine (8-aminoquinoline) are needed to prevent the secondary exoerythrocytic phase of the parasite. It controls the acute attacks of *P. falciparum* and its strains. Chloroquine is better than quinine in terms of potency and toxicity. It is given once a week as a suppressive agent. *P. falciparum* strains have developed resistance to chloroquine; the drawback of the compound has been reported.

Chloroquine interacts with the DNA of malarial parasites. This type of interaction also occurs with primaquine and quinine, but not with mefloquine. It has been significantly inhibiting the DNA polymerase. In infected erythrocytes, it has been interacting with aggregates of ferriprotoporphyrin IX (this compound is toxic, since it is a prooxidant and catalyzes the production of reactive oxygen species), which are released during the breakdown of hemoglobin.

Uses

- ✓ Chloroquine sulphate and phosphate are the official product and are used for the prophylaxis and treatment of malaria.

- ✓ Given alone or in combination with emetine hydrochloride for treatment of amoebic hepatitis.

- ✓ Used in the treatment of systemic amoebicide, in case of metronidazole is not useful for treatment.

- ✓ The compound is very much useful for the treatment of skin infections, rheumatoid arthritis, & giardiasis.

2.4.3 Amodiaquine

Historical Background

Amodiaquine was introduced in the late 1950s and shown to be a superior alternative to chloroquine. It is no more toxic than chloroquine, which was therapeutically used to treat uncomplicated *P. falciparum* malaria.

Chemical Structure: (Fig. 2.18)

Chemical Name: 4-((7-chloroquinolin-4-yl)amino)-2-((diethylamino)methyl)phenol

Structure-Activity Relationship

1. Chloro group at C-7, the tertiary amine and dialkyl side chain are required for antimalarial activity.

2. The phenolic group is essential for antimalarial activity.

3. Methylation of the phenyl group is destroying its antimalarial property

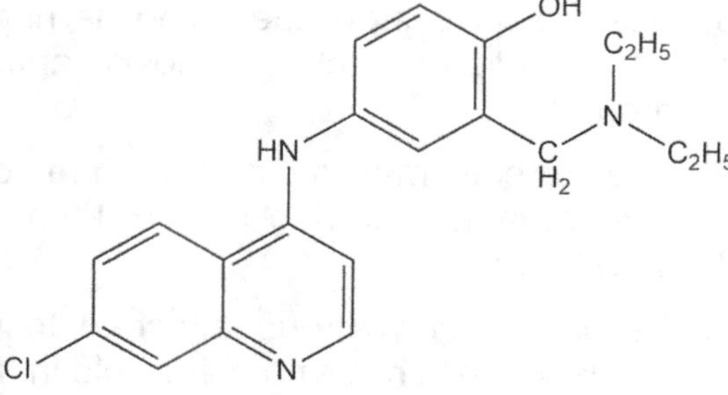

Fig. 2.18 Chemical structure of Amodiaquine.

Mechanism of Action

Amodiaquine is a 4-aminoquinoline with antimalarial activity and a mechanism of action similar to that of chloroquine. The activity of amodiaquine against some chloroquine-resistant strains of *P. falciparum*. While resistance to amodiaquine may limit its use. The artesunate–amodiaquine combination has proven very effective where responses to amodiaquine alone exceed 80%. It is 3-4 times more active than quinine.

It is thought to inhibit heme polymerase activity. This results in the accumulation of free heme, which is toxic to the parasites. The drug binds the free heme, preventing the parasite from converting it to a less toxic form. This drug-heme complex is toxic and disrupts membrane function.

Uses

✓ Used in combination with artesunate to treat uncomplicated *P. falciparum* malaria. It is also used in combination with sulfadoxine/pyrimethamine.

✓ Given for treatment of chloroquine-resistant *P. falciparum* strains of malaria.

✓ Amodiaquine hydrochloride is an official compound and is used once a week or daily for three days for the suppression of malaria.

2.4.4 Primaquine Phosphate

Historical Background

✓ 1891 - **P. Gutttmann** and **P. Ehrlich** examined the dye compounds on patients suffering from malaria.

✓ Methylene blue (dye) varients were tested antimalarial activity. In the chemical structure, the basic aliphatic chain (dialkylaminoalkylamino) showed high antimalarial activity.

✓ Quinine has also been proposed as another model antimalarial drug. The analogue of dialkylaminoalkylamino of 6-methoxyquinoline was prepared.

✓ Pamaquine was reported first synthetic antimalarial drug of this class and was found to be effective against tissue schizontocide.

✓ During world war II, many 8-aminoquinoline compounds were explored as pamaquine produce toxicity. As a result, pentaquine and primaquine were reported more potent and less toxic than pamaquine. In this class, primaquine is widely used as an antimalarial drug.

Chemical Structure: (Fig. 2.19)

Chemical Name:

N^4-(6-methoxyquinolin-8-yl)pentane-1,4-diaminephosphate   or   (*RS*)-8-(4-amino1-methylbutylamino)-6-methoxy-quinloline phosphate or (*RS*)-4-amino- 1-methylbutyl (6-methoxy-8-quinolyl) amine diphosphate

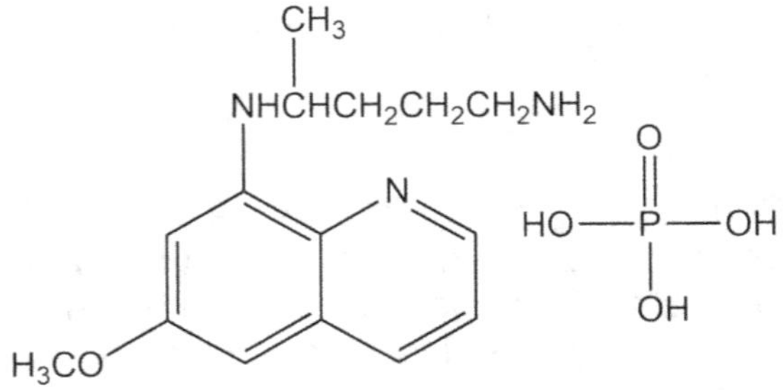

Structue-Activity Relationship

1. The presence of a 6-oxygen function in the quinoline ring has been shown to increase activity, the substitution of the 6-methoxy group in the ring retains its therapeutic activity against malarial parasites. Substitution of benzyloxy, methoxy group at C-2 have less active and less toxic than primaquine.

Fig. 2.19 Chemical structure of Primaquine phosphate.

2. Phenyl substitution at C-3 has lower activity and toxicity.

3. Methyl, ethyl and vinyl substituents at C-4 have equal to or slightly greater than that of primaquine. Methyl group at primaquine has been shown to possess significant activity against *Trypanosoma cruzi*.

4. Substitution of Phenylthio, anilino, or phenoxy groups at C-5 have retained the highest level of tissue *schizontocidal* activity.

5. Hydroxyl, methoxyl, 3-βhydroxyethoxyl at C-6 derivative compound have enhanced antimalarial activity but also increased toxicity.

6. Antimalarial activity will lose by the introduction of any groups at C- 7 of the quinoline ring.

7. **Multi substitution in the ring-** 2,4-dialkyl-6-methoxy -8-aminoquinoline analogue compounds were less active than primaquine. Similarly, 4-methyl-5-fluoro-primaquine compounds were produce very high activity but were also very toxic.

8. Optimal activity was obtained with 2-6 methylene groups between the two nitrogens of the side chain. Analogous groups with an even number of methylene groups were found to be slightly less active than those with an odd number.

9. Antimalarial activity did not improve with the introduction of heteroatoms into the basic side-chain of the compounds. It is also observed that antimalarial activity occurs when the 8-amino group is secondary and the terminal amine group is primary.

10. Stereochemistry

1. Stereoisomeric compounds have been examined for prophylactic antimalarial activity against *P. cynomolgi* in monkeys.

2. (+)- and (-)-primaquine possess identical chemical structure and are found to be similar to a racemic form of primaquine.

3. It has been observed that (-)-primaquine was 3-5 times more toxic than (+)-primaquine and about twice as toxic as racemic primaquine.

4. *d*-isomer of primaquine has been found twice active and low toxicity than *dl*-isomer in rhesus monkey.

5. Quinocide (Fig. 2.20) is a structural isomer of primaquine and found to be a similar mechanism of action & use to later compound.

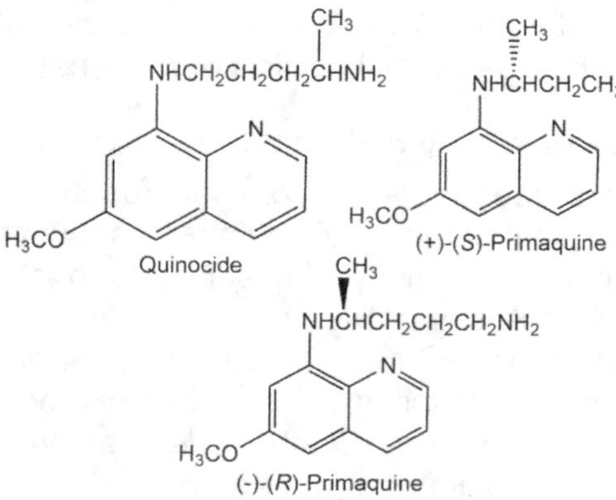

Mechanism of Action

Primaquine phosphate is a salt of primaquine, a synthetic compound with antimalarial properties. It binds and alters the properties of protozoal DNA. This agent eliminates tissue (exo-erythrocytic) malarial infection, preventing the development of the erythrocytic forms of the parasite, which are responsible for relapses in *Plasmodium vivax* and *ovale* malaria.

Fig. 2.20 Steroisomeric form of Primaquine.

Primaquine has *schizontocidal* activity. It has lethal action on primary and secondary exoerythrocytic forms of the parasite. It has also shown effectiveness against gametocytocidal activity in all four species, especially *P. falciparum*. It should not be given alone for the treatment of malaria. Its exact mechanism of action is not clear to understand.

Uses

- ✓ It is given for the treatment of *P. vivax* and other relapsing malaria.
- ✓ It has usually given with chloroquine in the treatment of malaria, in order to reduce the possibility of developing drug-resistant strains.
- ✓ It combines with clindamycin for the treatment of *Pneumocystis carinii* infection.

2.4.5 Pamaquine

Historical Background

- ✓ 1920 - The discovery of pamaquine was developed by replacing one of the methyl groups of methylene blue with a dialkylaminoalkyl chain by **Schoenhoefer, Schuleman,** and **Roehl.**

✓ 1924 - It was synthesised by **Schulemann, Schoenhoeffer,** and **Wingler**. Pamaquine was the first synthetic antimalarial compound among the 8-amino-quinoline class of compounds.

✓ 1926 - **Roehl** demonstrated that pamaquine was effective in treating malaria in birds, and later it was introduced in humans. Although it could not be used clinically due to its high toxicity it provides an important lead to developing better antimalarials. Pamaquine (Plasmochin) was first marketed in 1926.

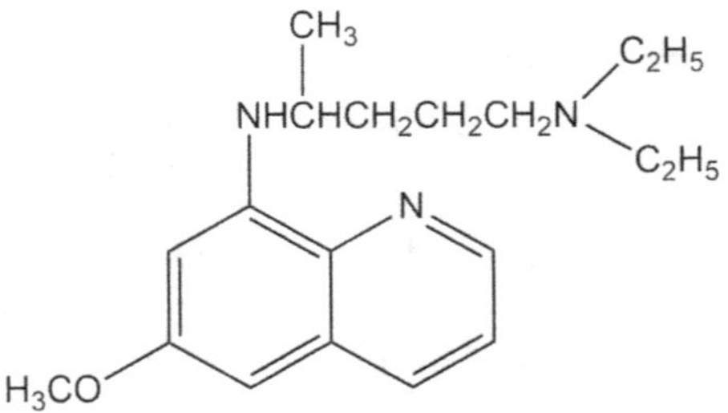
Fig.2.21 Chemical structure of Pamaquine.

✓ 1929 - The compound showed for the first time that it was possible to prevent relapses of *vivax* malaria.

Chemical Structure: (Fig. 2.21)

Chemical Name:

N^1,N^1-diethyl-N^4-(6-methoxyquinolin-8-yl) pentane-1,4-diamine or 8-(4-diethylamino-1 -methylbutylamino)-6-methoxyquinoline

Synthesis: (Fig. 2.22)

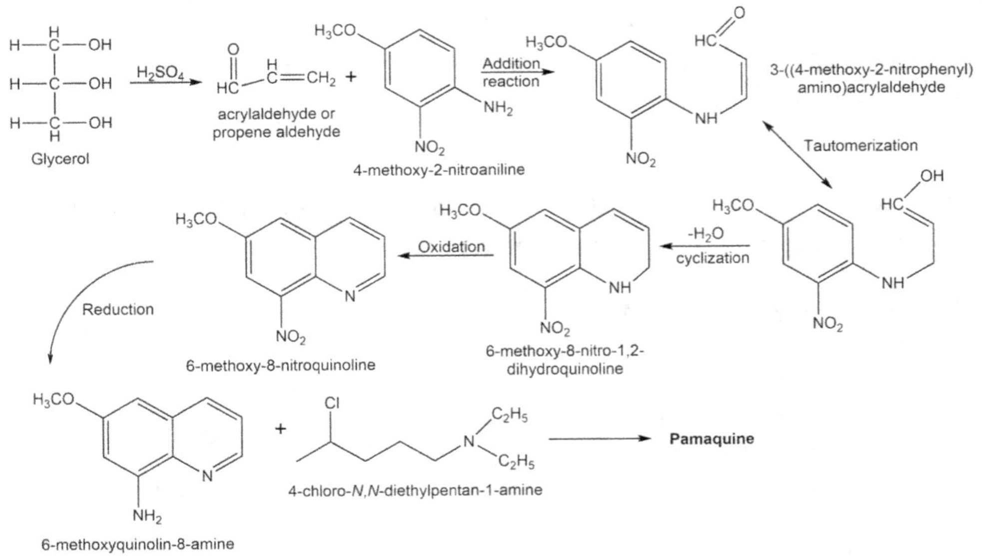

Fig. 2.22 Synthesis of Pamaquine.

1. Glycerol undergoes dehydration with H_2SO_4 (dehydrating agent) to produce acrylaldehyde or propene aldehyde.

2. Propene aldehyde undergo condensation with 4-methoxy-2-nitroaniline to form the product 3-((4-methoxy-2-nitrophenyl)amino)acrylaldehyde.

3. **Tautomerization**: Under favourable condition, the resultant product (3-((4-methoxy-2-nitrophenyl) amino)acrylaldehyde)(keto-form) converted to enol-form.

4. Enol form undergo cyclization and dehydration to form 6-methoxy-8-nitro-1,2-dihydroquinoline which further oxidised to form 6-methoxy-8-nitroquinoline.

5. The intermediate product undergoes a reduction process to form 6-methoxyquinolin-8-amine. The latter product was added with 4-chloro-N,N-diethylpentan-1-amine to form pamaquine.

Structure-Activity Relationship

1. All the pamaquine analogues proved to be inactive compounds.

2. Although pamaquine itself could not be used clinically due to high toxicity, it provided an important lead to developing better antimalarial such as primaquine.

Mechanism of Action

German researchers developed the first member (pamaquine) of the 8-aminoquinoline class in 1925. It was given special attention because of its efficiency against liver-stage parasites. It is capable of targeting pre-erythrocytic stages of *P. falciparum*, *P. vivax*, and *P. ovale*. It has excellent prophylactic activity. Even though it is not active against blood-stage parasites. It has been shown to inhibit the gametocyte stage of the parasite. Because of toxicological concerns, this compound was no longer employed clinically. The compound has led to the development of **tafenoquine,** which has a longer plasma half-life, less toxicity, and improved activities against both liver and blood-stage parasites. Pamaquine was reported in patients with glucose-6-phosphate dehydrogenase (G6PD) deficiency.

Uses

✓ It has extremely effective in the causal prophylactic treatment of malaria.

✓ Pamaquine naphthoate & Pamaquine embonate are salt products.

2.4.6 Quinacrine Hydrochloride

Historical Background

✓ There is a large number of acridine derivatives with basic side chains (9-aminoacridine class) that were prepared and tested in Germany.

✓ Out of which, quinacrine (mepacrine) was the first synthetic antimalarial drug discovered in 1932.

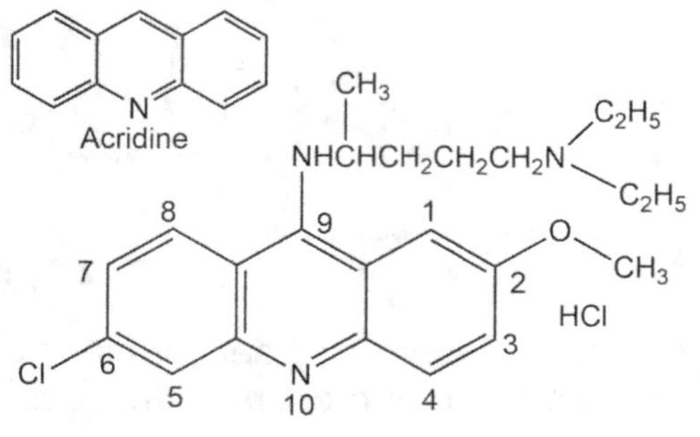

Fig. 2.23 Chemical structure of Quinacrine HCl.

Chemical Structure: (Fig. 2.23)

Chemical Name:

N^4-(6-chloro-2-methoxyacridin-9-yl)-N^1,N^1-diethylpentane-1,4-diamine

Structure-Activity Relationship

1. Quinacrine (mepacrine) (Fig. 2.23) is the first synthetic compound of the class & used before quinolines. In the chemical structure, an acridine ring (three member) is formed with an additional benzene ring fused with a quinoline (two member) nucleus. It is a fluorescent dye compound. In the past, it was used as an antiseptic for wound infection. Acrdiine has weak antiseptic and antibacterial properties.

2. An aliphatic chain at C-9, Cl group at C-2 & -CH3O group at C-6 of the acridine ring has become the compound as an antimalarial drug.

3. Methoxy group at C-6 is replaced by the ethoxy group in the ring increasing toxicity and interchange to C-2, the compound has a loss of antimalarial activity. The shifting of the methoxy group in either of any positions (C-1, 3, 5) has a loss of 50% antimalarial property.

4. Replacement of the Cl group with any other halogen group in the ring has lost antimalarial property.

5. An aliphatic chain at C-9 have no role in antimalarial activity. However, the aliphatic chain link with the aromatic ring has produced antimalarial properties.

6. An introduction of the -N atom at position 1 of the heterocyclic ring produce a product known as azacrine, which have possessed antimalarial activity.

7. Antimalarial activity has increased with the substitution of either the Cl or a cyano group in position 3, or the Cl atom in position 1. Placement of the halogens F or I, or of a methyl group, at the 3-position also increases potency but the same substituents in positions 2 and 4 diminish the activity.

8. Substitution of a 2-nitro group increased potency, while a 3-nitro group reduced activity. Methoxy or ethoxy group at C-7 of the ring does not affect potency but reduces the toxicity of the host.

9. The terminal secondary amine of the aliphatic chain is essential for antimalarial activity.

10. There are a number of 9-aminoacridines that were prepared and tested clinically, but none of them proved better than quinacrine.

Mechanism of Action

The exact mechanism of its antimalarial activity is unknown. It is supposed to act against a parasite cell membrane and inhibit DNA & RNA synthesis.

Uses

- ✓ Used in the treatment of malaria and protozoan and tapeworms of the *Taenia* and *Hymenolopis* species

- ✓ Given in petit mal epilepsy, cancer, and also effectively reduces inflammation related to rheumatoid arthritis and lupus erythematosus.

✓ The compound has low therapeutic activity. Hence, after the development of 4-aminoquinolines, they are rarely used in the treatment of malaria.

✓ Used as an anthelmintic for the treatment of giardiasis and leishmaniasis.

Drawback: After use, it develops yellow pigmentation in the skin and the appearance of yellow urine. These signs disappeared with the discontinuation of therapy.

2.4.7 Mefloquine

Historical Background

✓ 1970 - Mefloquine was developed at the **Walter Reed Army Institute of Research** (WRAIR) after the end of the Vietnam War. Mefloquine was screened out of a total of 250,000 antimalarial compounds.

✓ 1984 - The drug was first marketed under the name *Lariam* in Switzerland.

✓ 1994 - Severe psychiatric side effects were reported during prophylaxis and treatment with mefloquine.

✓ 2009 - Roche stopped marketing *Lariam* in the USA.

Chemical Structure: (Fig. 2.24)

Chemical Name: (2,8-bis(trifluoromethyl)quinolin-4-yl)(piperidin-2-yl)methanol or [2,8-Bis(trifluoromethyl)-quininolin-4-yl] [piperidin-2-yl] methanol

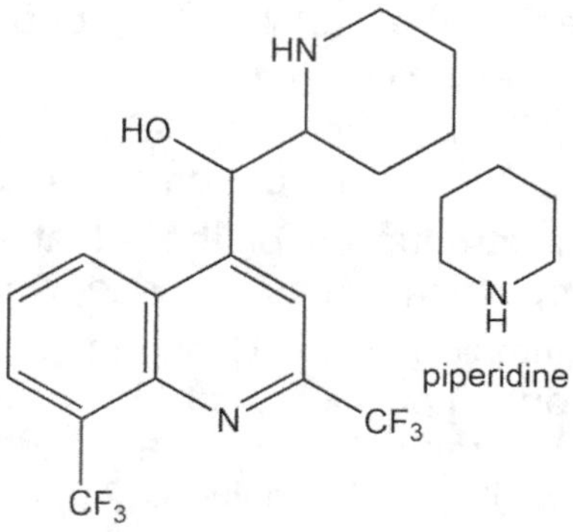

Fig. 2.24 Chemical structure of Mefloquine.

Structure-Activity Relationship

1. Mefloquine is an analog of quinine, and it differs from it in the side chain at C-4 of the quinoline ring contains a piperidine fragment instead of a quinuclidine fragment, and CF_3 groups are substituted at positions C-2 and C-8.

2. 2-pyridylmethanols substitution in place of 2-piperidylmethyl side chains of the aromatic ring has loses antimalarial activity.

3. A phenyl ring substitution at the position of C-2 of the quinoline ring retains antimalarial activity.

4. Substitution of methyl and ethyl, as well as acetylation of the piperidine ring and -OH groups in the structure, abolishes antimalarial activity.

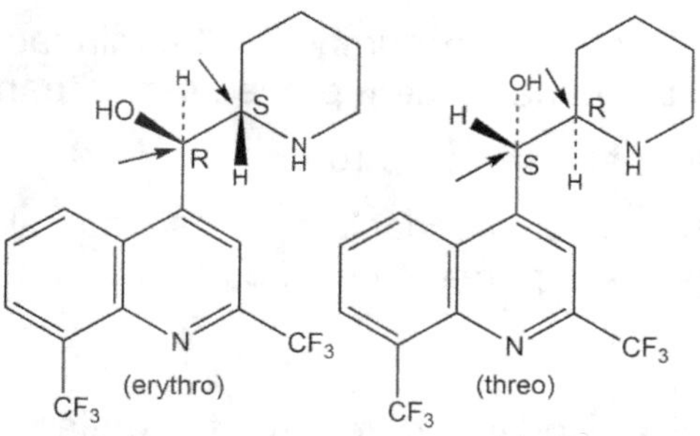

Fig. 2.25 Stereochemistry of Mefloquine.

5. Aziridine derived compound has lose its antimalarial property.

Stereochemistry

1. It is a racemate and consisting of two dissimilar asymmetric centers, exists in two racemic forms (*erythro* and *threo*) each of which is composed of a pair of enantiomers.

2. (-) and (+) *erythro* enantiomers have the 1*S*, 2*R* and 1*R*, 2*S* configurations and the (-) and (+) *threo* enantiomers the 1*S*, 2*S* and 1*R*, 2*R*, respectively.

3. *S*, *S* & *R*, *R* isomers are active compounds (Fig. 2.25).

Mechanism of Action

It acts on the host like quinine. It blocks the enzymatic synthesis of DNA and RNA. It is active against the asexual forms of the four species of *Plasmodium* and has some activity against the sexual forms (gametocytes) of *P. vivax*, *P. malariae,* and *P. ovale*. It is ineffective against gametocytes of *P. falciparum* and exoerythrocytic liver forms of *Plasmodium* species. It is extremely active against the blood *schizontocides P. vivax* and *P. falciparum*.

Another study suggests that mefloquine specifically binds the 80S ribosome of *P. falciparum*, inhibiting protein synthesis and causing subsequent *schizonticidal* development.

Uses

✓ It is given for the treatment of weak and moderate forms of malaria.

✓ Used to treat and prevent chloroquine resistance of malaria caused by *P. falciparum*

✓ Mefloquine HCl(salt) is given orally for the treatment of malaria.

2.5   Biguanides and Dihydro Triazines

Historical Background

✓ World war-II Period: In this era, researchers studied many types of chemical compounds including antibacterial agents such as sulphanilamides and bis(aminophenyl) sulphones. out of which, sulphapyrimidines were showing promising antimalarial activity.

✓ Several combinations of drugs were extensively studied for their antimalarial activity. Among them, Sulfadoxine (long acting sulphanilamide) and pyrimethamine, sulphadiazine, and pyrimethamine & dapsone, and pyrimethamine are the promising combinations of drugs that have been used for malarial treatment.

✓ In the meantime, antifolate inhibitors (sulphonamides and sulphones) drew much attention from researchers as they developed the compound as an antimalarial agent. These compounds have a much higher affinity for plasmodial dihydrofolate reductase, which takes part in the conversion of PABA to folic acid & further proceeds to DNA & RNA synthesis. The former process does not occur in mammals.

✓ In about 1940 — a research team at Wellcome Research Laboratories studied 2.4-diaminopyrimidiens (pyrimethamine) as an antifolate agent and found it to be an antagonist of folic acid synthesis in *Lactobacillus casei*. This led to the discovery of proguanil.

- ✓ **F.H.S Curd** & **F.L. Rose** of Imperial Chemical Industries developed **proguanil** as an antimalarial drug in the year 1948. Chloroproguanil; another antimalarial drug was included in B.P. in 1973.

- ✓ Here, Antifolate drugs such as cycloguanil pamoate, proguanil (biguanide class) & pyrimethamine (aminopyrimidine class) are discussed. These types of compounds are inhibiting plasmodial dihydrofolate reductase (an enzyme involved in the conversion of PABA to folic acid).

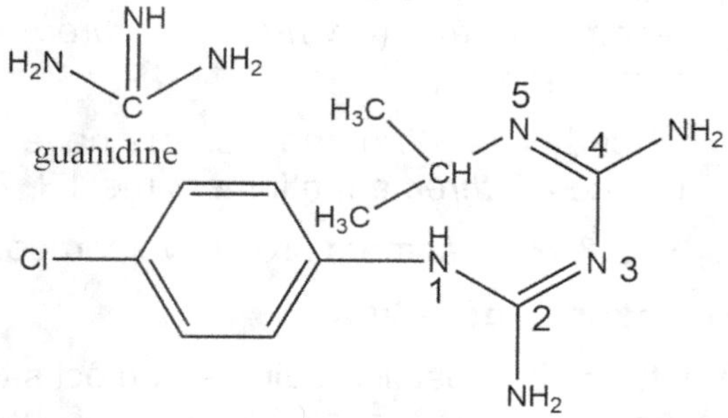

Fig. 2.26 Chemical structure of Proguanil.

2.5.1 Proguanil

Chemical Structure: (Fig. 2.26)

Chemical Name: (*Z*)-1-(4-chloro phenyl)- 2-((*Z*)-N'-isopropylcarbamimidoyl)guanidine or 1-(4-chlorophenyl)-5-isopropyl-biguani- dine

Structute-Activity Relationship

1. The antimalarial drug consists of a Cl-group in the benzene ring coupled with two basic guanidino groups. Proguanil and chloroguanide were found to be clinically effective by substituting the terminal guanidino group with simple alkali, isopropyl derivative.

2. The first substitution of N^1-aryl shows antimalarial activity. While the 2nd substitution reduces the activity.

3. Dihalogen substitution in positions C-3 & C-4 of the benzene ring possesses the potent compound.

4. Any alkyl substitution at N^1, C-2, or C-4 decreases the activity.

5. Replacement of the isopropyl group at N-5 with straight chain propyl group retains its activity.

6. The introduction of a shorter or longer alkyl chain at N-5 resulted in a decrease in activity.

Mechanism of Action

Proguanil (Prodrug) is a biguanide derivative compound that is converted to an active metabolite called cycloguanil pamoate (triazine metabolite). It inhibits plasmodial dihydrofolate reductase (DHFR) without harming host tissue, mainly through cycloguanil, which inhibits folate production in both pre-erythrocytic and erythrocytic parasites. Inhibition of DHFR prevents the parasite from recycling dihydrofolate back to tetrahydrofolate (THF). THF is required for DNA, amino acid synthesis, and methylation processes; thus, DHFR inhibition paralyzes the parasite. It is clinically effective against the *P. falciparum* parasite. It is also effective in suppressing the clinical attacks of *vivax* malaria.

It has a slower antimalarial effect compared with quinine. In *P. vivax*, it kills the asexual parasites in the RBC and controls the acute clinical stage. It has little or no activity against the exoerythrocytic stage of *P. vivax*.

Uses

✓ It is often used for the prevention and treatment of malaria, either alone or in combination with chloroquine.

✓ It can also be used in the prophylaxis and treatment of *P. falciparum* in combination with atovaquone.

✓ It is also effective in the treatment of multi-drug resistant forms of *P. falciparum*.

2.5.2 Cycloguanil Pamoate

Chemical Structure: (Fig. 2.27)

Chemical Name:

1-(4-chlorophenyl)-6,6-dimethyl-1,6-dihydro-1,3,5-triazine-2,4-diamine — Cycloguanil

4,4'-methyl- enebis(3-hydroxy-2-naphthoic acid) — Pamoate

Structure-Activity Relationship: see the drug proguanil.

Mechanism of Action

Cycloguanil inhibits plasmodial dihydrofolate reductase and is a metabolite product of the antimalarial drug proguanil.

It selectively inhibits the bifunctional dihydro folate reductase-thymidylate reductase of *Plasmodium*. Thus inhibiting DNA synthesis. It is active against pre-erythrocytic forms. It acts slowly on blood *schizontocide*. It also possesses some *sporontocidal* activity, which makes gametocytes non-infective to the mosquito.

Uses

It plays a important role in the early erythrocytic stages of all four *Plasmodium spp.* that causes human malaria and the primary hepatic stage of *P. falciparum*.

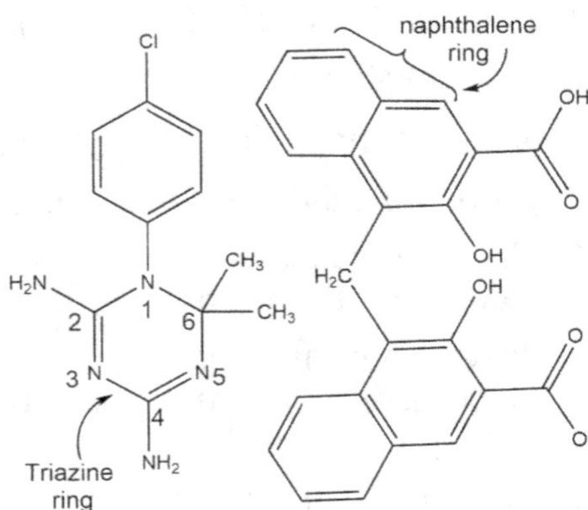

Fig.2.27 Chemical structure of Cycloguanil pamoate.

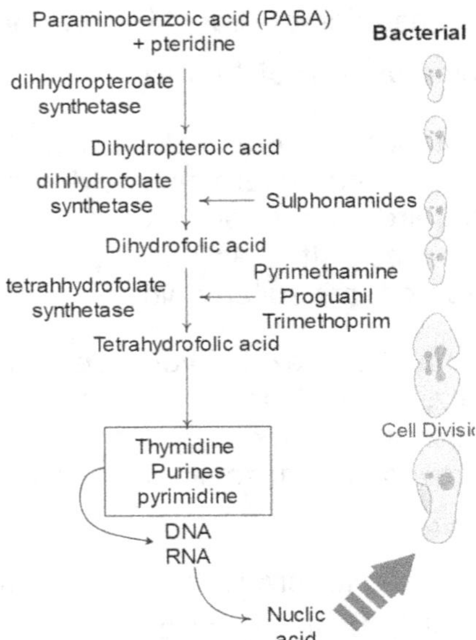

Fig. 2.29 Mechanism of antifolate drugs.

2.6 Miscellaneous

2.6.1 Pyrimethamine

Historical Background

- ✓ 1940 - Researchers of Wellcome Research Lab, USA were worked on aminopyrimidine class compounds & many of them identified as an antifolate agent.
- ✓ During the investigation, pyrimethamine was first reported as an antimalarial agent of aminopyrimidine class. Later, trimethoprim of this group was identified as both an antibacterial and antimalarial agent.

Chemical Structure: (Fig. 2.28)

Chemical Name:

5-(4-chlorophenyl)-6-ethyl pyrimidine -2,4- di amine

Structure-Activity Relationship

1. Amine functional group at C-2 & C-4 should be the primary state. The antimalarial activity of the compound may lose, If it changes to a secondary or tertiary state.

2. Insertion of methylene ($-CH_2-$) bridge in between aromatic and heteroaromatic rings decreases antimalarial property but increases antibacterial property (Ex. trimethoprim).

3. Replacement of aromatic ring by heteroaromatic ring has loses its activity. Substitution of the electron withdrawn group at the para position and donating group at the C-6 position of the aromatic ring must for activity.

4. An aromatic ring is directly linked with a pyrimidine ring for maximum activity. Insertion of C or N in between two rings decreases the activity.

Mechanism of Action

Pyrimethamine inhibits dihydrofolate reductase (DHFR), preventing the conversion of di- to tetra-hydrofolic acid, an important enzyme in nucleic acid synthesis which requires purine and pyrimidine synthesis (Fig. 2.29). This disrupts the parasite's DNA synthesis. It is active against both *P. falciparum* and *P. vivax* in combination with an appropriate sulfonamide.

It has been extensively used for the prophylaxis and treatment of chloroquine-resistant strains of *P. falciparum*. Pyrimethamine has a *schizonticidal* effect against malaria parasites in the blood and in some tissues. It doesn't kill gametocytes, but it does prevent the mosquito from sporogenesis.

Uses

- ✓ Used for preventing and treating malaria.
- ✓ It is used in combination with sulfadiazine to treat active toxoplasmosis (parasite infection - mild flu, muscle ache)
- ✓ A combination of pyrimethamine, sulfonamide, and quinine is given for the treatment of malaria and its chloroquine-resistant form of parasite

2.6.2 Artesunate

Historical Background

✓ 1977 - Liu Xu, a Chinese chemist developed Artesunate compound. It belongs to the artemisinins class of drugs, which are derived from the "qinghao," (Chinese name) or sweet wormwood plant (*Artemisia annua*). This is weed like plant growing large part of China, and It has been used for medicinal purposes for approximately 2000 years.

✓ In May 2020, it received FDA approval for medical use in the United States.

✓ Artemisinins belong to the sesquiterpene class compound. Structurally, it consists of lactone endoperoxide. These compounds are active against *P. vivax* as well as chloroquine-sensitive and chloroquine-resistant strains of *P. falciparum*. Many artemisinin compounds were screened and developed as antimalarial drugs.

✓ Among them, artemether, artether (lipid soluble) & sodium artesunate (water soluble) has been developed as an antimalarial drug.

✓ They are used in severe forms of malaria and chloroquine and multidrug-resistant strains of *P. falciparum*. They are usually used in conjunction with other antimalarial drugs in treatment of malaria or resistant strains.

✓ Artesunate is a semi-synthetic antimalarial drug derived from artemisinin.

Chemical Structure: (Fig. 2.30)

Chemical Name:

4-oxo-4-(((3R, 5aS,6R, 8aS,9R,10R, 12R, 12aR)-3, 6, 9- trimethyldecahydro-12H-3, 12-epoxy [1,2] dioxepino [4,3-i] isochromen-10-yl)oxy)butanoic acid

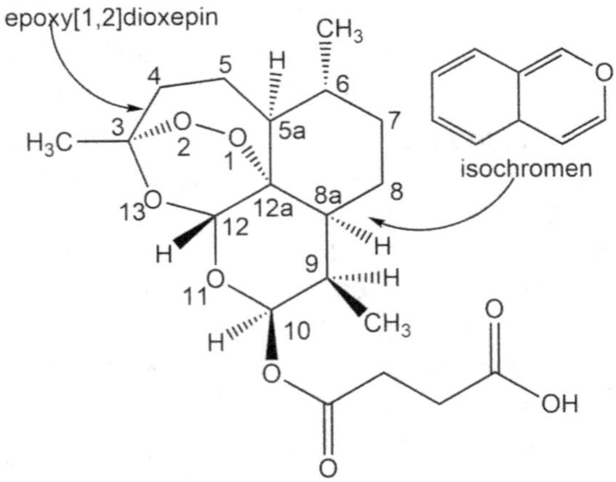

Fig. 2.30 Chemical structure of Artesunate.

Structure-Activity Relationship

1. Artemisinin is a 15-carbon molecule with an endoperoxide bridge that is essential for its anti-Plasmodium effect. Dihydroartemisinin, artemether, arteether, and artesunate (water soluble) are artemisinin derivatives.

2. Peroxide bridge and lactone ring are essential for antimalarial activity.

3. Removal of one or two methyl groups at C-3 & 6 does not affect the activity.

4. Reduction at C-1O of artemisinin to give dihydroartemisinin (seven times more potent than the parent compound *in vitro*), which acts as a prodrug. Which could be soluble in oil or water.

5. Methyl and ethyl substitution at C-10 produces a new antimalarial drug known as

artemether and arteether, which are lipid soluble. These are more potent than artemisinin.

6. Artemisone is a 2nd generation of artesunate. It has been shown to be effective against early-stage gametocytes as well as asexual stages of the parasite.

7. Artesunate oligomers have shown excellent *in vitro* plasmodial activity against chloroquine-resistant parasites. Among them, dimeric derivatives of artesunate were more active against *P. falciparum* than the trimers.

8. Sodium salts of artesunate were the most hydorphilic derivatives discovered. It has a lower activity than artimisin and is more susceptible to hydrolysis.

9. The substitution of an amino group with a carbonyl group could result in a remarkably effective antimalarial drug.

10. The lactone ring oxygen was replaced with nitrogen, yielding a molecule that was four times more active than artemisinin.

Mechanism of Action

Dihydroartemisinin is the active metabolite of artemisinin (Prodrug). Several mechanisms for artemisinin antimalarial activity have been hypothesised, including the creation of a carbon-centered radical, inhibition of heme group polymerization, development of free radicals, and change of malaria parasite membrane transport characteristics, which restrict nutrition flow.

Artesunate's mechanism of action remains unclear. Artesunate is a prodrug that rapidly converts to its active form, dihydroartemisinin (DHA). This process involves the hydrolysis of the 4-carbon ester group via the plasma esterase enzyme. It is hypothesized that the cleavage of the endoperoxide bridge in the pharmacophore of DHA generates reactive oxygen species (ROS), which increase oxidative stress and cause malarial protein damage via alkylation. In addition, artesunate potently inhibits the essential P. falciparum exported protein 1 (EXP1), a membrane glutathione S-transferase. As a result, the parasite's glutathione level is reduced.

Artesunate is fast-acting, effective against uncomplicated *P. falciparum* malaria, severe malaria, and blood-stage *P. vivax* infections, and has gametocidal activities. These compounds are generally given in combination with other long-acting antimalarial agents. Artesunate is involved in increased oxidant stress on the infected red blood cells.

Uses

✓ Used orally for the treatment of malaria & I.V. for severe malaria.

✓ Given a combination of drugs such as artesunate/mefloquine, artesunate/ pyronaridine, artesunate/amodiaquine, artesunate/ sulfadoxine–pyrimethamine and atovaquone–proguanil–artesunate, clindamycin (antibiotic)/artesunate for treatment of malaria.

✓ Sodium artesunate is a basic salt and is used in the treatment of simple and severe malaria.

2.6.3 Artemether

Historical Background

✓ Artemether has been studied since 1981, and in 1987, it was approved for use in the treatment of malaria.

✓ Artemether is an oil-soluble compound that is normally given intramuscularly.

Chemical Structure: (Fig. 2.31)

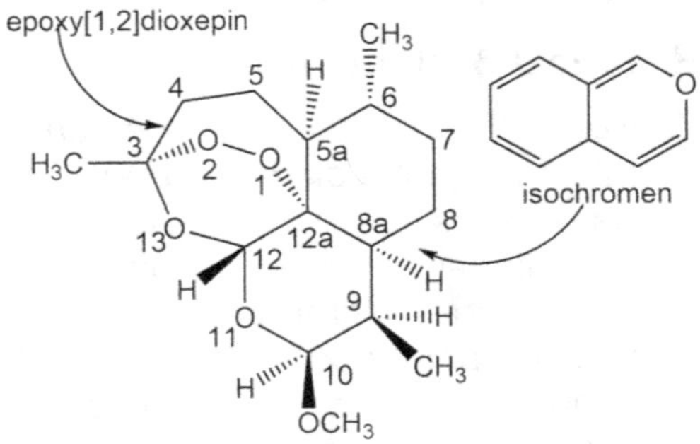

Chemical Name:

10-methoxy-3,6,9-trimethyldecahydro-12H-3, 12-epoxy[1,2]dioxepino[4,3-i]isochromene

Structure-Activity Relationship

1. Artemether is a methyl ether derivative of artemisinin. It is a prodrug of dihydroartemisinin,

Fig. 2.31 Chemical structure of Artemether.

2. Artemether would be more stable than artesunate if the ester linkage in the artesunate molecule was replaced with an ether linkage.

Mechanism of Action

Artemether (Prodrug) is metabolized rapidly into dihydroartemisinin after oral administration.

Artemether acts by interacting with heme, (a breakdown product of hemoglobin). As a result of this interaction, toxic oxygen, and carbon-centered radicals are formed. Thus, lesions and parasite growth may be minimized.

Artemether may cause oxidative and metabolic stress in cells by inhibiting antioxidant and metabolic enzymes involved in glutathione and glucose metabolism, according to one theory. The parasite may develop lesions as a result, preventing its growth. Another probable mode of action is that the drugs act by blocking an enzyme that regulates cellular calcium concentration, causing intracellular calcium deposition, which leads to cell death.

Artesunate and artemether have been demonstrated to be more effective than chloroquine and sulfadoxine/pyrimethamine in clearing parasites.

Uses

✓ Artemether is taken orally to treat malaria, and I. M. to treat severe malaria. It is used rather than quinine to treat severe malaria. It may not be as efficient as artesunate in adults.

✓ It is used in combination with lumefantrine (antimalarial agent) to treat multidrug-resistant falciparum malaria strains.

✓ It is used for the treatment of *P. falciparum* (chloroquine-resistant) or chloroquine-resistant *P. vivax* parasites.

✓ Artemether in combination with praziquantel to treat *schistosomiasis* trematode infections.

2.6.4 Atovoquone

Historical Background

✓ World War II Period - A shortage of quinine (antimalarial drug) prompted researchers to seek alternative antimalarial drugs. In this perspective, They were screened on number of hydroxynaphthoquinone derivative compounds, which were found to be more effective than quinine.

✓ Atovaquone (hydroxynapthoquinoneclass), was developed in 1990. It is the only drug in clinical use that targets the mitochondria of the parasite.

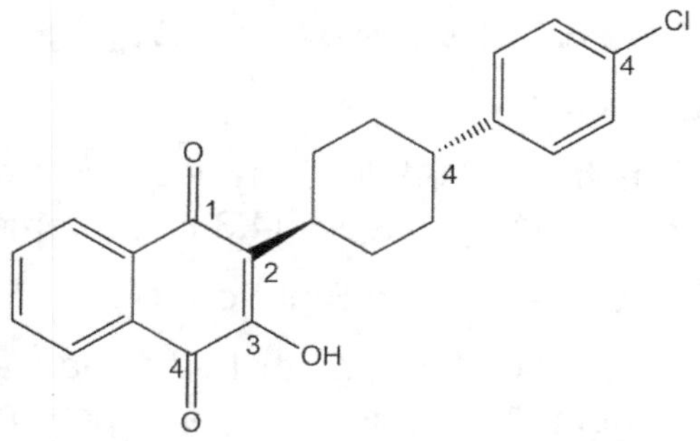

Fig. 2.32 Chemical structure of Atovaquone.

Chemical Structure: (Fig. 2.32)

Chemical Name:

2-((1r,4r)-4-(4-chlorophenyl)cyclohexyl)-3-hydroxynaphthalene-1,4-dione OR 2-[trans-4-(4-chlorophenyl)-cyclohexyl]-3-hydroxy-1,4-napthaquinone

Structure Activity Relationship

1. The quinoloid hydroxyl group is essential for activity, and its replacement with a range of substituents resulted in the loss of activity.

2. Substitution of the benzenoid ring resulted in a total or considerable loss of activity.

3. Higher activity was obtained by increasing the length of the isoalkyl chain at C-2, but only up to C9.

4. Substitution of branched alkyl side chains C-2, results twice as potent as its straight-chain or isoalkyl isomers.

5. The maximum number of carbons in the chain between C10-13, where the side chain comprised an aliphatic or aromatic ring/s at C-2, resulted in the highest activity of the compound.

6. The introduction of double bonds, halogens, or heteroatoms such as nitrogen or oxygen into the side chain decreased activity.

Mechanism of Action

Atovaquone has a lipophilic character and is closely related to the structure of ubiquinone (Coenzyme Q). Plasmodia can act specifically on complex III of the respiratory chain's mitochondrial electron transport and interfere with activities like ATP and pyrimidine production. As a result, pyrimidine synthesis is inhibited, DNA synthesis is prevented, and protozoal death occurs.

Furthermore, according to a recent study, atovaquone suppresses parasite purine production, resulting in mitochondrial dysfunction. In *P. falciparum*, atovaquone is also involved in the breakdown of the parasite's mitochondrial membrane potential.

Uses

✓ A fixed combination of atovaquone and proguanil is given orally in the treatment of mild to moderate attacks of chloroquine and multidrug-resistant *P. falciparum* malaria.

✓ It is active against the fungus *Pneumocystis carinii* and is used in the treatment of mild to moderate *P. carinii* pneumonia.

✓ It is frequently used in combination with oral azithromycin to treat *babesia*.

2.7 Prodrugs

Definition

1. A physiologically inactive molecule that can be converted into a therapeutically active chemical in the body.
2. Biologically inert drug molecule derivatives which undergo enzymatic and/or chemical conversion in *in vivo* to release the pharmacologically active parent drug.
3. Prodrugs are inactive compounds that are transformed into active drugs in the body.

2.7.1 Basic Concepts

Historical Background

✓ The first prodrug is believed to be sulfasalazine, which has two active metabolites in the colon: sulfapyridine and 5-aminosalicylic acid (5-ASA). Sulfasalazine was first approved in the United States in 1950 and is still used to treat autoimmune illnesses such as Crohn's disease and ulcerative colitis.

✓ Prodrugs are estimated to account for about 10% of all marketed pharmaceuticals, with a market share of 12% from 2008 to 2017. There were 249 novel molecular entities licensed during the period (2008-2017), with 31 of them being prodrugs.

Introduction

The process of discovering and developing new chemical entities (drugs) for the treatment of human illnesses and diseases is difficult, time-consuming, and expensive. Until recently, drug discovery was mostly an empirical process with a lot of accidental observation. Many of the therapeutic agents currently available to humans were discovered using empirical drug discovery approaches. Random biological screening of many chemical compounds obtained from synthetic or natural sources is the mainstay of the empirical approach. Compounds are then chosen based on favorable screening results and further developed from there.

In recent years, the growth of a considerable knowledge base in the biomedical sciences has aided drug discovery by allowing for a more rational approach to pharmacological intervention in pathophysiological processes. Regardless of how new lead compounds are discovered, their therapeutic potential must usually be optimized in the initial development and discovery process.

On the contrary, physical and chemical properties may threaten a novel drug's therapeutic efficacy. Furthermore, the new drug may interact negatively with the biological system, resulting in decreased therapeutic activity. Furthermore, the new drug's side effects may be so frequent and severe that its therapeutic value is also affected. Almost all drugs possess undesirable physicochemical and biological properties. Many drug molecules are discontinued due to poor pharmacokinetics or high toxicities. To optimize the medicinal properties of a newly discovered chemical entity, researchers/chemists can use a variety of strategies. Most of the time, therapeutically useful new drugs are made by making structural changes to the lead chemical or making structurally similar analogues based on known structure-activity relationships.

In some cases, therapeutic optimization may necessitate the development of a novel dosage form for the new drug, allowing it to be administered via a similar or different route than was originally employed.

The drug's physicochemical properties have had a significant impact on the onset, intensity, and duration of action. This has prompted researchers and chemists to build various types of prodrug strategies.

To overcome various limitations and barriers to reaching the target site, various types of prodrugs have been developed. The design of the prodrug is such that it will be rapidly converted to an active moiety after reaching its desired site.

Prodrug design is a typical novel drug development method that often enhances a drug's therapeutic value. Before the validation of the prodrug concept as a technique for new drug discovery and development in 1958. This type of drug was earlier referred to as "drug latentiation".

The prodrugs that were in use before the formal concept's recognition have been referred to as "accidental" or "empirical" prodrugs. Example. Chloral hydrate, a popular sedative compound that is transformed *in vivo* into its central nervous system (CNS) depressant activity, is an example of an unintentional prodrug. Also, methenamine, a commonly used antiseptic for the urinary tract, is a prodrug of the active antibacterial compound. Typically, derivatizing the parent drug produces a prodrug.

The Prodrug Approaches: The therapeutic efficacy of a drug molecule can be improved by eliminating undesirable properties while retaining desirable ones. This can be achieved by physical, biological, and chemical means.

The Biological Approaches involves changing the route of administration, which may or may not be acceptable to the patient. The **physical approach** involves changing the design of the dosage form of the drug, such as through controlled drug delivery. While the **chemical approach** is the design of prodrugs. This is the best approach for enhancing drug selectivity while minimizing toxicity.

Most prodrugs have two-dimensional structures that include a pharmacologically inactive promoter covalently linked to the parent drug structure. The complexity of the prodrug structure may extend from the simple ester derivates of a parent acid drug to the inclusion of the structural characteristics of the product, requiring the production of a parent species by specialised chemical or biological mechanisms.

In the design of a prodrug that must ensure that

1. A therapeutically useful prodrug is effectively converted into an active parent drug and a pharmacologically inactive compound.

2. Furthermore, the covalent connection between the promoiety and the parent drug must be stable enough to allow for dosage formulation of the prodrug and allow for separation at the proper time and site of action.

3. **The covalent link of the prodrug':** It shall undergo chemical or enzymatic breakdown at the required site and/or time in the bioenvironment.

4. The relative strength of the covalent bonding between promoiety and parent drug can be changed so that bioactivation of the prodrug happens at a specified location in the body.

5. Any groups in the prodrug that have been cleaved (split) from the molecules are non-toxic.

6. The most efficient, stable, safe, and acceptable form of prodrug should be able to overcome physical, chemical, and biological approach barriers.

Types of Prodrug

1. **Bipartite:** Most prodrugs have bipartite structures, which include a pharmacologically inactive promoiety that is covalently connected to the parent drug.

2. **Tripartite:** Tripartite prodrugs have three parts: two inactive and one active. The body's natural processes can then break down the inactive components, making the drug's active ingredients available. So, tripartite prodrugs are better for drug delivery.

3. **Mutual prodrugs:** These are formed by combining two active drug structures so that each functions as a prodrug for the other. Mutual prodrugs may be especially useful in treating patients when the pharmacological actions of the parent drugs are compatible, i.e., synergistic or additive in action.

4. **Polymeric prodrugs:** A parent drug is bonded to a polymer to form polymeric prodrugs. This prodrug design technique is frequently used to provide timed release of the parent drug *in vivo*.

Purpose of prodrug: (Fig. 2.33)

1. A prodrug is more cost-effective than developing a new chemical entity to replace the existing drug.
2. It makes a novel lead compound more therapeutically useful.
3. It improves the safety or efficacy of the existing drugs.

Limitations of New or Existing Therapeutic Drug (Fig. 2.33)

- New or existing drugs usually lead to challenges in three phases: pharmaceuticals, biopharmaceutics, and pharmacodynamics phase.
- The pharmaceutical phase refers to the pre-absorption of the physical and chemical nature of the drug. It also includes both dosage forms and challenges at the site of administration.
- Absorption, distribution, biotransformation, and excretion of the drugs are all included in the biopharmaceutic phase.
- The pharmacodynamic phase describes the effects of drugs and their mechanisms.
- Problems related to any of these drug action phases may lead to either subtherapeutic or toxic drug therapy for patients.

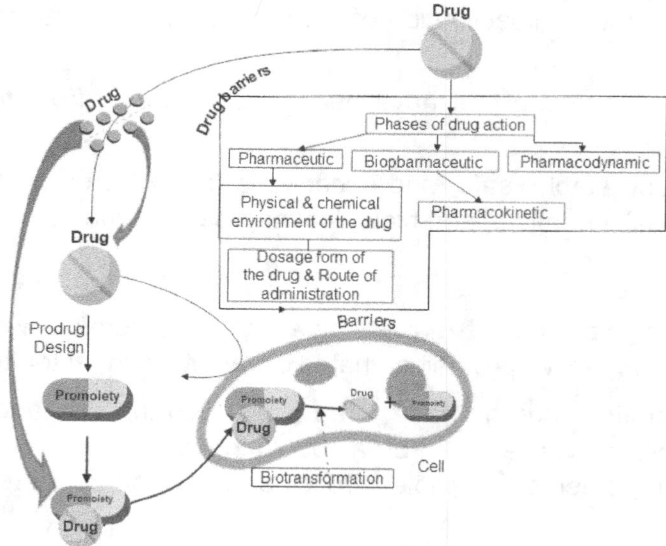

Fig.2.33 The Prodrug concept.

2.7.2 Application of Prodrugs Design

In recent years, the application (Fig.2.34) of prodrugs to the creation of new chemical entities has grown more creative and complicated. The most significant contribution of the prodrug idea to developing novel drugs is the ability to safeguard tested chemical compounds. Otherwise, it would not be commercialized due to pharmaceutical, biopharmaceutical, or pharmacodynamic defects.

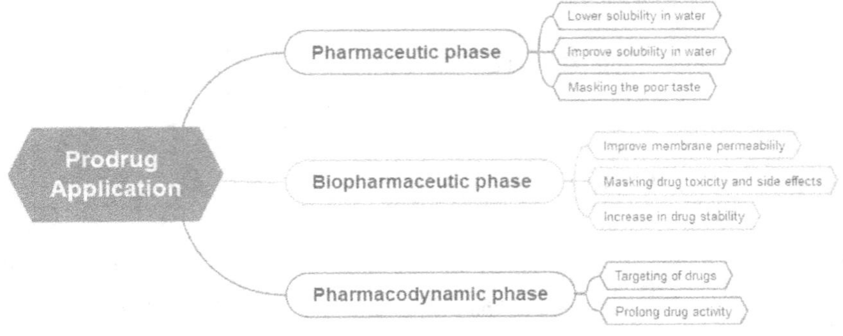

Fig. 2.34 Application of Prodrug.

Prodrug design has shown useful in expanding the therapeutic range and safety of current medications, as well as assisting the development and commercialization of newly discovered chemical compounds. major applications of the prodrug strategy, including improving oral absorption, improving aqueous solubility, enhancing lipophilicity, enhancing active transport as well as achieving site-selective delivery.

Prodrugs are increasingly being used to improve diverse drug properties, and their influence and development are expected to increase. Irrespective of the specific approach or purpose, the prodrug must take a step towards activating the free parent drug, which can then exert a specific pharmacological effect.

1. Prodrug with low water solubility properties

Some drugs have an unbelievably bad flavour. The problem can be solved in this situation by lowering the water's solubility characteristics. As an example, the palmitate ester can be used to mask the bitter taste of the antibiotic **chloramphenicol** (Fig. 2.35). Because chloramphenicol doesn't dissolve well in water, adding a highly lipophilic moiety (a long chain of fatty acids) to its structure makes it less soluble in water and tasteless.

2. Prodrug with an increase in water solubility properties

Prodrugs have been used to make drugs more water-soluble. This is especially beneficial for injectable types of compounds, where it allows for larger concentrations and smaller quantities of the drug. For example, **chloramphenicol succinate ester** (Fig.2.35), a prodrug that increases its water solubility character due to the presence of an additional carboxylic acid. When the esterified salt is hydrolyzed, chloramphenicol is released along with succinic acid. The later form of the released product is naturally present in the body.

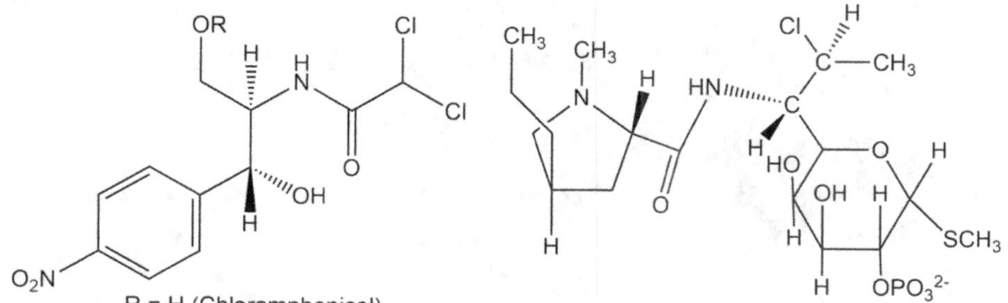

R = H (Chloramphenicol)
R = (-CO(CH$_2$)$_{14}$CH$_3$) (chloramphenicol palmitate)
R = (-CO(CH$_2$)$_2$COOH) (chloramphenicol succinate)

Clindamycin phosphate

Fig. 2.35 Prodrug of Chloramphenicol & Clindamycin.

Because of the drug's low solubility at the injection site, prodrugs that promote water solubility are effective in reducing the pain associated with some injections. For example, **clindamycin** (Fig.2.35), an antibacterial antibiotic, is painful to inject. However, this can be prevented by employing a phosphate ester prodrug, which has a substantially higher solubility due to the ionic phosphate group.

3. Prodrug with an increase in lipid solubility property

By esterifying the hormone with a suitable carboxylic acid, a prodrug of hydrocortisone can be made that dissolves better in lipids (Fig. 2.36). The obtained prodrug can then be dissolved in a suitable lipid solvent and subsequently, injected directly into skeletal muscle tissue (IM).

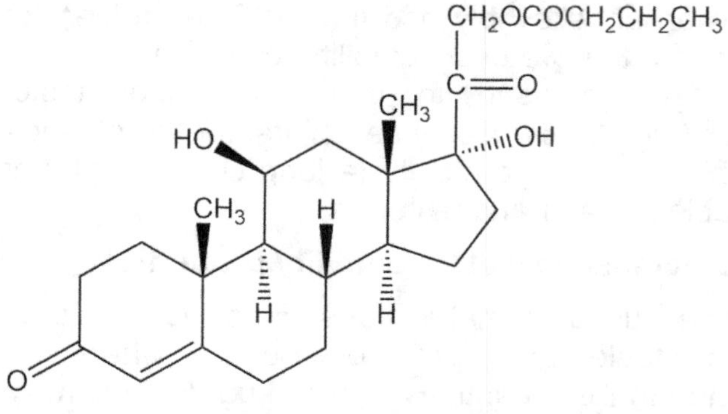

Fig.2.36 Prodrug of Hydrocortisone 21-butyrate.

Following that, the body receives a long-term supply of hormonal activity from the oil's slow release of hydrocortisone and subsequent hydrolytic activation.

4. Prodrugs that improve chemical stability

The antibacterial agent ampicillin decomposes in a concentrated aqueous solution. The antibiotic undergoes auto aminolysis, which is an intermolecular nucleophilic reaction between the α-NH$_2$ group on one molecule's side chain and the β-lactam function (four-membered ring) of a second molecule. Therefore, antibiotic activity is lost due to auto aminolysis.

Hetacillin (Fig. 2.37) is a prodrug that prevents this reaction by enclosing the inappropriate α-NH in a ring. Hetacillin decomposes slowly to release ampicillin and acetone after administering the drug. Cyclopropane carboxyl acid esters are being explored as possible prodrugs of acyclovir to increase the chemical stability of antiviral drugs in solution.

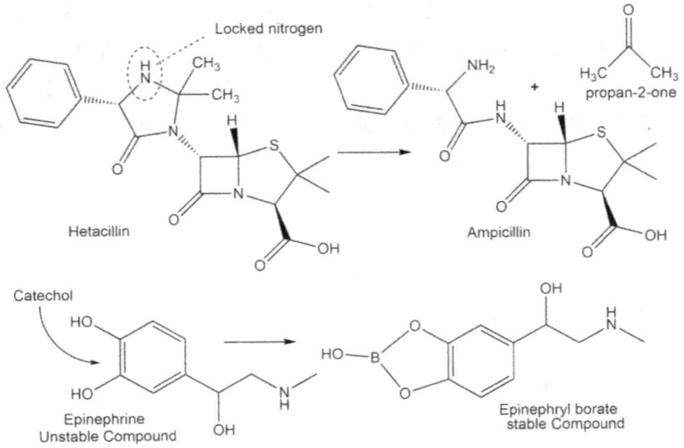

Fig.2.37 Prodrug of Hetacillin & Epinephryl borate.

For many years, **epinephrine** (Fig. 2.37) has been employed as a therapeutic agent. The catechol moiety within this hormone's structure undergoes relatively easy oxidation. So, it has limited its therapeutic efficacy. Converting epinephrine to its borate prodrug makes it easier to make aqueous solutions of the drug, which can be used to give epinephrine for the treatment of specific ocular disorders.

5. Prodrug to improve the permeability of the membrane

The most common application of the prodrug technique in novel drug design and development has been to improve a parent drug's behaviour when it is encountered in a living system. When a complex molecule form of a drug is exposed to a biological system, it encounters several barriers that prevent it from reaching its desired therapeutic site. These barriers include aqueous environments such as gastrointestinal contents, blood, and extracellular fluid, as well as lipid barriers such as gastrointestinal membranes, cell membranes, and the blood-brain barrier. Other barriers could be enzymatic, causing the drug to be bio-inactivated before it reaches its therapeutic site of action.

Epinephrine (adrenaline) (Fig. 2.38) has long been used ophthalmically to treat glaucoma, a disorder characterized by abnormally high intraocular pressure that is triggered by a fluid build-up in the eye. When epinephrine is injected into the eye, it causes an increase in fluid outflow as well as a decrease in pressure. The therapeutic response is required by relatively high concentrations of epinephrine (2 %) because it is difficult for this polar drug to penetrate its intraocular site and also develop metabolic inactivation in the ocular tissue. The application of high doses (2%) of epinephrine to the eye raises the risk of ocular tissue irritation as well as adverse cardiovascular effects. Diesterification of epinephrine's (the prodrug's) phenolic hydroxyl groups using trimethyl acetic (pivalic) acid (Dipivefrin) enhances the parent drug's lipophilicity, which aids intraocular transport of the prodrug and enables the therapeutic drug concentration to decrease to 0.1%. Dipivefrin (the prodrug) is bioactivated at the site of action by ocular esterase enzymes, which release the therapeutic amounts of the parent drug, epinephrine. **Dipivefrin** users have shown fewer adverse effects. The prodrug improves the parent drug's chemical (oxidation process) and biochemical (metabolic inactivation) stability, as well as its delivery to the site of action.

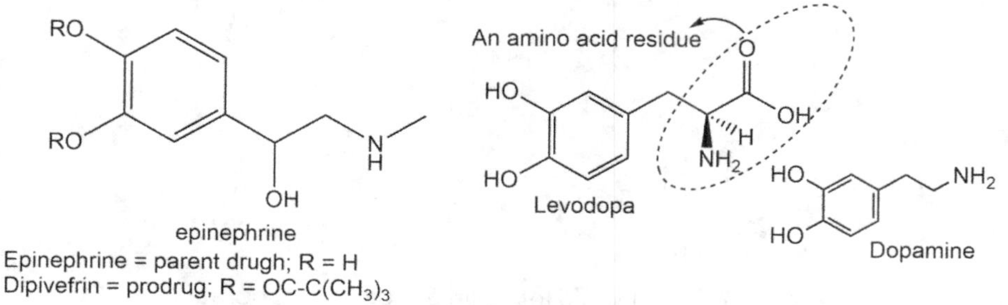

Fig. 2.38 Prodrug of Dipivefrin & levodopa.

Parkinson's disease (PD) is treated with **levodopa** (Fig.2.38), which is a prodrug for the neurotransmitter dopamine. A deficiency of dopamine in the brain causes PD. Dopamine is unable to pass the blood-brain barrier because it is too polar. Levodopa is a much more polar prodrug. However, it contains an amino acid in its chemical structure. Amino acid transport proteins recognize levodopa and transfer it across the cell membrane. A decarboxylase enzyme in the brain eliminates the acid group and produces dopamine.

6. Prodrugs to extend the duration of drug activity

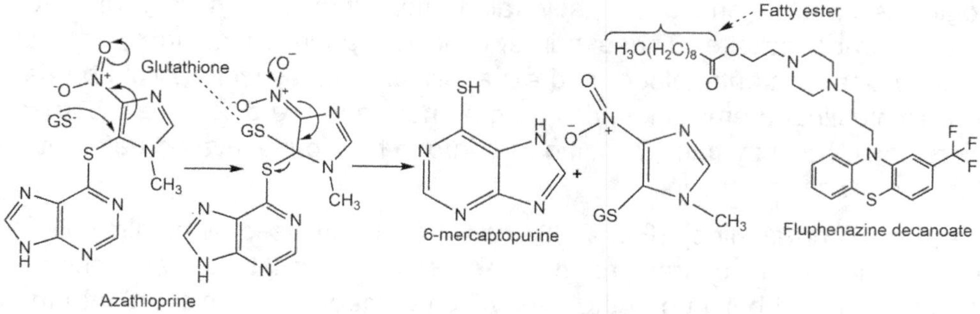

Fig. 2.39 Prodrug of azathioprine & Fluphenazine decanoate.

Prodrugs are occasionally altered so that they convert slowly to an active drug in the body, and thus improve the drug's effectiveness. For example, 6-mercaptopurine reduces the immunological response of the body, which makes it effective for transplant protection. Unfortunately, the drug is excreted too quickly from the body. The prodrug **azathioprine** (Fig.2.39) has the advantage of being slowly transformed into 6-mercaptopurine by glutathione activation, allowing for more prolonged activity. The rate of conversion can be changed depending on the heterocyclic group's ability to draw electrons. The faster the breakdown, the greater the electron-drawing power. Because the NO_2 group is strongly electron-withdrawing on the heterocyclic ring, it is present to ensure an efficient conversion to 6-mercaptopurine. The electron-withdrawing substituent (this center is an electron-rich carbanion or an alkoxide (RO-) anion) acts as a stabiliser.

Fluphenazine decanoate (prodrug) (Fig. 2.39) is an esterified compound with increased lipophilicity character. It is used to extend the duration of action of the antipsychotic drug fluphenazine. The prodrug is given intramuscularly and gradually diffuses from adipose tissue into the bloodstream, where it is rapidly hydrolyzed.

7. **Drug toxicity and adverse effects/side effects are concealed by prodrugs**

The prodrug concept has also been applied to lower toxicity and adverse reactions. Drugs used for treating joint pain are good choices for safer drug development due to their strong gastrointestinal irritant properties. This irritating effect can lead to illness, from nausea to peptic ulceration on the gastrointestinal wall.

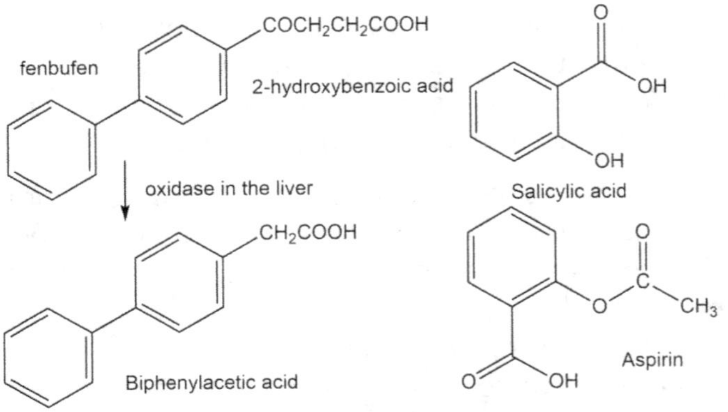

Fig.2.40 Prodrug of Biphenyl acetic acid & aspirin.

In this therapeutic class, prodrug design aims to create a pharmacologically inactive precursor to the antiarthritic drug. As a result, when the prodrug is taken orally, the gastrointestinal system is protected from the parent drug's toxicity.

The prodrug is absorbed and then bioactivated by normal metabolic mechanisms to deliver the antiarthritic drug to its therapeutic locations. For example, **biphenyl acetic acid** (Fig. 2.40), a prodrug of fenbufen, has been shown in studies to be significantly less ulcerogenic than other antiarthritic agents.

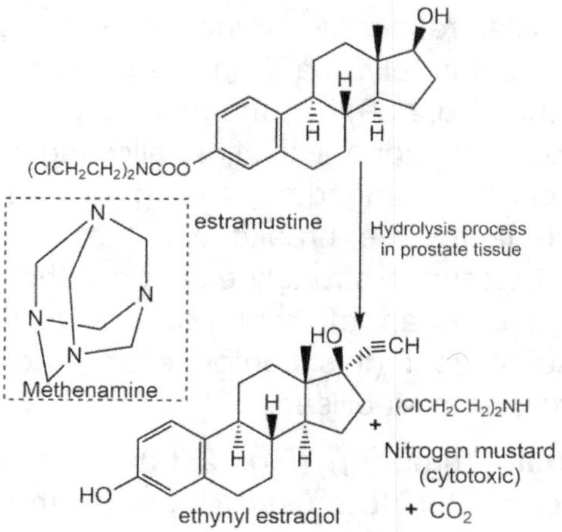

Fig.2.41 Prodrug of Estramustine & methenamine.

Drug side effects can be avoided by taking prodrugs. For instance, salicylic acid performs well as a pain reliever. However, the free phenolic acid group causes gastric bleeding. This is altered by concealing phenol as an ester (aspirin) (Fig. 2.40). **Aspirin** (the prodrug) is then hydrolysed by esterase to release the effective drug.

8. Drug-targeting prodrugs

The approach of site-specific drug delivery is a popular procedure used in the research and development of cancer drugs. The purpose of this strategy is to deliver anticancer drugs selectively to cancer cells, where they can show their lethal effects while protecting normal cells from these drugs' effects.

Estramustine (Fig. 2.41), a commonly used drug to treat prostate cancer, was developed to incorporate the components of a naturally occurring oestrogen, estradiol. The chemical structure contains a cytotoxic moiety (the nitrogen group) that kills cancer cells. The mechanism of estramustine is aimed at involving selective transmission to the prostatic tissue. The drug's cytotoxic nitrogen species is very firm and targets a protein which is found in large quantities in this tissue. Therefore, normal cells are ultimately immune to the cytotoxic effects of the drug due to the high levels of this protein.

At a pH of greater than 5, **methenamine** (Fig. 2.41) is a stable, inactive compound. In an acidic pH, however, the compound spontaneously degrades to form formaldehyde. The antibacterial property of formaldehyde is beneficial in the case of UTI. The normal pH of the blood is slightly alkaline. The drug passes through the body unaltered. When the compound is excreted through the urinary tract, it comes into contact with acidic urine, where it degrades to form formaldehyde, which has antibacterial properties against UTIs. Therefore, where it is necessary, it breaks down.

9. Externally activated prodrugs

Prodrugs are often metabolized in the body to form active compounds. A "sleeping agent" is an alternative to the prodrug approach. This is an inert molecule that is only transformed into an effective compound when it is exposed to an external stimulus. In cancer treatment, the use of photosensitizing agents (such as porphyrins or chlorins) is known as photodynamic therapy. These drugs aggregate within cells and have some selectivity for tumor cells when given intravenously. The effects of the agents themselves are limited, but if the cancer cells are exposed to light, porphyrins become excited and react with highly toxic singlet oxygen and molecular oxygen.

10. Miscellaneous

Prodrugs help to resolve problems like acid sensitivity, poor membrane permeability, the toxicity of medications, bad taste, and the short duration of action of the chemical compound. In this regard, the researcher/chemist can use knowledge of the prodrug to alter drug metabolic processes to his or her benefit.

The prodrug approach makes progress and achieves success in supplying effective medications for several diseases. Kinetics and thermodynamics have been extensively researched and demonstrated to be effective for biological systems (active receptor sites, enzyme sites, etc.) with biomedicinal interests. It still needs the use of sophisticated computational drug design methods. The active location of receptors and enzymes has become increasingly characterised by quantum mechanics (such as *ab initio*, semiempirical, and functional theory of density (DFT)) and molecular mechanics (MMs), including docking. These commonly used methods have been shown to be effective tools for calculating structure energy for accurate drug prediction.

The prodrug concept has had the most significant impact on the return of usable drugs to the market because of pharmaceutical, biopharmaceutical, or pharmacodynamic deficits. Prodrug design has provided new therapeutic possibilities and safety, as well as a platform for new drug discoveries. The prodrug concept is expected to continue to play a pivotal role in the development of novel therapeutic medicines in the future.

Prodrugs are being employed more and more to help improve drug properties, and this trend is predicted to continue. Different linkers/spacers are predicted to be used in future prodrug design and synthesis to improve drug transport, targeting, and control of the active parent drug's release. New computational methods aid in the optimization of prodrugs and increase the efficiency of the drug development process. Prodrug use is increasing and is likely to continue to grow.

CHAPTER 3

ANTI-TUBERCULAR AGENTS
URINARY TRACT ANTI-INFECTIVE AGENTS
ANTIVIRAL AGENTS

3.1 Anti-Tubercular Agents

Historical Background

Tuberculosis (TB) is one of the world's top 10 leading causes of death. The current death rate is about 193 per 100,000 people. 95% of tuberculosis cases are reported in developing nations. HIV (human immunodeficiency virus)-positive people are 20 to 30 times more likely to develop tuberculosis. In 2019 alone, 10 million individuals were infected, with 1.4 million claiming to have died due to tuberculosis. In 2017, adults accounted for 90% of all reported cases, with male patients accounting for 64% of all cases. Two-thirds of the tuberculosis cases occurred in eight countries: India (27%), China (9%), Indonesia (8%), the Philippines (6%), Pakistan (5%), Nigeria (4%), and South Africa (3%). People who have HIV, malnutrition, diabetes, or who smoke tobacco are more prone to infection. Tobacco use is responsible for nearly 8% of all TB cases worldwide.

Individuals with tuberculosis can infect more than 15 people in a single year. TB can also be spread through close contact, like most other infectious diseases. When HIV-positive people get infected with tuberculosis, the death rate rises to nearly 100%. When an infected person sneezes in a crowded environment, the virus spreads through the air. Even if a person only inhales a few of those germs, they will most likely become infected. Despite this, it is equally contagious among people of all ages, including children, throughout the world. However, TB remains a major threat to human health, and it is more than necessary to raise awareness about the disease. Tuberculosis, as deadly as it may make you feel, can be treated and cured—or at least controlled. Multidrug-resistant tuberculosis (MDR-TB) is one of the most difficult diseases to treat for healthcare providers all over the world.

Infections with *Mycobacterium* species result in the development of chronic diseases such as tuberculosis and leprosy. *Mycobacteria* are intermediate forms of bacteria and fungi. It is an aerobic, acid-fast bacterium. It is either gram+ve or gram-ve bacteria. *M. tuberculosis*, or *M. bovis*, causes tuberculosis. On rare occasions, *M. africanum* causes human TB. Numerous cases of tuberculosis show nodular bodies or tubercles, thus the name "tuberculosis". This disease may affect nearly any part of the body, and the most affected site is the lungs. Miliary tuberculosis is a severe and rapidly deadly form of tuberculosis.

64

Coughs with sputum and blood, chest pains, weakness, weight loss, fever, and night sweats are all common symptoms of TB. The Xpert MTB/RIF, Xpert Ultra, and Truenat assays are WHO-recommended rapid tests. It is difficult and expensive to diagnose multi-drug resistant (MDR) and other forms of resistant TB, as well as HIV-associated TB. Children with tuberculosis are very difficult to identify.

MDR-TB continues to be a public health crisis and a health security risk. In 2019, 2 million people worldwide were diagnosed with multidrug- or rifampicin-resistant tuberculosis. From 2000-2019, approximately 60 million lives were saved by TB diagnosis and treatment. It is a fact that a number of strains have developed resistance to a variety of currently available drugs. Chronic disease, patent adherence, therapeutic toxicity, and the emergence of microbial resistance are the key challenges in treating these diseases.

TB is curable and treatable. Active, drug-susceptible tuberculosis is treated with a 6-month course of four antituberculosis drugs, as well as information and assistance from a healthcare professional or trained worker. TB diagnosis and treatment have saved approximately 63 million lives since 2000.

Definition: It is a chemical substance which is effective against tuberculosis (a communicable bacterial infection that normally affects the lungs).

Classification of Anti-Tubercular Drugs

The patient's disease status—whether it is active or dormant—determines the drug combination and length of therapy. MDR-TB (multidrug-resistant tuberculosis) is defined by its resistance to the first-line (isoniazid and rifampin) antimicrobial agents. Rifampin, isoniazid, pyrazinamide, and ethambutol are anti-tubercular drugs that have been approved by the USFDA to treat TB. MDR-TB therapy is advancing at a rapid pace, and recommendations are constantly changing. Kanamycin, capreomycin, and amikacin are commonly used second-line drugs for MDR-TB. Fluoroquinolones such as levofloxacin, moxifloxacin, and gatifloxacin are also frequently used as second-line agents when first-line agents develop resistance. Pretomanid, in combination with bedaquiline and linezolid, was recently approved by the USFDA for the treatment of multidrug-resistant tuberculosis.

Synthetic drugs and antibiotics are the two types of drugs used to treat tuberculosis.

1. **First line drug**: Isoniazid, rifamycin, pyrazinamide, ethambutol, and streptomycin are the first-line/major drugs used to treat drug-sensitive tuberculosis (TB). They produce the highest degree of effect with less toxicity.
2. **Second line drug**: Reserve/second-line drugs are amikacin, capreomycin, ciprofloxacin, cycloserine, ethionamide, kanamycin, ofloxacin, p-aminosalicylic acid, and protionamide for the treatment of drug-sensitive (DS) and multidrug-resistant (MDR) tuberculosis. These drugs are less effective against the tuberculosis vector than first-line agents and are more toxic to humans. They are used by patients who have developed resistance to first-line tuberculosis drugs.

3. **Third line drug**: Amoxicillin/clavulanate, clarithromycin, clofazimine, imipenem, and linezolid are examples of third-line medicines that may be effective but have unclear or unproven efficacy against tuberculosis.

4. **Miscellaneous drug**: bedaquiline,& delamanid.

3.2 Synthetic Anti-Tubercular Agents

Historical Background

✓ In the past, many synthetic compounds have been tested for antitubercular effects. Researchers have found aminosalicylic acid, isoniazid, pyrazinamide, thioacetazone, ethionamide, protionamide, and ethambutol to be prominent synthetic drugs. In a further study, the rationale and attributes of the development of anti-TB drugs could also be explored.

✓ The initial testing is performed in mice that are infected by the *M. tuberculosis* (H37 Rv) human virulent strain, and active compounds are examined in rhesus monkeys, whose TB is similar to that of humans.

✓ Dapsone, or bis (4-aminophenyl) sulphone, was the first synthetic antimycobacterial drug discovered. In experimental tuberculosis, it was found to have chemotherapeutic properties. Clinical trials of the drug revealed that high doses have toxic effects. Now, dapsone is widely used as an antileprotic drug.

✓ 1940- **Frederick Bernheim**, a biochemist from the United States, invented aspirin, and **Jorgen Lehman** used the same procedure to produce para-aminosalicylic acid, reported as the first synthetic anti-tuberculosis drug.

✓ 1941 - **F. Bernheim** observed that benzoate and salicylate ions (aspirin) induced increased oxygen absorption by *tubercle bacilli*, which prompted a search for antagonists among benzoic and salicylic acid derivatives.

✓ 1946 - **J. Lehmann** observed that *p*-aminosalicylic acid (PAS) has a high tuberculostatic effect, even though it does not reduce *tubercle bacilli's* oxygen consumption. Clearly, the reasoning for its design has not been justified during this period.

✓ However, it was also observed that p-aminosalicylic acid has antibacterial activity that is countered by *p*-aminobenzoic acid. Perhaps *p*-aminosalicylic acid acts by inhibiting the biosynthesis of *mycobactin*, an iron ionophore (a chemical capable of transporting certain ions across a cell's lipid membrane) found in the mycobacterial cell wall.

✓ The tuberculostatic activity was revealed in the thiosemicarbazone molecule using a Sulfathiazole model approach. This research led to the development of thiacetazone, an antitubercular drug. The drug was used to control the TB epidemic in Germany after World War II. Clinically, it produces a toxic effect. Until the advent of hydrazides, this compound was the most common in clinical use.

✓ **V. Chorine** found the tuberculostatic activity of nicotinamide in 1945, which was later validated by other researchers in 1948.

✓ 1952 - **S. Kushner** and his colleagues discovered pyrazinamide, a non-vitamin heterocyclic analog of nicotinamide that is being studied as an antitubercular drug. Likewise, isonicotinic acid-containing compounds were also tuberculostatic without possessing vitamin like properties. Thioisonicotinamide was shown to have a potent tuberculostatic & toxic effect. After that, ethionamide and propionamide derivatives were developed for clinical use.

✓ One of the most well-known incidents in medicinal chemistry is the accidental discovery of isoniazid. The chemical compound is much more effective than streptomycin.

✓ Ethambutol, a clinically effective antitubercular drug, was produced by structural modifications of *N, N'*-diisopropylethylenediamine. It has excellent structural and steric properties.

✓ The new delamanid drug was introduced in 2012 for the treatment of MDR-TB. Bedaquiline is also used when no other treatment is available to treat drug-resistant TB.

3.2.1 Isoniazid

Historical Background

✓ **Meyer** and **Malley** developed isoniazid in 1912. The antibacterial property was unknown to them. **Hans Offe** and **Werner Siefken** at Bayer AG synthesized hydrazine derivatives, and isoniazid (the intermediate) was identified. Following a series of tests in 1950, they found a good antituberculosis effect.

✓ In 1953, the drug isoniazid was approved for use in the treatment of tuberculosis.

Chemical Structure: (Fig. 3.1)

Chemical Name:

Isonicotinohydrazide; Isonicotinylhydrazine OR isonicotinic acid hydrazide

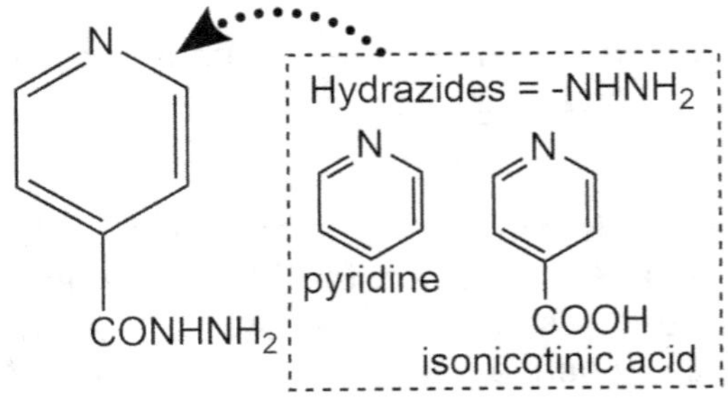

Fig.3.1 Chemical structure of Isoniazid.

Synthesis

1. First method: (Fig. 3.2)

2. It can be prepared from 4-methylpyridine (γ-picoline) by condensing ethyl isonicotinate with hydrazine in the final step of the process.

3. Second method: (Fig. 3.2)

4. The ethyl ester of isonicotinic acid is mixed with hydrazine to produce isoniazid.

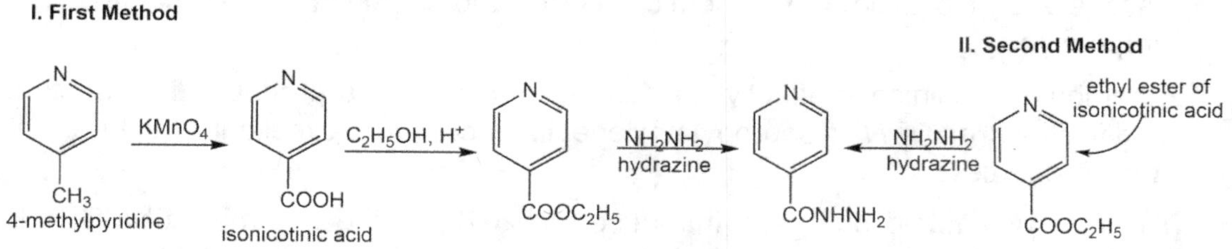

I. First Method

II. Second Method

Fig.3.2 Synthesis of Isoniazid.

Structure-Activity Relationship

1. Antitubercular activity requires the pyridine ring and the hydrazine group. The N^1 nitrogen atom in the side chain of hydrazine should remain unsubstituted.

2. Variable antitubercular activity results from N^1 and N^2 substitutions. N^2 nitrogen may be substituted with an acetyl group at N^2, resulting in acetyl isoniazid, which is an inactive compound.

3. The replacement by other aromatic rings, such as benzene or piperidine, or thiazole, of the pyridine nucleus decreased anti-tubercular activity.

4. Iproniazid is synthesized when an isopropyl group replaces only the hydrogen of the terminal amino group of isoniazid. It was originally designed as an antituberculosis antibiotic, but it is currently used as a psychomotor stimulant. Iproniazid was discovered in the 1950s and has a chemical structure that is quite similar to isoniazid.

5. Although numerous derivatives have been synthesized, none have shown activity superior to the parent medication.

Mechanism of Action

Because of its bioavailability, isoniazid is a popular tuberculosis drug. It invades the *tubercle bacilli* directly after absorption. Isoniazid has now been hydrolyzed to produce isonicotinic acid and hydrazine. The coenzyme NAD^+ is responsible for the synthesis of fatty acids, which protect the *tubercle bacilli's* cell wall from acid attack and the immune system. Isonicotinic acid, rather than nicotinic acid, is stored in *tubercle bacilli* NAD^+. Because the NAD^+ complex has been altered, it can no longer produce fatty acids, and the tubercle bacilli become vulnerable to acid and the human immune system, allowing them to be digested or die on their own. As a result, it appears that isoniazid is both tuberculostatic (it inhibits germ growth) and tuberculocidal (it kills germs) in nature.

The antimicrobial activities of isoniazid (INH) are selective for mycobacteria, perhaps because they can inhibit mycolic acid synthesis, which affects cell wall synthesis and produces a bactericidal effect. Mycolic acids are crucial components of the mycobacterium cell wall. INH also interferes with the synthesis and/or metabolism of lipids, carbohydrates, DNA, and nicotinamide adenine dinucleotide (NAD). The sensitive non-tubercular *mycobacteria* are *M. kansasii* and *M. xenopi*, but the *M. avium complex* is often INH-resistant.

Isoniazid, ethionamide, and prothionamide all belong to this drug class. The catalase peroxidase (KatG) enzyme activates isoniazid. Due to mutations in the katG, most katG-resistant isoniazid has occurred. Isoniazid's active species appears to have several cellular targets. Isoniazid is thought to work on InhA, which is an NADH-dependent enoyl acyl carrier protein reductase involved in making mycolic acid. The activated species forms an association with the NAD radical, likely an isonicotinic acyl radical. The end product, called isonicotinic acyl-NADH aggregate (INA), binds to InhA and stops *M. tuberculosis* from making mycolic acid.

INH is effective against both intracellular and extracellular *M. tuberculosis*. INH is bacteriostatic for "resting" *bacilli* but bactericidal for actively dividing *bacilli*. When used alone, INH resistance develops quickly. Resistance may not be an issue when used solely for prevention purposes. For INH-susceptible isolates, the minimum inhibitory concentration (MIC) of *M. tuberculosis* ranges between 0.03 - 0.125 μg/mL.

Uses

✓ It is used as a first-line treatment for pulmonary and extrapulmonary tuberculosis.

✓ Used in conjunction with rifampicin and pyrazinamide in the treatment of tuberculosis, but is used alone in prophylaxis treatment.

✓ It can be administered orally, intramuscularly, & intravenously as well.

✓ When pyridoxine is used with isoniazid, the drug's side effects could be reduced.

3.2.2 Ethionamide

Historical Background

✓ Researchers were looking for more effective derivatives of nicotinamide for the treatment of tuberculosis when they discovered INH's anti-TB efficacy in 1952. In subsequent trials, ethionamide and prothionamide were also found to have effective anti-TB properties. These two drugs are primarily used to treat MDR-TB and patients who cannot tolerate first-line anti-TB drugs.

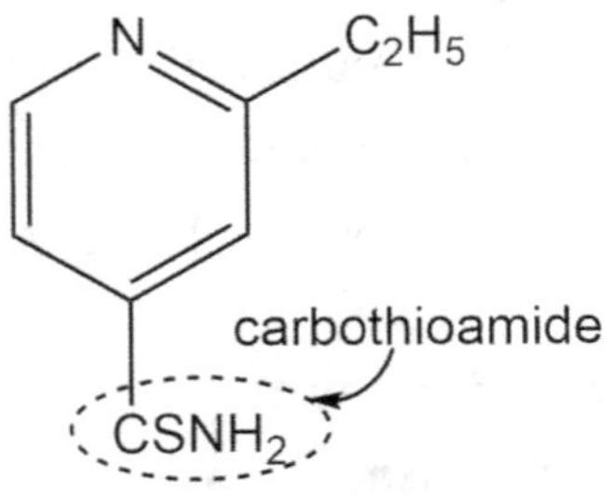

Fig.3.3 Chemical structure of Ethionamide.

✓ Ethionamide was developed in 1956 and received FDA approval for medicinal use in 1965. It is listed on the WHO's Essential Medicines List.

Chemical Structure: (Fig. 3.3)

Chemical Name: 2-ethylpyridine-4-carbothioamide; ethyl isonicotine acid thioamide

Structure-Activity Relationship

1. The common therapies for tuberculosis are isoniazid and ethionamide; ethionamide is the structural analogue of isoniazid. As a result, the metabolism, toxicity, and molecular targets of these two drugs are remarkably similar. Ethionamide, on the other hand, is a disubstituted drug, with S replacing O.

2. By substituting an ethyl group at C-2, the lipophilicity of the compound was increased.

3. It is less active *in vitro* but more active *in vivo*.

Mechanism of Action

Ethionamide inhibits the synthesis of mycolic acid, a saturated fatty acid present in the bacterial cell wall. As a result, the bacterial cell wall is disrupted, and the cell is ultimately digested. Ethionamide's activity may be bacteriostatic or bactericidal, depending on the drug's concentration at the site of infection and the organism's susceptibility.

Ethionamide's main target is also thought to be InhA (an NADH-dependent enoyl acyl carrier protein reductase involved in the synthesis of mycolic acid). The enzyme EthA, on the other hand, is responsible for the activation of this drug. It also inhibits the synthesis of peptides. Isoniazid, ethionamide, and prothionamide resistance are mostly caused by mutations in the activation enzymes (catalase-peroxidase (KatG) or EthA (an enzyme that can activate ethionamide)) or their molecular targets (InhA).

Ethionamide is active against *M. tuberculosis* and *M. leprae* but does not affect other bacteria. It promotes phagocytosis at the site of tuberculous inflammation, thereby accelerating its decay. However, it usually causes gastrointestinal adverse effects as well as a hepatotoxic effect.

Uses

✓ It is used for the treatment of TB. It is used in combination with other antituberculosis drugs when primary treatments fail or cannot be used.

✓ It should not be used alone.

✓ It has been employed in the treatment of leprosy in some cases.

3.2.3 Ethambutol

Historical Background

Ethambutol was discovered in 1961, observed in the American Cyanamid Lederle Laboratories, and tested in animals after it was shown to be stereospecific.

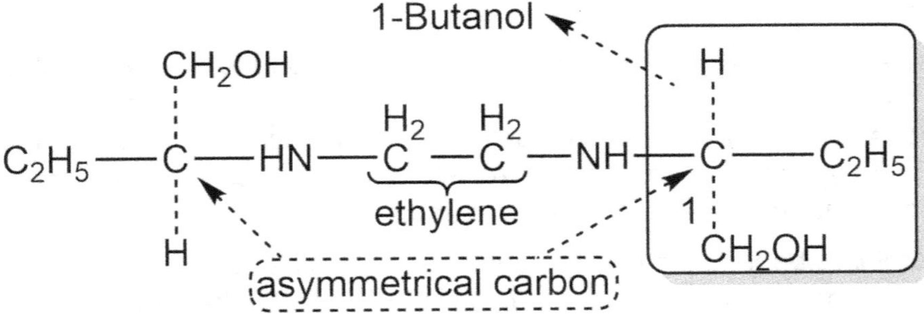

Fig.3.4 Chemical structure of Ethambutol.

Chemical Structure: (Fig. 3.4)

Chemical Name:

N,N'-ethylenbis-(2-aminobutan-1-ol); *N,N'*-bis(1-hydroxymethylpropyl)ethylenediamine

Structure Activity Relationship

1. Antimicrobial action is dependent on the presence of two amino moieties. A decrease in activity occurs when the length of the ethylene diamine chain lengthens. Increases in the size of the *N*-substituent result in a decrease in inactivity.

2. The presence of short, branched alkyl groups on the nitrogen atom also affects antimycobacterial activity. The replacement of either amino group results in a loss of activity.

3. The antimycobacterial activity was abolished when amino moieties were replaced with acetyl, sulphonyl, or nitrosyl moieties.

4. Heteroatoms such as oxygen or sulfur were substituted for the ethylene moiety, and inactive derivatives were formed.

5. The hydroxyl group must be the primary alcohol. When hydroxyl groups were replaced with -OCH_3 or -OC_2H_5 groups, the activity was equivalent to that of the parent drug. Removing hydroxyl groups results in a decline in activity.

6. While substituting methoxy or ethoxy for hydroxyl groups retains activity, substituting aromatic groups (phenyl, pyridine) results in activity loss.

Stereochemistry

1. Ethambutol's mode of action against *M. tuberculosis* is characterized by stereospecificity; it is active only against one of the four enantiomers, (*S, S*)-ethambutol. This series was improved using combinatorial synthesis. It gave rise to a new molecule, a highly lipophilic compound with a different mode of action than ethambutol.

2. Stereoisomers revealed that the dextro (*S, S*) form was 12 times more active than the meso form, whereas the levo form of the compound was completely inactive.

Mechanism of Action

It is unclear exactly how ethambutol works against *tubercle bacilli*, but it appears to inhibit the mycolic acid reorganisation process in *mycobacteria*. At elevated concentrations, ethambutol is bacteriostatic and bactericidal against M. *tuberculosis*. When ethambutol is administered alone, resistant strains are easily produced. It inhibits *tubercle bacilli* that are resistant to isoniazid and streptomycin.

Ethambutol is a bacteriostatic drug that is only effective against M. *tuberculosis* and has little effect on non-replicating organisms. Ethambutol has the main function of preventing the emergence of drug resistance in combination therapies. It blocks the enzyme arabinosyl transferase, for which the embA and embB genes appear to be ethambutol's main targets.

When mycolic acids bind to the 5'-hydroxyl groups of arabinogalactan D-arabinose residues in the cell wall, they form the mycolyl-arabinogalactan-peptidoglycan complex. By blocking the enzyme arabinosyl transferase from working, ethambutol affects the production of arabinogalactan, which makes the cell wall more permeable.

Uses

- ✓ Ethambutol is a drug that is primarily used to treat tuberculosis.
- ✓ Ethambutol hydrochloride is used to treat both pulmonary and extrapulmonary tuberculosis, along with other drugs like isoniazid, rifampicin, and pyrazinamide.
- ✓ It is also effective against M. *avium* complex and M. *kansasii*.
- ✓ 15 to 25 mg/kg once a day is the adult dosage.

3.2.4 Pyrazinamide

Historical Background

Although pyrazinamide was discovered and patented in 1936, it was not used to treat tuberculosis until 1952. It was surprising because, although it has no activity against tuberculosis *in vitro*, it was unexpectedly found to be effective in treating tuberculosis *in vivo*.

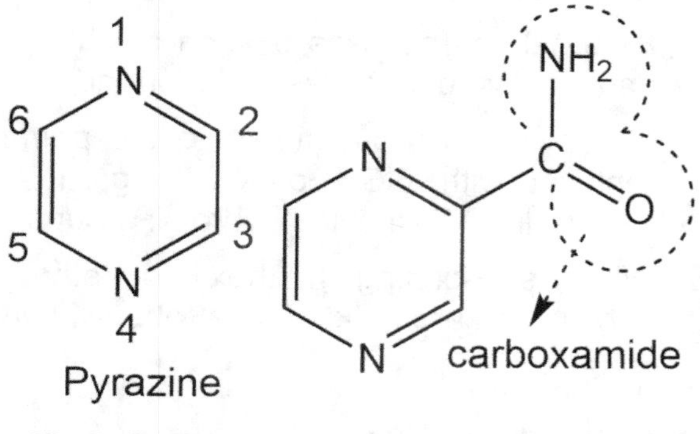

Fig.3.5 Chemical structure of Pyrazinamide.

Lederle and Merck's experiments with mice confirmed pyrazinamide's ability to kill tuberculosis, and later, it was used immediately in humans.

Chemical Structure: (Fig. 3.5)

Chemical Name: Pyrazine-2-carboxamide;

Structure-Activity Relationship

1. It has a pyrazine ring, which is a six-membered heterocyclic ring comprising two nitrogen atoms separated by two carbon atoms. To obtain optimum activity, the 2-amino side group is required.

2. The substance became less active when the pyrazine ring was substituted with an alternate heterocyclic ring, such as pyridine or pyrimidine.

3. Mono-substituted derivatives of the pyrazine ring are more active than di-substituted derivatives.

4. The activity is reduced when "N" is replaced with "C" (nicotinoyl). Any additional change in the ring will result in a loss of activity.

5. 5-chloropyrazinamide is a structural analogue of pyrazinamide, but it does not appear to have antitubercular activity. This compound may serve as the basis for new chemical compounds with different therapeutic activities.

6. It's a prodrug that the body converts to pyrazinoic acid.

Mechanism of Action

Pyrazinamide is commonly used as a bacteriostatic agent. Although the role of pyrazinamide against intracellular organisms is unknown, it is thought to be more active at an acidic pH (e.g., within macrophages) and against dormant or semi-dormant microorganisms. It enters the bacterium through passive transport, and pyrazinamidase converts it into pyrazinoic acid, which is the drug's active component. It may also inhibit *M. tuberculosis's* fatty acid synthetase I enzyme.

When used in conjunction with other antibiotics, pyrazinamide appears to have the effect of increasing the sterilizing effect of isoniazid and rifampin.

Uses

Pyrazinamide has a unique role in the treatment of multidrug-resistant tuberculosis (MDR-TB) in both first- and second-line regimens, as well as in the treatment of drug-resistant tuberculosis.

3.2.5 *p*-Aminosalicylic acid

Historical Background

✓ *p*-aminosalicylic acid (PAS), once a popular component of TB therapy, is now used as a second-line agent. Its use has been greatly reduced as a result of bacterial resistance and severe side effects.

✓ **Seidel** and **Bittner** invented PAS in 1902. **Jörgen Lehmann**, a Swedish chemist, rediscovered salicylic acid after learning that tuberculosis bacteria keenly metabolized it to salicylic acid.

✓ Late in 1944, **Lehmann** tried PAS as an oral TB therapy for the first time on a patient who showed a remarkable recovery from TB. However, the drug has made people resistant to TB.

✓ In 1948, researchers at the Medical Research Council of the United Kingdom demonstrated that combining streptomycin and PAS was superior to either drug alone, establishing the principle of combination therapy for tuberculosis.

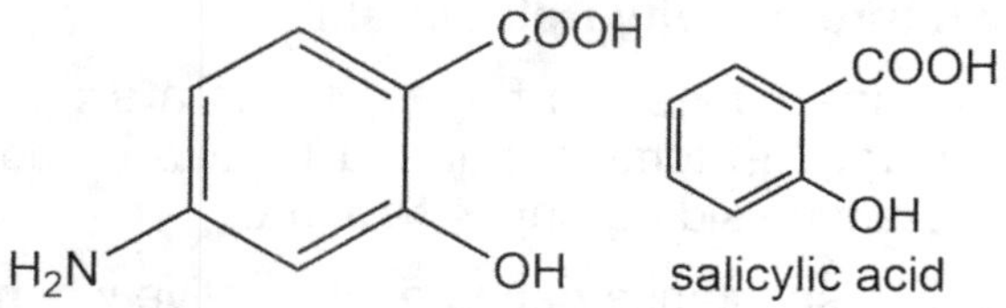

Fig.3.6 Chemical structure of *P*-amino salicylic acid.

Chemical Structure: (Fig. 3.6)

Chemical Name: 4-amino-2-hydroxybenzoic acid; *p*-Aminosalicylic acid

Synthesis: (Fig. 3.7)

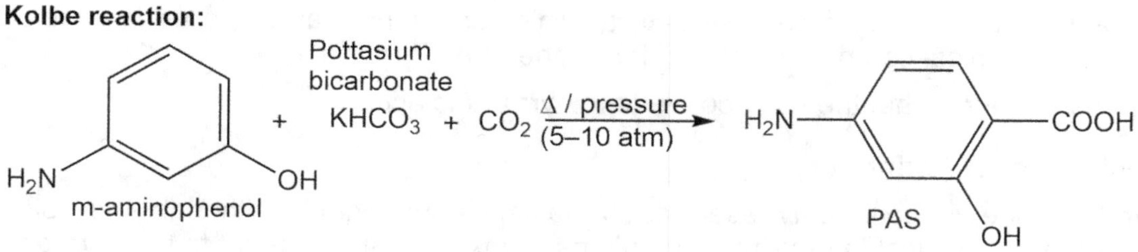

Kolbe reaction:

Fig.3.7 Synthesis of PAS.

1. The Kolbe reaction is used to prepare PAS.

2. It is a reaction in which m-aminophenol reacts directly with potassium bicarbonate and carbon dioxide while being heated at a moderate pressure of 5–10 atm.

Structure-Activity Relationship

1. The -COOH and NH_2 groups should be in a para position for maximum activity.

2. The -OH group can be in either an ortho or a meta-position, but while in the ortho position, they possess the maximum activity.

3. When an alkyl group or a -Cl ion replaces the $-NH_2$ group, its activity decreases.

4. When -COOH is transformed into an amide or ester molecule, it loses its activity.

Mechanism of Action

PAS's mechanism of action is still unknown. It is a structural analogue of p-aminobenzoic acid and inhibits folic acid synthesis by targeting dihydrofolate reductase and/or iron reduction by inhibiting mycobactin. It is incorporated into the folate pathway by dihydropteroate synthase (DHPS) and dihydrofolate synthase (DHFS) to produce hydroxyl dihydrofolate antimetabolite, which inhibits the enzymatic activity of dihydrofolate reductase (DHFR).

PAS is bacteriostatic and has highly specific antimicrobial activity; microorganisms other than *M. tuberculosis* are unaffected. Its antituberculosis activity is relatively low when compared to other antituberculosis drugs. When PAS is used alone, microbes develop resistance quickly.

Uses

✓ PAS and its salts (sodium aminosalicylate) are used as "second-line" treatments for MDR *M. tuberculosis.*

✓ It may aid in the prevention of resistance to other medications, particularly INH and streptomycin.

✓ It can be used in conjunction with isoniazid and streptomycin for the treatment of tuberculosis.

✓ It's not as good as isoniazid or streptomycin. It produces nephrotoxic and hepatotoxic effects, so it's only used in exceptional cases.

3.3 Anti-Tubercular Antibiotics

Historical Background

1909–1910-**Paul Ehrlich** showed that a "magic bullet" (a drug substance) could kill microorganisms without harming their human host.

Between 1940 and 1960, the antibiotic golden era gave birth to the majority of known anti-TB drugs.

Antibiotics, including penicillin, were not used to treat diseases until nearly a decade after **Alexander Fleming** discovered them in 1929. In the year 1908, prontosil (a sulpha drug) was first synthesized by German chemist **Gerhard Domagk**. Prontosil produces the active metabolite, sulphonamides. Later, sulphonamide was considered the first modern miracle drug. Despite the use of penicillin and sulpha drugs, however, no success was had in combating tuberculosis.

During the 1940s and 1960s, after the discovery of streptomycin, there was a great wave of new drug discovery research. **Schatz, Bugie**, and **Waksman** in Rutgers, New Jersey, discovered streptomycin, which was first reported in January 1944.

During the 1950s, the antibiotics rifampicin and rifamycin were discovered in Italy as part of a study into the antibiotic properties of *Nocardia mediterranei*. Rifampin was first used in clinical practice in 1966, and by the early 1970s, it had become essential in all tuberculosis treatment.

3.3.1 Rifampicin

Historical Background

✓ In 1957, **Piero Sensi** and **Maria Teresa Timbal** collected and examined a soil sample from a pine forest on the French Riviera, France, at the research facility of Lepetit Pharmaceuticals in Milan, Italy. They found a new bacterium (*Streptomyces mediterranei*) and developed an antimicrobial drug known as rifamycin.

✓ The term rifamycins (formerly rifomycins) was derived from the title of a popular French crime novel, "**Rififi**" (about a jewel heist and opposing gangs).

✓ After two years of research on rifamycins, a more stable semisynthetic compound known as rifampicin (rifampin) was developed in 1965. Rifampicin was licensed by the FDA in 1971 and commercialized in Italy in 1968.

Rifampicin (rifampin) is a broad-spectrum, semi-synthetic antibiotic. It consists of a macrocyclic ring which is connected to two nonadjacent (ansa) locations of an aromatic nucleus. As a result, they've been termed ansamycins.

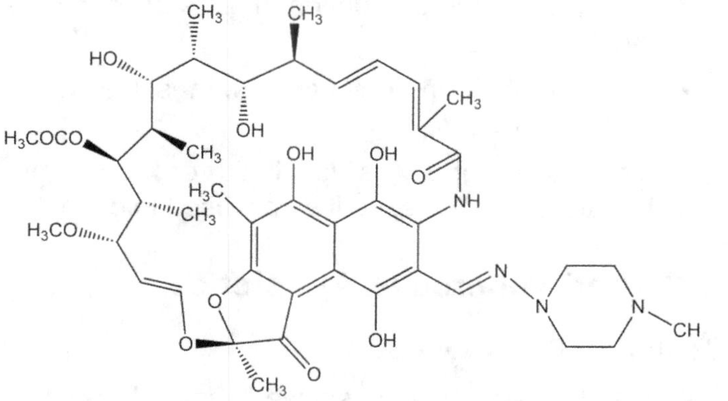

1963-1981-Several hundred semisynthetic rifamycins were prepared. Many compounds in this group have low potency, low solubility, poor bioavailability, and a short half-life. The early members of the family generally do not get much attention as medicinal agents. Hence, the native rifamycins were structurally modified, resulting in numerous very powerful and orally accessible derivatives being produced.

Fig.3.8 Chemical structure of Rifampicin.

Rifamycin B, O, S, SV, and X are the most studied members of the rifamycin family. Rifamycin S is a quinone class that is found in rifamycin B and rifamycin O solutions. Rifamycin SV, like rifamycin B, is a semisynthetic antibiotic. Certain *S. mediterranei* mutants can also be used to make rifamycin SV.

Recently, rifampicin, rifapentine, and rifabutin are three semisynthetic chemicals now in clinical use. Rifapentine and rifabutin, two of the newest members, have shown certain advantages over rifampicin, such as a longer half-life, a lower risk of drug-drug interactions, and/or efficacy against some rifampicin-resistant strains.

Chemical Structure: (Fig. 3.8)

Rifampicin is a semisynthetic derivative of rifamicin B, which is a macrolactam antibiotic and one of more than five antibiotics made from a mixture of rifamicins A, B, C, D, and E called a rifamicin complex. The rifamicin complex is produced by *actinomycetes* known as *Streptomyces mediteranei* (*Nocardia mediteranei*).

Chemical Name:

5,6,9,17,19-pentahydroxy-23-methoxy-2,4,12,16,18,20,22-heptamethyl-8-(4-methylpiperazin1-yliminomethyl)-1,11-dioxo-2,7-(epoxypentadeca-1,11,13-trienimino)-1,2-dihydronaphtho[2,1-b] furan-21-yl acetate.

Structure-Activity Relationship

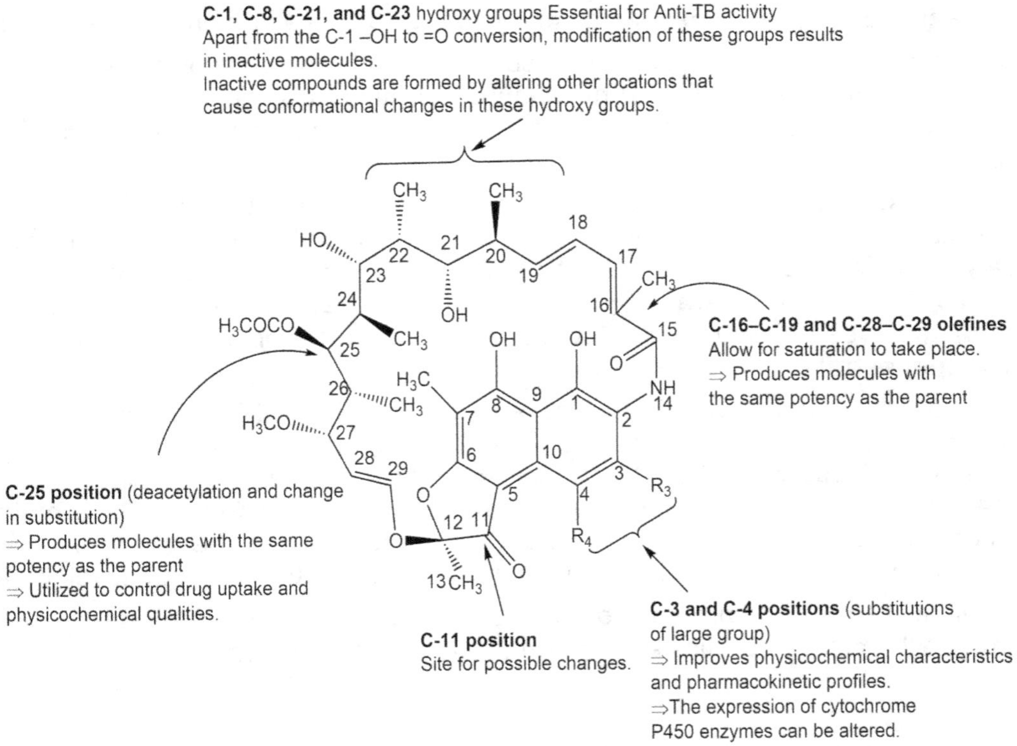

Fig.3.9 SAR of Rifampicin.

A wide range of rifamycin derivatives have been derived from naturally occurring rifamycins. The following assumptions about the structure-activity relationship (SAR) can be drawn from the compounds (Fig. 3.9):

1. The antibacterial action of rifamycin is dependent on four hydroxy groups situated at C-1, C-8, C-21, and C-23. Any changes to these hydroxy groups (except for the position at C-1 –OH to = O conversion) result in molecules with a decrease in activity. Additionally, other changes that altered the conformation of these hydroxy groups resulted in inactive compounds. These groups are crucial for binding to DNA-dependent RNA polymerase attachment (DDRP) via hydrogen bonding. Any modification in the skeletal system that disrupts such interactions will result in compounds with lower binding affinity.

2. The activity of the macro ring gradually decreases when the double bonds in the ring are in a reduction state. Additionally, opening the macro ring yields inactive compounds.

3. Saturation of one or more of the double bonds at the positions of C-16/C-17, C-18/C-19, and C-28/C-29 results in compounds with similar or slightly lower activity than their parent compounds. In terms of potency, these modifications do not provide a significant advantage over the parent compounds.

4. Inactive chemicals are formed when C-21 and/or C-23 are acetylated. Rifamycin metabolites are produced during the deacetylation process at position C-25. In general, these hydroxyl-derived compounds (C-25) are as potent as their parents.

5. Any acetyl group substitution results in potent compounds with varying physicochemical properties. Any changes to this position, however, could be considered "temporary" because the ester groups attached to this position are easily hydrolyzed *in vivo*.

6. The most important rifamycin derivatives are formed with C-3 and C-4 modifications. Substitution at C-3 or C-4 yields antibacterial compounds with varying degrees of antibacterial action. These positions of the compound have an affinity for RNA polymerase (RNAP). Modification at the C-3 and C-4 positions often improves physicochemical and pharmacokinetic properties and bacterial cell wall permeability.

7. Rifampicin is a potent and orally active compound derived from 3-formyl rifamycin SV. The rifampicin series was further modified to yield rifapentine, a cyclopentyl analogue. Rifapentine has a longer half-life than rifamycin. The joining of C-3 and C-4 resulted in the formation of rifabutin. Compared to rifampicin, this molecule has better tissue penetration and less cytochrome P_{450} enzyme induction. Rifalazil is a newer member of the rifamycin family and is currently in clinical development.

8. Rifampicin's C-11 carbonyl group is a potential site for modulating the physicochemical properties and pharmacokinetics of the drug.

Mechanism of Action

Rifamycin is a highly effective inhibitor of RNA polymerase (RNAP). Rifampicin binds to the b subunit of the RNA channel in a deep pocket about 12 A distant from the active center. When the transcript reaches two to three nucleotides in length, the drug blocks the path of the lengthening RNA. Rifamycin resistance is widespread and caused by mutations in the RNAP b subunit's rifamycin-binding region.

Rifamycin binds to the β-subunit of bacterial DNA-dependent RNA polymerase (DDRP) and is particularly effective against rapidly dividing intracellular and extracellular bacteria. Rifampin is effective against DDRP from both gram-+ve and gram-ve bacteria, but it is less effective against infections caused by gram-negative bacteria due to rifampin's low penetration of their cell walls. When DDRP is inhibited, the commencement of RNA synthesis chain formation is blocked. The naphthalene ring of rifamycin is thought to form a π-π bond with an aromatic amino acid ring in the DDRP protein. The DDRP is a metalloenzyme with two zinc atoms in it. The oxygens at positions C-1 and C-8 of rifamycin can bind to a zinc atom, which makes it stick to DDRP better. The oxygens at positions C-21 and C-23, on the other hand, form strong hydrogen bonds with DDRP. Rifamycin binds to DDRP and suppresses the production of RNA. Rifampin has been shown to prevent full-length transcripts from elongating, although it does not affect transcription. Resistance develops when a mutation in the gene responsible for the β-subunit of the RNA polymerase occurs, causing the antibiotic to lose its capacity to bind to the RNA polymerase.

Rifamycin is effective against gram-positive and gram-ve bacteria, as well as *M. tuberculosis* and *M. leprae*. By inhibiting DNA-dependent RNA polymerase, the activity is bactericidal and interferes with nucleic acid synthesis. Rifamycin sodium and rifampicin are the two official drugs. Rifamycin sodium is presently only used in a few cases. Rifampicin is a key component of tuberculosis and leprosy treatment regimens, as well as other illnesses.

Rifampicin is antibacterial because it inhibits the synthesis of RNA. It inhibits DNA-dependent RNA polymerase by interfering with the chain's initial development, not by destroying it. Rifampicin does not bind to the mammalian RNA polymerase nucleus and thus does not affect the corresponding RNA synthesis. It can also inhibit mitochondrial RNA synthesis.

Uses

✓ It is the most effective treatment for tuberculosis, both pulmonary and non-pulmonary, including tuberculosis meningitis, *M. avium* complex, and leprosy.

✓ It is used to treat tuberculosis in conjunction with isoniazid and pyrazinamide.

✓ In the treatment of leprosy, it is used with dapsone and clofazimine.

✓ It is also used to treat *brucellosis*, *Staphylococcal endocarditis*, and *meningococcal* and *Haemophilus influenzae* meningitis.

3.3.2 Rifabutin

Historical Background

✓ Semi-synthetic antibiotics have shown promise in the past. Rifabutin (mycobutin), a derivative of rifamycin S, is one such drug. It is beneficial for preventing MAC (*Mycobacterium avium complex*) infections in HIV-positive people.

✓ Scientists at the Italian pharmaceutical company Achifar discovered rifabutin in 1975.

✓ In the early 1990s, this company's Adria Laboratories division applied for USFDA approval of rifabutin under the brand name Mycobutin, and the drug received USFDA approval in December 1992.

Chemical Structure: (Fig. 3.10)

Chemical Name

1',4-didehydro-1-deoxy-1,4-dihydro-5'-(2-methylpropyl)-1-oxorifamycin OR 6,16,18,20-tetrahydroxy-1'-isobutyl-14-methoxy-7,9,15,17,19,21,25-heptamethyl-spiro[9,4-(epoxy-pentadeca[1,11,13]trienimino)-2H-furo[2',3':7,8]naphth[1,2-d]imidazole-2,4'-piperidine]-5,10,26-(3H,9H)-trione-16-acetate

Structure-Activity Relationship

1. Bridging the C-3 and C-4 positions of rifampicin results in the formation of rifabutin.

2. In comparison to rifampicin, this chemical has better tissue penetration and less cytochrome P_{450} enzyme stimulation.

Mechanism of Action

Rifabutin is an antibiotic that inhibits the activity of DNA-dependent RNA polymerase in susceptible cells. It particularly interacts with bacterial RNA polymerase but does not inhibit mammalian RNA polymerase. It is bactericidal and has a broad spectrum of activity against most gram-positive and gram-negative bacteria (including *Pseudomonas aeruginosa*) and *Mycobacterium tuberculosis*. Because of the rapid emergence of resistant bacteria, use is limited to mycobacterial infections.

Rifabutin has a higher tissue level of availability, is lower in cytochrome P_{450} initiation, and is active against some rifampicin-resistant bacteria.

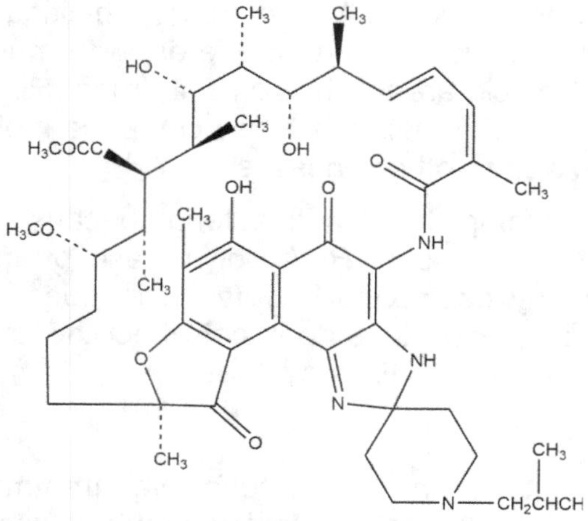

Fig.3.10 Chemical structure of Rifabutin.

Uses

- ✓ It's used to treat tuberculosis as well as to prevent and treat *M. avium* complex infections.

- ✓ It's usually given to those patients who can't take rifampin, such as those who have TB and HIV co-infections.

3.3.3 Cycloserine

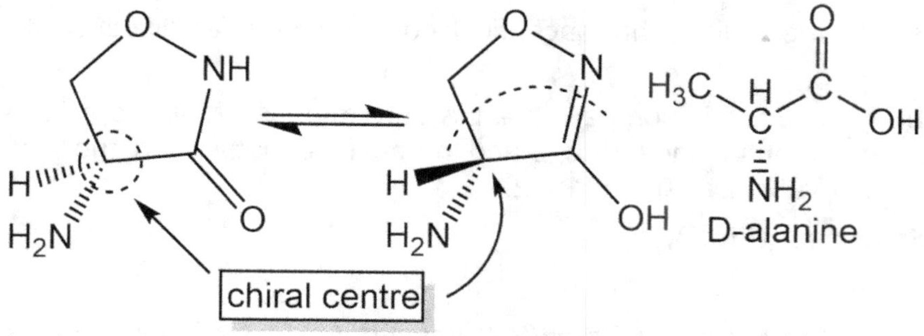

Fig.3.11 Chemical structure of Cycloserine.

Historical Background

Cycloserine is a natural product that was isolated from *Streptomyces orchidaceus,* or *S. garyphyllus,* in 1955. It has antibacterial properties against both Gram-+ve and Gram-ve bacteria. It is only marginally active against *M. tuberculosis* and is primarily used to treat MDR-TB. Due to its low activity and frequent side effects, the use of cycloserine is limited.

Several antibiotics are derived from amino acids; some are derived from a single amino acid, while others are made up of two amino acid units, and there is also a large category of polypeptide antibiotics.

Cycloserine is a structural homolog of D-alanine, an essential amino acid.

Chemical Structure: (Fig. 3.11)

Chemical Name: 4-aminoisoxazolidin-3-one

Structure-Activity Relationship

1. Although the structure of cycloserine is basic, few analogues have been found to preserve useful antibacterial action.
2. The amine group (C-4) must be present for enzyme recognition since cycloserine is an amino acid substitute for D-alanine. As a result, removing the C-4 amine functionality causes the antibacterial action to be lost. In these circumstances, it's ideal to leave the amine unsubstituted; alkylation or acylation significantly reduces or eliminates the action.
3. The D-configuration of this lone chiral center is necessary for its antibacterial properties.
4. The isoxazolidone ring system is also important for antibacterial activity, as it is the appropriate heteroatom substitution pattern.
5. Replacement of either cyclic nitrogen or oxygen atoms decreases inactivity. It most likely destroys the ring's planarity, which is required for enzyme recognition. Similarly, the breaking of the ring and/or the place of bond breakdown are usually diminished by inactivity. The significant exception is O-carbamoyl-n-serine, which is an alanine racemase inhibitor that also has antibacterial effects.
6. The position at the C-5 center remains unsubstituted. But few groups have been tolerated in this position in terms of antibacterial activity. Small size substituents (e.g., methyl) and ideally no heteroatoms/functional groups appear to be the requirements for this position.
7. Cycloserine has not been improved upon by any structural modifications, and no such agent has yet been developed. However, researchers will likely continue to investigate novel amino acid substitutes other than serine/cycloserine as potential chemotherapeutic agents.

Sterochemistry: (Fig. 3.12)

1. Cycloserine is a D-serine (non-essential amino acid) derivative. D-configuration is the chemically active form.

2. D-Cycloserine (DCS) is a naturally occurring antibiotic with high oral bioavailability and antibacterial activity against both Gram-+ve and Gram–ve bacteria.

Fig.3.12 Sterochemistry of Cycloserine.

3. D-Cycloserine inhibits the activity of two enzymes that are important for the biosynthesis of cell walls: 1) L-alanine racemase, which is needed to convert D-alanine to L-alanine; and 2) D-ala-D-ala-ligase, which is needed for mycobacteria to make the D-ala-D-ala dipeptide. Cycloserine in its D-form is required for peptidoglycan crosslinking.

4. It is a reserve drug for the treatment of tuberculosis (MDR-TB).

Mechanism of Action: (Fig. 3.13)

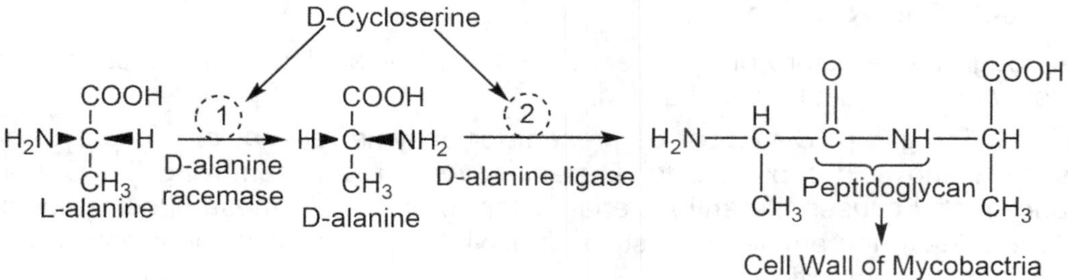

Fig. 3.13 Mechanism of Cycloserine.

Cycloserine is an antibiotic with a broad spectrum of activity. Its activity against *M. tuberculosis* is especially interesting. When cycloserine is used alone, resistance develops quickly.

D-cycloserine is considered the active form of the drug. It inhibits two important enzymes in mycobacteria. They are D-alanine racemase and D-alanine ligase. D-alanine is a component of the mycobacterial cell wall's peptidoglycan portion. Mycobacteria are capable of synthesizing D-alanine from naturally occurring L-alanine via the enzyme D-alanine racemase. Under the influence of D-alanine ligase, the resulting D-alanine is coupled to itself to form a D-alanine–D-alanine complex, which is then incorporated into the mycobacterial cell wall's peptidoglycan portion. D-cycloserine has a structural similarity to D-alanine, so it competitively inhibits D-alanine binding to both of these enzymes and incorporation into the peptidoglycan portion. Resistance to D-cycloserine is linked to D-alanine racemase overexpression.

Uses

Cycloserine is used to treat individuals with chronic tuberculosis who have failed to respond to treatment with the first group of drugs. As a result, it is only approved for the treatment of multidrug-resistant and severely drug-resistant *M. tuberculosis* strains.

3.3.4 Streptomycin

Historical Background

Aminoglycosides are a class of antibiotics that are widely used due to their broad-spectrum activity. Streptomycin is the first agent in this class. Streptomycin, kanamycin, and amikacin are the three drugs in this class that are currently used to treat tuberculosis.

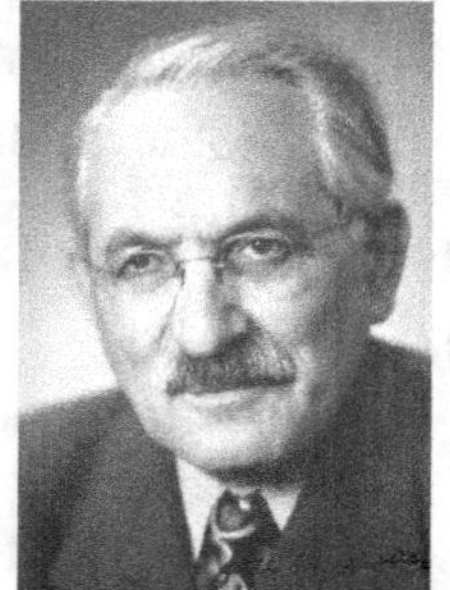

Fig. 3.14 Selman Abraham Waksman.

Streptomycin and kanamycin are natural antibiotics, while amikacin is a semisynthetic antibiotic derived from kanamycin.

The idea that a "chemical agent from microbes" could cure tuberculosis and other infectious diseases was first proposed by **Dr. Robert Koch's** colleague, **Paul Ehrlich**. Ehrlich developed a toxin-based treatment and won the Nobel Prize for it. In 1928, **Alexander Fleming**, a Scottish scientist, discovered a type of mould called *penicillium* that could be purified and used to treat bacterial infections. Penicillin was the first modern antibiotic.

Selman A. Waksman's (Fig. 3.14) research on soil microbiology led to the discovery of streptomycin, an antibiotic to treat tuberculosis. Waksman grew up in Priluka, Ukraine, and moved to America in 1910. Waksman worked in soil microbiology at Rutgers University, USA, where he mentored graduate students Rene Dubos, H. Boyd Woodruff, and Albert Schatz. To combat infections resistant to Fleming's penicillin, Schatz isolated a soil-borne bacterium called *Streptomyces griseus*. On October 19, 1943, **Albert Schatzhe** and **Waksman** refined streptomycin for the first time.

S. A. Waksman was awarded the Nobel Prize in Physiology or Medicine in 1952 for "discovering" streptomycin, the first antibiotic effective against tuberculosis.

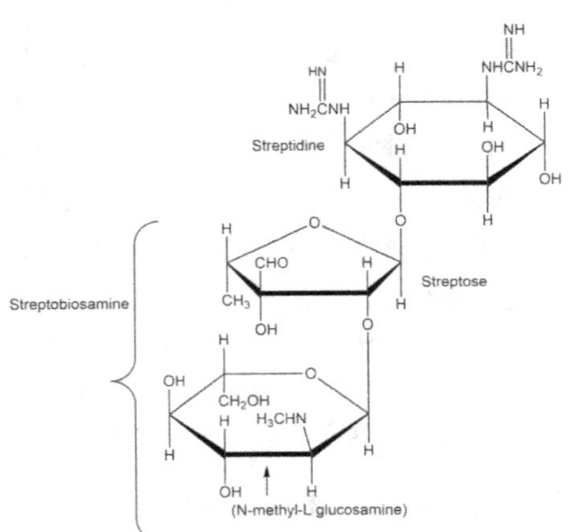

Fig.3.15 Chemical structure of Streptomyci.

Waksman and his laboratory staff discovered several antibiotics, including actinomycin, clavacin, streptothricin, streptomycin, neomycin, fradicin, candicidin, and candidin.

Among them, streptomycin (Fig. 3.15) and neomycin have found widespread use in the treatment of a variety of infectious disorders.

Chemical Structure: (Fig. 3.15)

Chemical Name:

2,4-diguanidino-3,5,6-trihydroxycyclohexyl-5-deoxy-2-O-(2-deoxy-2-methylamino- α -L-glucopyranosyl)-3-C-hydroxymethyl-β-L-lyxo-pentofuranoside

Chemistry

1. Streptomycin has an aldehydic carbonyl group and is a triacidic base. Streptidine (the diguanidinyl molecule corresponding to streptamine), streptose, and N-methyl-L-glucosamine are the three structural units of the aminoglycoside, which are linked together by glycosidic connections.

2. When hydrolyzed under suitable conditions, streptomycin produces diacidic-base streptidine.

3. On alkaline hydrolysis, the streptidine is transformed first into a urea derivative, then into the diamine streptamine (Fig. 3.16). It is a meso molecule (it contains several chiral centers and is optically inactive). Streptamine's absolute stereochemistry is similar to that of the 2-deoxystreptamine unit, which is found in neomycins and kanamycins.

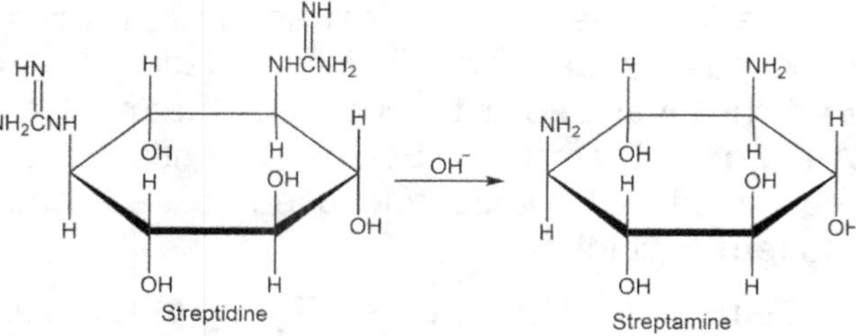

Fig. 3.16 Chemical reaction of Streptomycin.

4. After mild methanolysis (CH_3OH/HCl), streptomycin gives off streptidine and methyl streptobiosaminide, and dimethyl acetal.

5. Dihydrostreptomycin is a semisynthetic antibiotic. It is prepared by reducing streptomycin. It is also a naturally occurring antibiotic that was isolated from *Streptomyces humidas*. Dihydrostreptomycin is no longer used in humans since it is more ototoxic than streptomycin, yet it is still used in veterinary medicine.

Structure-Activity Relationship

1. There are currently about a dozen naturally occurring and semisynthetic aminoglycosides available for treating various bacterial infections. Streptomycin is the only aminoglycoside with a streptidine group; all other aminoglycosides have a 2-deoxystreptamine moiety.

2. Amikacin is slightly more effective against *M. tuberculosis* than streptomycin and kanamycin among all aminoglycosides. Other members of the class are inactive against *M. tuberculosis*.

3. In place of the primary amines in 2-deoxystreptamine, it has an axial hydroxyl group at C-2 and two highly basic guanidino groups at C-1 and C-3.

4. Another molecular feature, the α-hydroxy aldehyde moiety, is a center of instability, so streptomycin cannot be sterilized by autoclaving, so streptomycin sulfate solutions that require sterilization are made through ultrafiltration.

5. It is well known that *N*-acetylation and *O*-phosphorylation are the main causes of streptomycin resistance. It is no longer often used as a single agent.

Mechanism of Action

In many ways, the specific antibacterial mechanism of aminoglycosides is unknown, and it cannot be concluded from a single mechanism of action. The aminoglycosides primarily inhibit bacterial protein biosynthesis, but they also have effects on the bacterial cell membrane. The importance of both phenomena in the overall antibacterial action of these agents has been recognized in modern times.

Streptomycin is active against *tubercle bacilli*, which are found extracellularly, but not against tubercle bacilli found inside infected cells. It acts as a protein synthesis inhibitor by binding to the 16S rRNA and preventing the genome chain from being translated into proteins.

Streptomycin is an aminoglycoside antibiotic that acts by binding to the 30S ribosomal subunit of bacteria, causing t-RNA misreading and preventing the organism from biosynthesising proteins which are necessary for bacterial growth.

Streptomycin is an aminoglycoside antibiotic which binds irreversibly to the bacterial 30S ribosomal subunit's 16S rRNA and S12 protein. As a result, it disrupts the formation of the initiation complex between mRNA and the bacterial ribosome, thus preventing protein synthesis from starting. Additionally, it causes premature termination of translation due to gene mutations and misreading of the mRNA template. This leads to bacterial cell death.

Uses

- ✓ Its primary use is in the treatment of tuberculosis, where it is used in conjunction with other antimycobacterial agents.

- ✓ It has been used in combination with penicillin to treat endocarditis as an alternative to gentamicin.

- ✓ It is used to treat bacterial endocarditis (inflammation of the endocardium), peritonitis (redness and swelling (inflammation) of the lining of the abdomen), meningitis (inflammation of the meninges), urinary tract infections, and gastric infections.

- ✓ It can be used to treat plague and tularemia (a disease that can infect animals and people).

3.3.5 Capreomycin Sulphate

Historical Background

Capreomycin was an antibiotic developed in the United States in 1960 and first used in a clinic in 1968. It was first used for tuberculosis in 1979.

Capreomycin is a polypeptide antibiotic that works similarly to aminoglycosides in terms of modes of action, pharmacokinetics, potency, and toxicity. It has an elevated level of nephrotoxicity and ototoxicity.

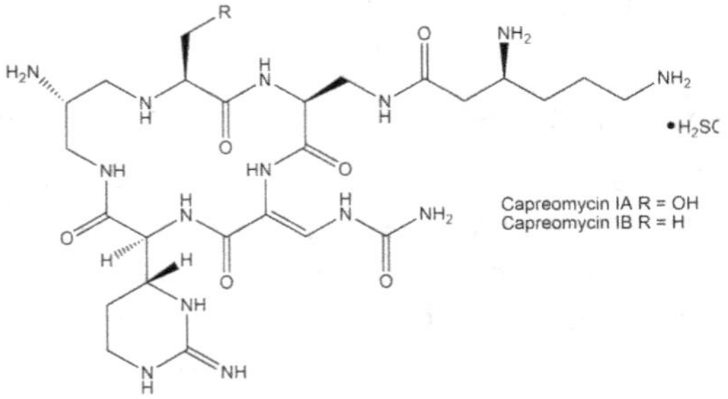

Capreomycin IA R = OH
Capreomycin IB R = H

Fig. 3.17 Chemical structure of Capreomycin sulphate.

Capreomycin is a semisynthetic antibiotic isolated from *Streptomyces capreolus* culture fluid.

Capreomycin is a mixture of four cyclic polypeptides (IA, IB, IIA, and IIB), 90% of which are capreomycin IA (R = OH) and IB (R = H).

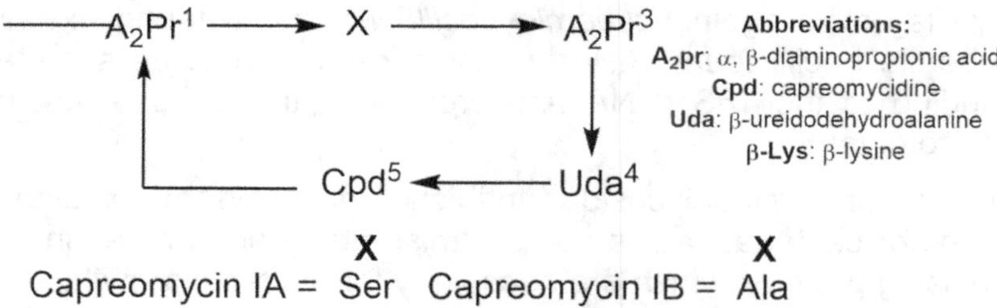

Fig. 3.18 The cyclic moieties of capreomycin structures.

Chemical Structure: (Fig. 3.17)

Structure-Activity Relationship

1. All amino acid components have L-configurations.

2. The similar antibacterial activity of capreomycin IB (pseudocapreomycin IB) to natural capreomycin IA (Fig. 3.18).

Mechanism of Action

Its mechanism of action is not fully understood, but it acts as a potent inhibitor of protein synthesis, particularly that dependent on mRNA at the 70S ribosome. It also prevents chain elongation by binding to the 50S or 30S ribosomal subunits.

Capreomycin is a cyclic polypeptide antibiotic that has antitubercular properties. Although the exact mechanism by which capreomycin acts is unknown, this agent may bind to the 50S subunit of the 70S ribosome in bacteria. This causes interference with the translational start complex, mRNA misreading, and, finally, protein synthesis suppression. Capreomycin also binds to the components of bacterial cell walls, blocking cell wall production.

Comparative MOA in between Aminoglycosides and Polypeptide antibiotics

Capreomycin can be used to treat MDR-TB as a second-line treatment. Capreomycin and aminoglycosides differ from each other in that they have anaerobic activity against *M. tuberculosis*. Anaerobic conditions increase capreomycin's efficacy against *M. tuberculosis*, whereas aminoglycosides have no effect on *M. tuberculosis*. This difference could be explained by changes in drug transport: aminoglycosides require active absorption, which slows dramatically under anaerobic conditions, whereas capreomycin could be carried by a different mechanism that is still active under these circumstances.

Uses

✓ The drug should not be used alone; rather, it should be used in combination with other antituberculosis agents to treat TB.

✓ It is used when the main drugs (isoniazid, rifampin, ethambutol, aminosalicylic acid, and streptomycin) don't work, cause side effects, or have *tubercle bacilli* that are resistant to them.

✓ It is used as a second-line treatment for drug-resistant tuberculosis.

✓ It has been linked to kidney and liver damage, hearing loss, and allergic reactions.

3.4 Urinary Tract Anti-Infective Agents

Definition: Urinary anti-infectives are drugs that are used to treat or prevent infections of the urinary tract. The urinary tract consists of a tube that carries urine from the kidneys to the outside of the body.

When disease-causing organisms enter the urinary tract from other areas of the body or from the outside, the bladder, urethra, and other components of the urinary tract can become infected. Such infections are treated with urinary anti-infective agents.

Causative Agent

Infections of the urinary tract are particularly frequent among women. *Escherichia coli* is a common pathogen that causes infection. Infections caused by *Staphylococcus saprophyticus* are prevalent in young women. *Staphylococcus epidermidis*, *enterococci*, and *Pseudomonas* species are among the additional infectious bacteria involved in urinary tract infections.

Urinary tract infections are less common in men and frequently occur because of genitourinary system abnormalities such as prostatic enlargement. *Neisseria gonorrhoeae* is one of the most common pathogens that cause infected urethritis in men. *Chlamydia trachomatis* and *Ureaplasma urealyticum* can also cause urethritis that is not caused by *gonococci*. Urethritis (inflammation of the urethra) is frequently accompanied by *epididymitis*.

3.5 Quinolones

Historical Background

✓ Antibiotics, sulphonamides, quinolones, trimethoprim, and urinary tract antiseptics are commonly used to treat urinary tract infections.

✓ Nalidixic acid, a naphthyridine agent, was identified as an antibacterial agent in 1940.

✓ Following that, 4-quinolone compounds such as oxolinic acid and cinoxacin were produced, which showed improved action against a small number of gram-ve bacteria.

✓ In Japan, parallel developments led to the discovery of 7-piperazine-substituted molecules such as pipemidic acid, which had little antibacterial action.

✓ Fluoroquinolones (ciprofloxacin, ofloxacin, and levofloxacin) have become a major class of synthetic antibiotics with antibacterial activity since they were introduced in the mid-1980s.

✓ The synthesis of temafloxacin, which had four to eight times the activity of ciprofloxacin, was the next breakthrough in the early 1990s. However, only a few months after its launch, it was withdrawn due to toxicity.

✓ Furthermore, the development of many other antibacterial substances, including sparfloxacin, sitafloxacin, trovafloxacin, clinafloxacin, and grepafloxacin, has been halted due to substantial adverse effects.

✓ Fortunately, the 8-methoxyquinolines moxifloxacin and gatifloxacin have filled this therapeutic need, as they are immensely powerful, therapeutically effective, and appear to be free of substantial or unexpected toxicity. Nowadays, 8-methoxyquinoline derivatives are the preferred agents. The continued development of the naphthyridine subclass, particularly gemifloxacin, which has a 10-fold increase in antibacterial activity, is another step forward.

Classification

A Chemical and Functional Classification of Quinolones and Fluoroquinolones

A. First-generation compounds:

    I.   4-quinolones Ex. nalidixic acid, oxolinic acid

B. Second-generation compounds:

    II.   6-Fluoroquinolones-7-piperazinyl   Ex.   levofloxacin,   ciprofloxacin, norfloxacin, ofloxacin, pefloxacin, enoxacin

    III.   6,8-difluoro-7-piperazinyl Ex. lomefloxacin

    IV.   6-fluoro-8–chloro-7-pyrrolodinyl Ex. sparfloxacin

    V.   6,8-difluoro-7-dimethylpiperazinyl Ex. grepafloxacin

C. Third-generation compounds:

    VI.   6-fluoro-8-methoxy-7-azabicyclo Ex. moxifloxacin

    VII.   6-fluoro-8-methoxy-7-piperazinyl Ex. gatifloxacin

    VIII.   6-fluoro-7-methoximinonaphthyridone Ex. gemifloxacin

Structure-Activity Relationships of Quinolones: (Fig. 3.19)

1. The biological action of quinolone antibacterial drugs is dependent on their structural requirements. An N-substituted 4-oxo-1,4-dihydroquinoline with an acidic function at the C-3 position is the most important property.

2. When this simple heterocyclic assemblage is broken, the antibacterial activity of the compound is lost.

3. Inactive derivatives result from replacing the nitrogen atom at position 1 with oxygen, sulfur, or carbon (the methylene group). The quinoline system is essential.

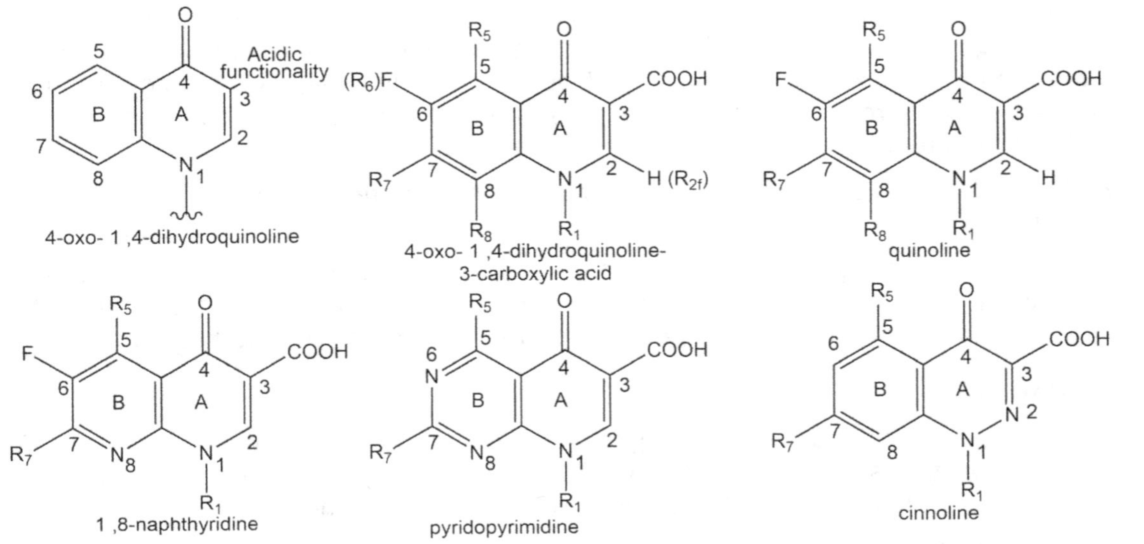

Fig. 3.19 SAR of quinolones structure.

1. Antibacterial activity is lost when the aromatic (B) ring system is modified. However, (B) ring benzene isosteres (molecules or ions with similar shapes and often electronic properties), such as 2,3-fused thiophene, can provide compounds with antibacterial activity.

2. Any change to the 4-oxo moiety has resulted in a loss of antibacterial action.

3. For gyrase inhibition and antibacterial activity, an acidic group, usually a carboxylic acid linked to the C-3 center, is required.

4. In terms of antibacterial action, specific heteroatom alterations inside this quinolone nucleus are well tolerated. In fact, including nitrogen at positions 2, 6, or 8 can result in compounds with antibacterial properties.

5. The cinnoline heterocycle is created by replacing carbon with nitrogen at position 2. The prototypic aza-quinolone with this heterocyclic nucleus is cinoxacin (Figure 7.2). Pyridopyrimidine heterocycles such as pipemidic acid and piromidic acid are formed when nitrogen is incorporated at positions 6 and 8.

6. The inclusion of nitrogen at position 8 yields the 1,8 naphthyridine heterocycle found in the powerful drug enoxacin.

7. Active molecules can be made from isomeric 1,5-naphthyridines and 1,6-naphthyridines, but 1,7-naphthyridine analogues are largely inactive.

8. The pyridopyrazine heterocyclic system is formed by including nitrogen at positions 5 and 8, and analogues have significant antibacterial activity.

Substituents at N-1:

1. The quinolone nucleus in the N-1 position was predominantly determined by steric considerations.

2. The highest antibacterial activity found in this series is found in an ethyl moiety or a group of comparable size. This property is found in many well-known quinolones, including norfloxacin, enoxacin, and pefloxacin. Similarly, a fluoroethyl group is present in fleroxacin, an aminomethyl group is present in amifloxacin, and a methoxy group is present in miloxacin at N-1.

3. Both the quinolone and 1,8-naphthyridine families showed excellent antibacterial activity *in vitro*.

4. The cyclopropyl group is still one of the first N-1 moieties to be investigated while developing novel quinolone antibacterial drugs today. Ciprofloxacin belongs to this group and is the most widely used quinolone antibiotic on the market today.

Substituents at C-2:

1. It appears that replacing hydrogen at C-2 has not been beneficial either. For instance, the antibacterial activity of the compound decreases when methyl or hydroxyl groups are substituted at C-2 of the quinolone ring.

2. Antibacterial action has been established when a sulfur atom is directly attached to the C-2 location.

Substituents at C-3:

1. In terms of antibacterial action, a free carboxylic acid at the C-3 position or a C-2, C-3 fused isothiazolone ring is suitable.

2. Other acidic groups, such as sulfonic acid and phosphonic acid, as well as esterification, result in the loss of antibacterial action.

Substituents at C-4:

1. The antibacterial activity of the quinolone nucleus appears to be dependent on the oxo group at the C-4 position. The antibacterial activity is lost when a 4-thioxo group or a 4-sulfonyl group is substituted at the C-4 position.

Substituents at C-5:

The steric configuration appears to be the main factor influencing substitution at C-5 of a quinolone. Only methyl or similar-sized alkyl substitutions at the C-5 position are helpful. Larger groups of substitutions result in a loss of antibacterial action. In terms of potency and activity spectrum, several C-5 methylated quinolones appear to be promising compounds.

In the case of several quinolone derivatives, the addition of an amino group at the C-5 position is beneficial for antibacterial activity. The amino group at C-5 of the quinolone ring has been alkylated or acylated and has shown only moderate antibacterial activity.

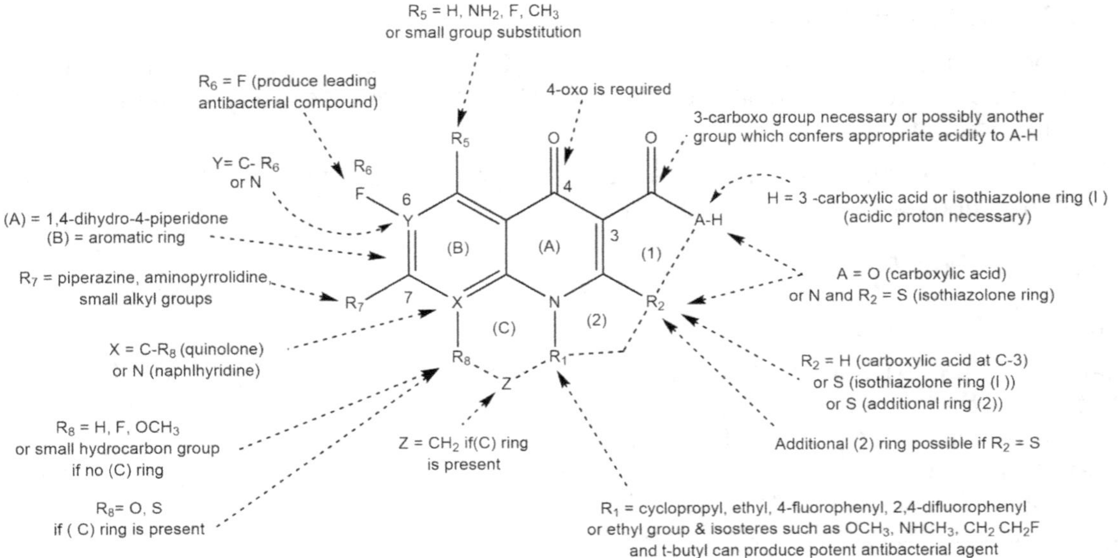

Fig. 3.20 SAR of quinolone nucleus that gives possible antibacterial activity.

Substituents at C-6:

1. The addition of a fluorine atom to the C-6 position of a quinolone has shown both gyrase inhibitory and antibacterial action.

2. In terms of antibacterial action, chloro, bromo, methyl, or cyano group substituents at the C-6 position are allowed, although the resultant compounds have shown less activity than C-6 fluoroquinolone compounds.

Substituents at C-7:

1. Small groups (like methyl or amino), heteroatoms (like alkyloxy, alkylamino, or alkylthio), or halogens (like chloro) make less active compounds. Adding a piperazine group to the C-7 position enhances antibacterial activity.

2. In terms of antibacterial action, other heterocyclic systems such as thiazole, imidazole, pyrrole, and pyridine can be useful for C-7 substituents.

3. In comparison to piperazinyl analogues, aminopyrrolidine groups at C-7 have better antibacterial action, although they are insoluble.

Substituents at C-8:

1. The substitution of lipophilic groups such as fluoro, trifluoromethyl, and methoxy groups in C-8 has now received attention due to an increase in antibacterial activity.

2. For antibacterial activity, alkylation at the C-8 position, particularly if the substituent is lipophilic or contains small groups (methyl), is allowed. Vinylic, propargylic, and methyl groups can provide molecules with minor antibacterial activities. While amino, hydroxyl, or nitro groups in this position abolish antibacterial activity.

C-1, C-8 bridged variations:

1. The joining of the N-1 groups to the C-8 position is a favourable change. Flumequine and ofloxacin are two examples of oxazine derivatives that have such modifications.

2. Other changes, such as piperazinyl fused ring systems, can also result in compounds with higher antibacterial activity (Fig.3.20).

3.5.1 Nalidixic Acid

Historical Background

Nalidixic acid (NA) is the first quinolone antibiotic that has been used to treat urinary tract infections for a long time. In 1962, **George Lesher** and colleagues discovered synthetic quinolone (nalidixic acid) antibiotics as a byproduct of chloroquine synthesis. It has a narrow spectrum of activity against gram-ve bacteria.

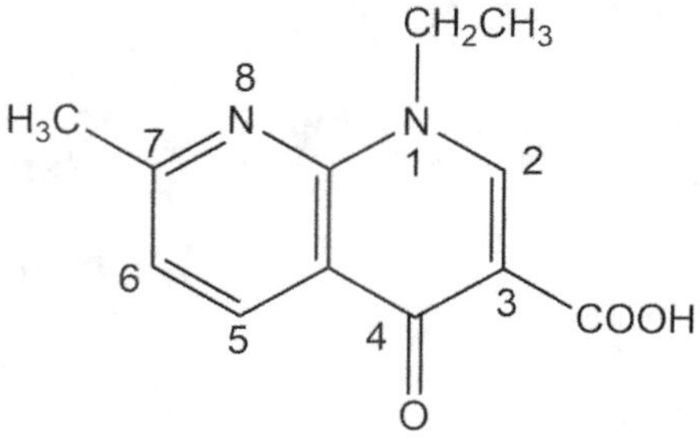

Fig. 3.21 Chemical structure of Nalidixic Acid.

Compounds such as oxolinic acid, cinoxacin, and pipemidic acid, which were introduced into the clinic in the 1970s, performed somewhat better than nalidixic acid.

Chemical structure: (Fig. 3.21)

Chemical name:

1-ethyl-7-methyl-4-oxo-1,4-dihydro-1,8-naphthyridine-3-carboxylic acid

Mechanism of Action

It checks the replication and repair of DNA in bacteria. It prevents both gram-positive and gram-negative bacteria by inhibiting DNA gyrase. It also inhibits the start of the translation process by inhibiting the development of the 70S ribosomal initiation complex in developing bacteria by binding to the 50S ribosomal subunit.

Uses

✓ It is commonly used to treat urinary tract infections.

✓ It is also employed in the treatment of pyelonephritis (kidney infection), urethritis (swelling, irritation, or inflammation of the urethra), prostatitis (pain or burning sensation during urinating (dysuria), and difficulties urinating), as well as gastrointestinal tract infections.

3.5.2 Norfloxacin

Historical Background

Norfloxacin was discovered in 1979 by the pharmaceutical company, Kyorin Seiyaku Kabushiki Kaisha, in Tokyo, Japan.

It is the first in a series of fluorinated quinolones, as well as the first drug with a piperazine substituent among quinolone derivatives. It served as a model for enoxacin, pefloxacin, and ciprofloxacin, all of which are now widely used quinolones with significant oral activity. When compared to earlier nonfluorinated derivatives, these chemicals have a broader spectrum of antibacterial action and better pharmacokinetic features.

Chemical Structure: (Fig. 3.22)

Chemical Name:

1-ethyl-6-fluoro-4-oxo-7- (piperazin-1-yl) -1, 4-dihydroquinoline-3-carboxylic acid

Mechanism of Action:

Norfloxacin is a broad-spectrum antibiotic that is effective against both gram-+ve and gram-ve bacteria. These compounds are believed to block the A subunit of the enzyme DNA gyrase (a number of bacteria have DNA gyrase). DNA gyrase comprises type II topoisomerase and topoisomerase IV, enzymes required for bacterial DNA separation, thereby inhibiting cell division. It binds to the substrate DNA but not to DNA gyrase.

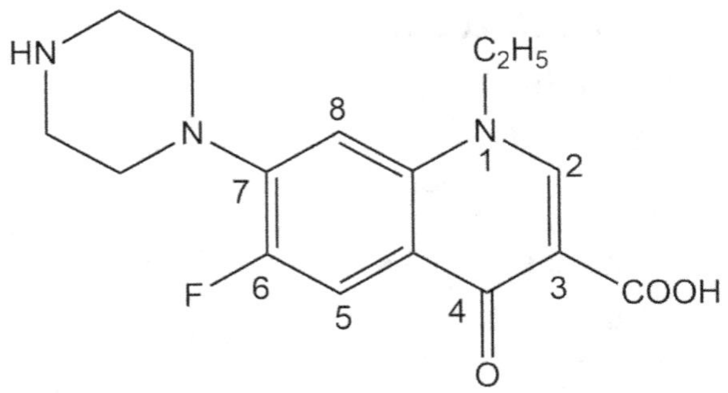

Fig. 3.22 Chemical structure of Norfloxacin.

Uses

It is utilized to treat urinary tract infections, prostate infections, and stomach infections, although it is also used to treat gonorrhea.

3.5.3 Enoxacin

Historical Background

Enoxacin, an analogue of nalidixic acid, was discovered in 1980 and found to have a broader spectrum of activity against gram-ve and gram-+ve bacteria.

Chemically, it is a pyridonecarboxylic acid derivative compound.

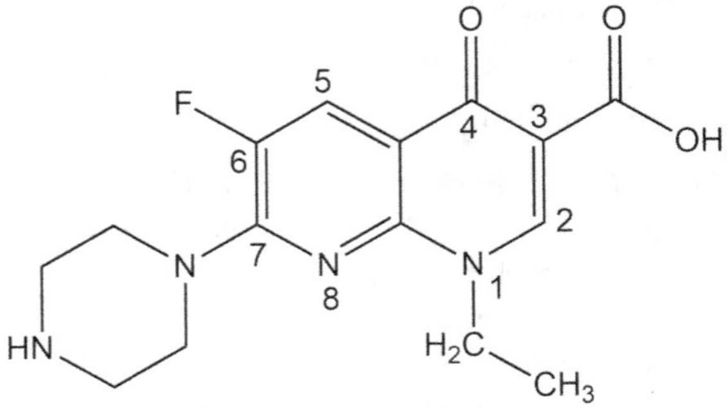

Fig. 3.23 Chemical structure of Enoxacin.

Chemical Structure: (Fig. 3.23)

Chemical Name:

1-ethyl-6-fluoro-4-oxo-7-(piperazin-1-yl)-1,4-dihydro-1,8-naphthyridine-3-carboxylic acid

Mechanism of action:

Enoxacin is an antibiotic that belongs to the quinolone/fluoroquinolone family. Enoxacin is antibacterial, and its mechanism of action is to prevent bacterial DNA replication by binding to the enzyme DNA gyrase. This type of enzyme helps uncoil DNA strands. Fuhrer, the enzyme, is required to copy one DNA double helix into two. Enoxacin is a broad-spectrum antibiotic that kills gram-+ve as well as gram-ve bacteria.

Uses

- ✓ It's used to treat infections of the urinary tract and gonorrhea.
- ✓ It is equally effective in the treatment of genital tract, skin, and soft tissue infections.

3.5.4 Ciprofloxacin

Historical Background

- ✓ Ciprofloxacin, also known as Cipro, is one of the most commonly prescribed antibiotics for bacterial infections in the world. It belongs to the antibacterial class of fluoroquinolone compounds.

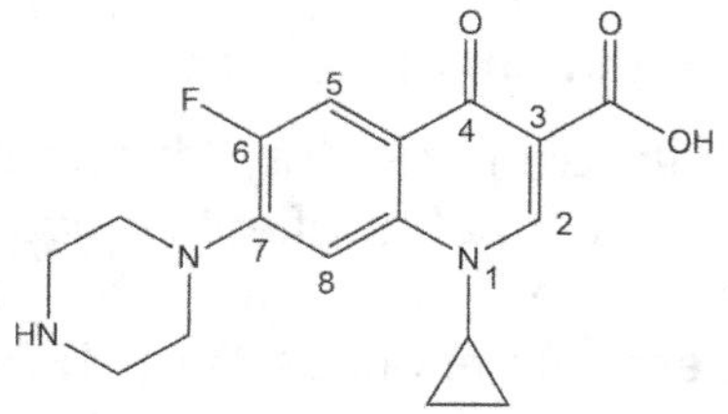

Fig. 3.24 Chemical structure of Ciprofloxacin.

- ✓ In the 1980s, scientists at Bayer Pharmaceuticals learned that substituting a cyclopropyl group in place of the ethyl group in the norfloxacin structure. The resulting product has substantially increased its gram-ve bactericidal action.

- ✓ In 1987, the US FDA approved the oral form of ciprofloxacin, and in 1991, the intravenous form.

- ✓ Ciprofloxacin has been widely used as a low-cost, broad-spectrum antibiotic. It is listed on the WHO's Essential Medicines List.

Chemical structure: (Fig. 3.24)

Chemical Name:

1-cyclopropyl-6-fluoro-4-oxo-7-(piperazin-1-yl)-1,4-dihydroquinoline-3-carboxylic acid

Synthesis: (Fig. 3.25)

1. Ciprofloxacin is synthesized via acylation of 2,4,5-trifluorobenzoyl chloride with ethyl-3-(dimethylamino) acrylate, yielding an acrylate derivative compound.

2. The acrylate product is then treated at low temperatures with cyclopropylamine to make an intermediate called ethyl-3-(cyclopropylamino)-2-(2,4,5-trifluorobenzoyl) acrylate.

3. Following that, the intermediate product is cyclized with dimethylsulfoxide (DMSO) at 150°C to produce a naphthalene-2-carboxylate derivative compound.

4. Then, a naphthalene-2-carboxylate derivative compound is made by cyclizing the intermediate product with dimethylsulfoxide (DMSO) at 150°C.

5. To make ciprofloxacin HCl salt, the end product is treated with alkali (NaOH) and acid (HCl) at appropriate temperatures.

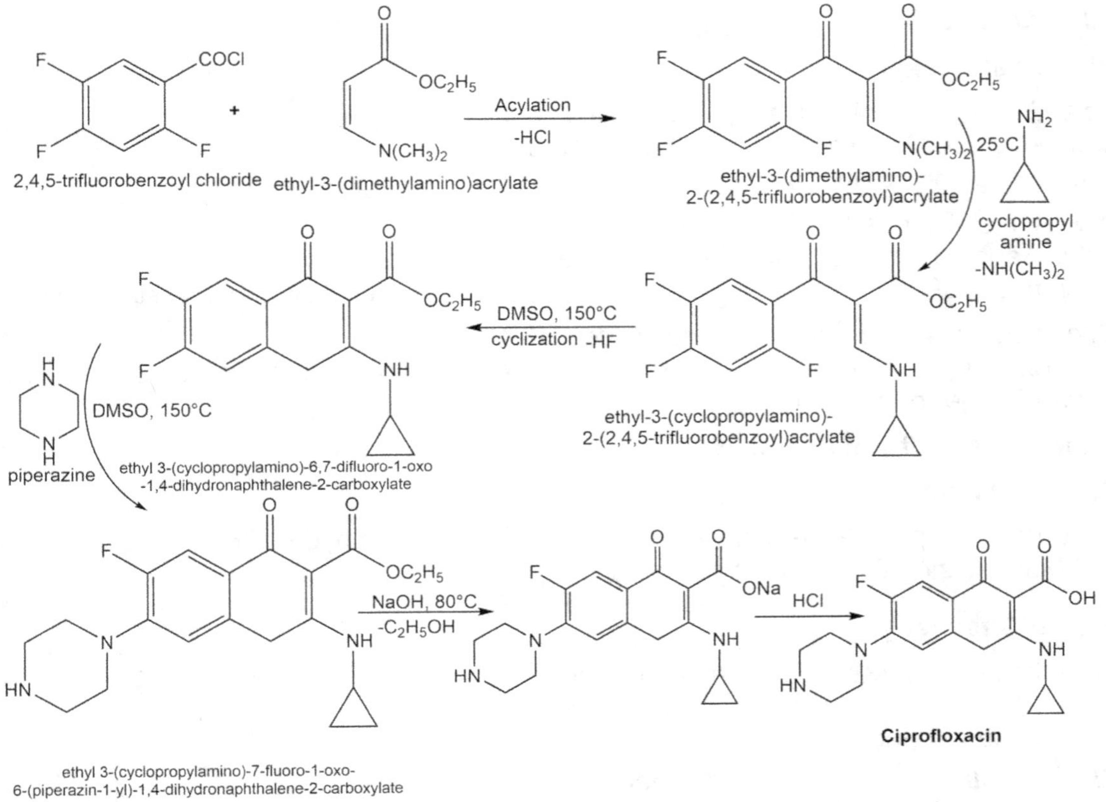

Fig. 3.25 Synthesis of Ciprofloxacin.

Mechanism of Action

Ciprofloxacin is a bactericidal antibiotic belonging to the fluoroquinolone class. It prevents DNA replication by inhibiting the enzymes bacterial DNA topoisomerase and DNA-gyrase. It is the most effective drug that acts against gram-ve bacteria (such as *E. coli*, *Salmonella spp.*, *Shigella spp.*, and *Neisseria*). Some gram-+ve bacteria are also susceptible to ciprofloxacin. Oral ciprofloxacin has a bioavailability of 70 to 80 percent. It has been among the few oral antibiotics that can treat infections with *P. aeruginosa*.

Uses

- ✓ It has been used to treat a variety of illnesses, including typhoid and paratyphoid fever, urinary tract, eye, bones, joints, and skin infections.
- ✓ It's also used in the treatment of the respiratory tract, biliary tract infections, and inflammatory diseases of the abdominal cavity and organs.
- ✓ It can also be employed to treat bacterial prostatitis (prostate gland inflammation), uncomplicated gonorrhea, and pulmonary infections.
- ✓ It works well for acute infectious diarrhoea and enteritis (inflammation of the intestines).

3.5.5 Ofloxacin

Historical Background

Scientists at Daiichi Seiyaku, Japan, designed and developed ofloxacin, a second-generation fluoroquinolone compound.

It was first licensed for oral use in Japan in 1985 and received USFDA approval in December 1990.

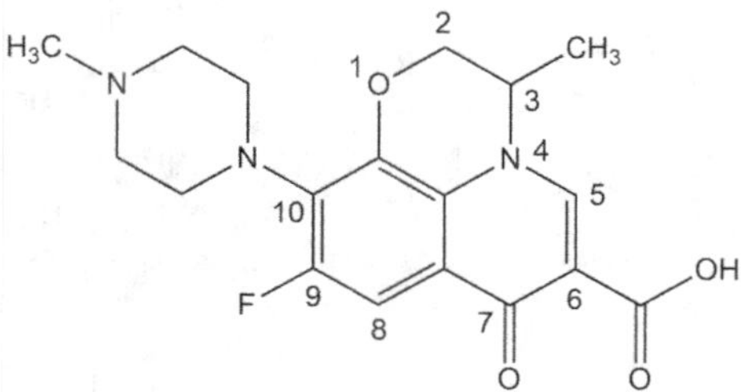

Fig. 3.26 Chemical structure of Ofloxacin.

Ofloxacin is a racemic combination of 50% levofloxacin (the physiologically active component) and 50% dextrofloxacin, which is its "mirror image" or enantiomer.

Chemical structure: (Fig. 3.26)

Chemical name:

9-Fluoro-3-methyl-10- (4-methyl-1-piperazinyl)-7-oxo-2,3-dihydro- 7H- pyrido [1,2,3-de] [1,4]benzoxazine-6-carboxylic acid

Stereo-Chemistry

1. Ofloxacin possesses a tricyclic ring and is an oxazine derivative compound (Fig.3.27).

2. *In vitro*, the (*S*)-enantiomer of ofloxacin is significantly more effective than the (*R*)-enantiomer (8–64 times for most species).

3. The discovery of the (*S*)-enantiomer of ofloxacin (levofloxacin) has resulted in the development of several novel compounds.

Fig. 3.27 Stereo configuration of Ofloxacin.

Mechanism of Action

Ofloxacin, like other second-generation fluoroquinolone drugs, is a broad-spectrum antibacterial with bactericidal properties. It performs this by interacting with and inhibiting the enzyme bacterial topoisomerase II (DNA gyrase). The DNA gyrase relaxes the supercoiled DNA structure. Another enzyme, topoisomerase IV, separates connected daughter chromosomes after replication. These inhibitory actions disrupt DNA replication, transcription, and repair, blocking bacterial cell division.

Uses

✓ It has a similar antibacterial action to ciprofloxacin. It is used to treat lower respiratory tract infections, skin infections, urinary tract infections, prostatitis, and sexually transmitted disorders (gonorrhea).

✓ It's also used to treat infections of the ears, throat, nose, soft tissue, bones, and joints.

✓ It is employed in the treatment of infective-inflammatory disorders of the abdominal cavity organs (kidneys, urinary tract) and pelvic minor organs (genitalia).

✓ It's used to treat chlamydial as well as mycobacterial infections like leprosy.

3.5.6 Lomefloxacin

Historical Background

Lomefloxacin is a difluorinated quinolone with a 3-methyl piperazine moiety. It can be taken orally and is effective against a broad range of gram-negative and gram-positive bacteria.

Chemical structure: (Fig. 3.28)

Chemical Name:

1-ethyl-6,8-difluoro-7-(3-methylpiperazin-1-yl)-4-oxo-1,4-dihydroquinoline-3-carboxylic acid

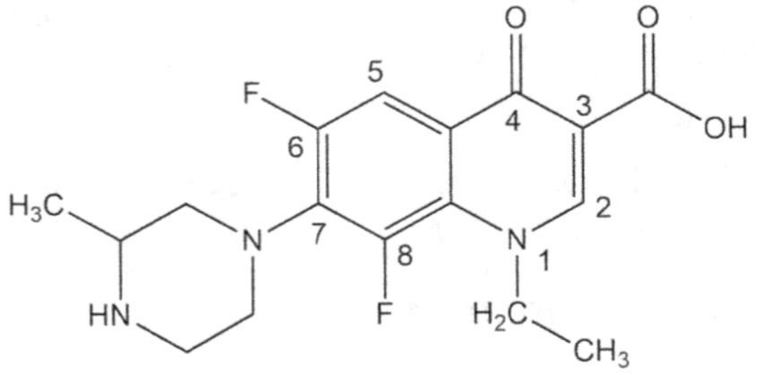

Mechanism of Action

The bactericidal action of lomefloxacin interferes with the functioning of the bacterial enzymes DNA gyrase and topoisomerase IV. Both enzymes are involved in bacterial DNA transcription and replication. For gram-ve bacteria,

Fig. 3.28 Chemical structure of Lomefloxacin.

DNA gyrase appears to be the principal target of quinolones. In gram-+ve bacteria, topoisomerase IV appears to be the preferred target. When these two topoisomerases are inhibited, the bacterial chromosome undergoes strand breakage, supercoiling, and resealing. This inhibits the transcription and replication of DNA.

Uses

✓ It is beneficial for treating chronic bronchitis and infections of the urinary tract.

✓ It's also used to prevent urinary tract infections in those who are undergoing surgery.

3.5.7 Sparfloxacin

Historical Background

Sparfloxacin is a fluoroquinolone antibiotic of the third generation with a broad spectrum of activity. Its key advantage over earlier fluoroquinolones is enhanced activity against gram-positive bacteria. It was withdrawn from the market in 2001 because it was more phototoxic than other fluoroquinolones.

Chemical Structure: (Fig. 3.29)

Chemical Name

5-amino-1-cyclopropyl-7-((3R,5S)-3,5-dimethylpiperazin-1-yl)-6,8-difluoro-4-oxo-1,4-dihydroquinoline-3-carboxylic acid

Mechanism of Action

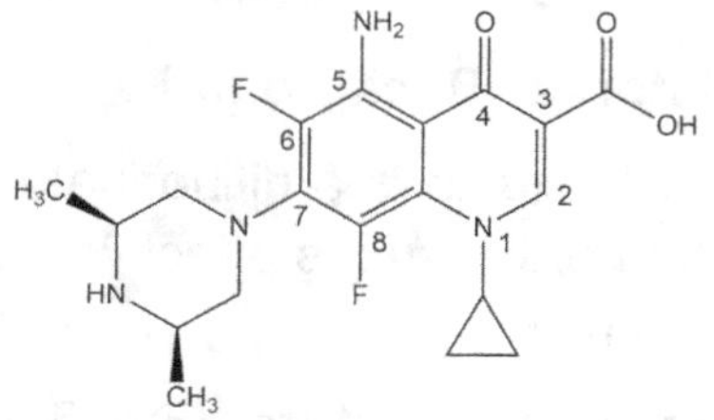

Inhibition of DNA gyrase activity is one of the mechanisms through which Sparfloxacin interferes with DNA synthesis in bacteria. Its primary target is DNA gyrase (topoisomerase II), while its secondary target is topoisomerase IV (also known as parC). Sparfloxacin, on the other hand, targets topoisomerase IV rather than DNA gyrase. Thereby inhibiting DNA replication and transcription in bacteria. Individual fluoroquinolones may differ in their antibacterial efficacy due to their varied affinity for their intrinsic action against certain target enzymes. The addition of fluorine or methoxy at position 8 protects topoisomerase IV from mutations.

Fig. 3.29 Chemical structure of Sparfloxacin.

Uses

It is a helpful treatment for people with sinusitis, chronic bronchitis from susceptible organisms, and pneumonia.

3.5.8 Gatifloxacin

Historical Background

1. Bristol-Myers Squibb, USA, introduced gatifloxacin for respiratory tract infections in 1999. Kyorin Pharmaceutical Co., Ltd. of Tokyo, Japan, developed it.

2. It is a fourth-generation fluoroquinolone antibacterial agent. It has a broader spectrum of antibacterial activity than previous quinolones, such as ciprofloxacin. It is effective against a wide range of gram-positive and gram-negative organisms.

3. Only an ophthalmic solution of gatifloxacin is currently available in the United States and Canada.

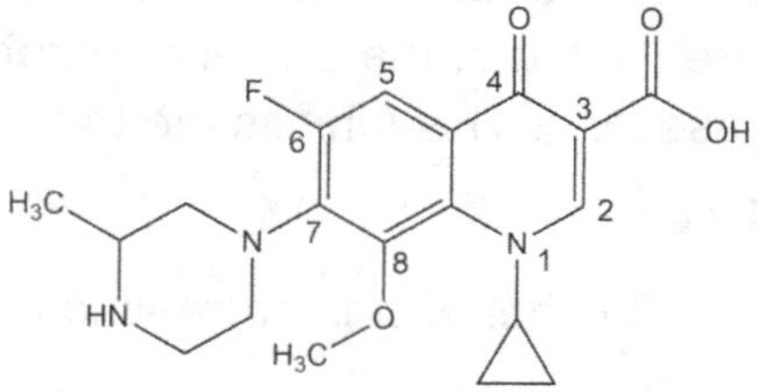

Fig.3.30 Chemical structure of Gatifloxacin.

4. Because of the severe side effects of gatifloxacin, India banned its manufacture, sale, and distribution in 2011.

Chemical structure: (Fig. 3.30)

Chemical Name:

1-cyclopropyl-6-fluoro-8-methoxy-7-(3-methylpiperazin-1-yl)-4-oxo-1,4-dihydroquinoline-3-carboxylic acid

Mechanism of Action

Gatifloxacin inhibits the enzymes topoisomerase II (DNA gyrase) and topoisomerase IV, which are necessary for bacterial DNA replication, transcription, repair, and recombination. The bacterial DNA gyrase is required for DNA replication. DNA gyrase is a member of the topoisomerase enzyme family, which is involved in the regulation of DNA topological transitions. The methoxy group is considered to be involved in the binding of the DNA–DNA gyrase complex to the DNA–topoisomerase complex, thus decreasing the chance of high-level resistance.

Uses

The ophthalmic solution of gatifloxacin is used to treat bacterial eye infections.

3.5.9 Moxifloxacin

Historical Background

In 1999, the USFDA approved moxifloxacin for use in the United States to treat certain bacterial illnesses. Bayer A.G. first patented it (a United States patent) in 1991.

Chemical Structure: (Fig. 3.31)

Chemical Name:

1-cyclopropyl-6-fluoro-8-methoxy-7-(octahydro-6H-pyrrolo [3,4-b] pyridin-6-yl) -4-oxo-1, 4-dihydroquinoline-3-carboxylic acid

Mechanism of Action

Moxifloxacin is an antibiotic with a broad spectrum of activity. It is effective against both gram-+ve and gram-ve bacteria. It inhibits DNA gyrase, a type II topoisomerase, and topoisomerase IV. These two enzymes are required for the separation of bacterial DNA, thereby preventing cell replication.

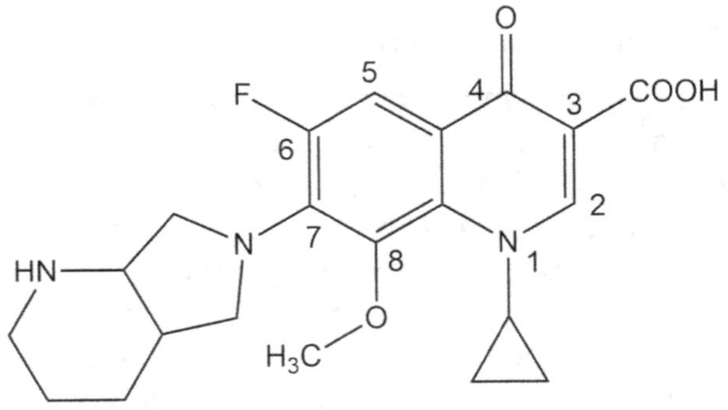

Fig. 3.31 Chemical structure of Moxifloxacin.

Uses

It treats a variety of bacterial illnesses, including pneumonia, conjunctivitis, endocarditis, TB, and sinusitis.

Mechanism of Quinolones

The quinolone class of drugs is active against DNA topoisomerases, particularly topoisomerase II, also known as DNA gyrase, and topoisomerase IV. DNA gyrase is needed for DNA replication, transcription, and repair, while topoisomerase IV is needed for the segregation of chromosomal DNA during cell division. DNA gyrase is therefore projected to be a more essential target in the non-replicating state. Quinolones are dual-action antibiotics that inhibit both DNA gyrase and topoisomerase IV.

3.6 Miscellaneous

Nitrofurantoin and hexamine are two other drugs used as urinary tract antiseptics. Nitroheterocycles have attracted the attention of researchers as potential chemotherapeutic agents. For example, nitrofurantoin was first introduced in 1952 as an orally active anti-infective agent for treating urinary tract infections. It's effective against both gram-positive and gram-negative bacteria in the urinary system.

Classification of drugs:

1. Nitrofurans derivative compounds Ex. Furazolidine, Nitrofurantoin

2. Hexamine compounds Ex. Methanamine

3.6.1 Furazolidone

Historical Background

Furazolidone is a metabolite of nitrofurantoin. It is effective against both gram-+ve and gram-ve bacteria. However, it also has antitrichomonal action. Furazolidone is more active against gram-negative microorganisms and is less toxic as compared with nitrofurazone and nitrofurantoin.

Chemical Structure: (Fig. 3.32)

Chemical Name: 3-(5-nitrofurfuryliden)amino-2-oxazolidinone

Mechanism of Action

The mechanism of action of furazolidone against bacteria and sensitive protozoa (including *Giardia* and *trichomonads*) remains unknown. Although it appears to be an inhibition of oxidative reactions, such as the decarboxylation of pyruvate to acetyl coenzyme A, which lowers available energy for important cellular functions of microbes, Additionally, it is believed that the nitro group of furazolidone undergoes reductive metabolism within the cell, generating reactive compounds that bind to parasite DNA and inhibit replication and transcription.

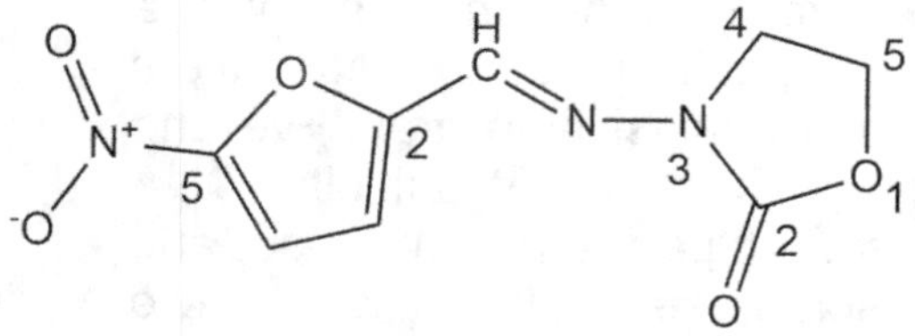

Fig. 3.32 Chemical structure of Furazolidone.

Uses

✓ Furazolidone is an antibacterial and antiprotozoal drug. It is used to treat giardiasis, diarrhea, and gastroenteritis.

✓ It is primarily used to treat infections of the urinary tract such as pyelitis (inflammation of the renal pelvis), pyelonephritis (inflammation of the kidney), cystitis (inflammation of the urinary bladder), and urethritis (inflammation of the urethra).

3.6.2 Nitrofurantoin

Historical Background

Kenyon J. Hayes of the now-defunct Eaton Laboratories received the first US patent for the manufacture of nitrofurantoin in 1952. It was first used to treat urinary tract infections in 1953 as an antibacterial drug. **Benjamin E. Blass** called nitrofurantoin "a remarkably successful drug" in his 2015 book Basic Principles of Drug Discovery and Development.

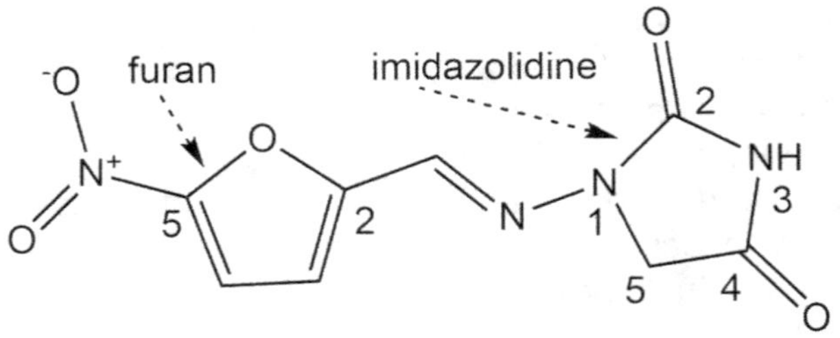

Fig. 3.33 Chemical structure of Nitrofurantoin.

Chemical Structure: (Fig. 3.33)

Chemical Name:

1-(((5-nitrofuran-2-yl) methylene) amino)imidazolidine-2,4-dione

Synthesis: (Fig. 3.34)

1. It is synthesized by reacting chloroacetic acid with hydrazine to produce hydrazinoacetic acid.

2. Hydrazinoacetic acid reacting with potassium cyanate gives semicarbazidoacetic acid, or 3,4-diamino-4-oxobutanoic acid.

3. Semicarbazidoacetic acid, which upon heating undergoes cyclization to form 1-aminoimidazolidine-2,4-dione (1-aminohydantoin).

4. The resultant product further reacts with diacetylacetal of 5-nitrofurfurol (5-nitrofur-furaldehyde diacetate) under appropriate conditions ($CH_3COOH/H_2SO_4/C_2H_5OH$) to give the desired nitrofurantoin.

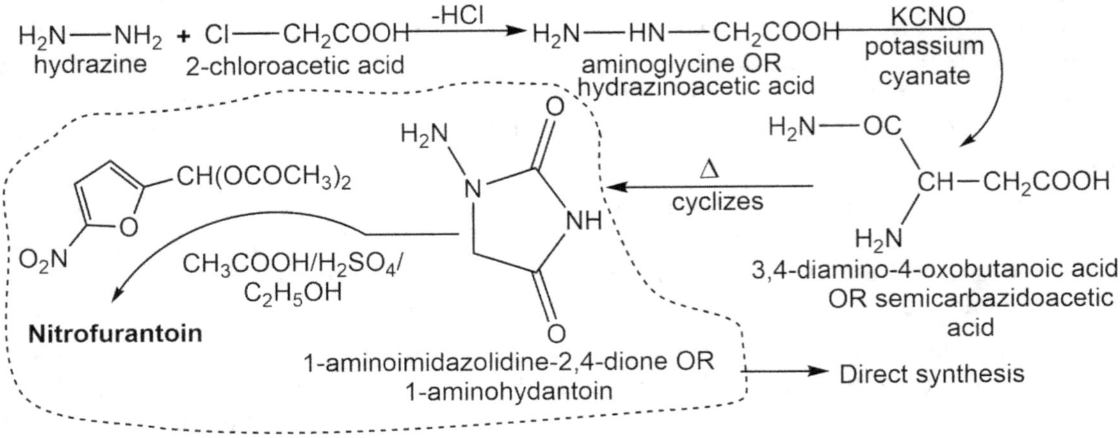

Fig. 3.34 Synthesis of Nitrofurantoin.

Mechanism of Action

The mechanism of the antibacterial activity of nitrofurantoin remains unclear, but it is thought to involve changes to ribosomal proteins and other intracellular structures. It is activated inside bacteria by being reduced (the reduction process) to form an unstable metabolite by the flavoprotein nitrofurantoin reductase, which disrupts ribosomal RNA, DNA, and other intracellular components. It is bactericidal, particularly against bacteria found in acidic urine. Nitrofurantoin is effective against the majority of gram-positive bacteria, including *E. coli*.

Uses

It is used in the treatment of lower urinary tract infections, including cystitis and kidney infections.

3.6.3 Methanamine

Historical Background

The US FDA approved methylamine in 1967 for people 12 years of age and older. It is found in all living organisms and in relatively high concentrations in plant foods, such as carrots and tea. It is a salt (methenamine mandelate and methenamine hippurate) that eventually converts to formaldehyde and exhibits an antimicrobial effect in the urine.

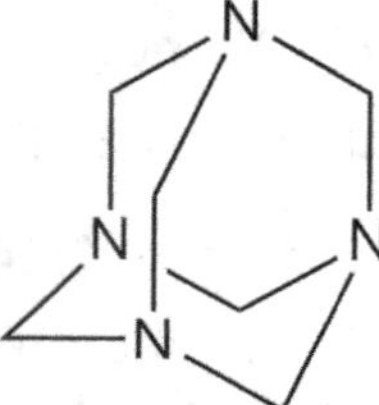

Fig. 3.35 Chemical structure of Methanamine.

Chemical structure: (Fig. 3.35)

Chemical Name:

1,3,5,7-tetraazaadamantane; 1,3,5,7-tetraazatricyclo [3.3.1.1 ^{3,7}]decane

Mechanism of Action

In the acidic environment of the urine, formaldehyde is the primary metabolite of methenamine. Formaldehyde has nonspecific antibacterial activity by denaturing bacterial proteins and nucleic acids. The concentration of formaldehyde >25 mg/ml is considered bactericidal. In this study, bacteria are not resistant to formaldehyde in an acidic environment, and at a suitable concentration, formaldehyde acts as an antiseptic.

In vitro, formaldehyde has been found to inhibit a wide range of gram-positive, gram-negative, and anaerobic bacteria, including *Proteus spp.* However, urease-producing bacteria, such as *Proteus* sp., can make urine alkaline *in vivo*, which prevents methenamine from being converted to formaldehyde.

Methenamine's antibacterial properties are linked to the hydrolysis of methenamine salts into ammonia and formaldehyde in acidic urine. The pH of the urine and the amount of methenamine in the urine determine the amount of formaldehyde in the urine. Urinary formaldehyde concentrations are related to antimicrobial action in urine. Although keeping a low urine pH (below 6) is required to obtain bactericidal formaldehyde concentrations. The link between treatment efficacy and low urinary pH has not been proven on every occasion.

Uses

Used as methenamine hippurate or methenamine mandelate for suppressive treatment of chronic urinary tract infections.

3.7 Antiviral Agents

Definition: Antiviral agents are chemical substances that prevent the transmission of viruses, such as by preventing genome replication, preventing virus entry into host cells, or reducing viral protein synthesis or viral assembly.

Infections caused by viruses are becoming more prevalent. Viruses are thought to be responsible for approximately 60% of human illnesses, while bacterial infections are thought to be responsible for about 15%. Common colds, influenza, bronchitis, hepatitis, herpes, poliomyelitis, gastroenteritis, rabies, chickenpox, smallpox, measles, mumps, yellow fever, and AIDS (acquired immune deficiency syndrome) are some of the most well-known viral disorders. They have the potential to cause blindness, deafness, paralysis, mental retardation, and different birth abnormalities cases of sclerosis (abnormal hardening of body tissue), Hodgkin's disease, Down's syndrome, cancer, and schizophrenia are thought to be caused by viruses.

Structure of Viruses

Viruses (**Fig.**3.36) are obligatory (they cannot reproduce outside their host), parasites, and considerably simpler organisms than bacteria. They are heavily dependent on the host cell for nutrition and reproduction. They are composed of protein components (called capsids) and nucleic acids. A basic viral particle is a single nucleoprotein molecule made up of double- or single-stranded ribonucleic acid (RNA) or deoxyribonucleic acid (DNA) molecules chemically attached to a large protein molecule. A virus can have either RNA or DNA, but not both at the same time. Protein molecules form a protective membrane. As a result, viruses can be thought of as protein-coated nucleic acid inserts. The nuclear material carries codes for viral reproduction. In some viruses, there is an outer envelope that is made up of lipids or polysaccharides in addition to the protein coat.

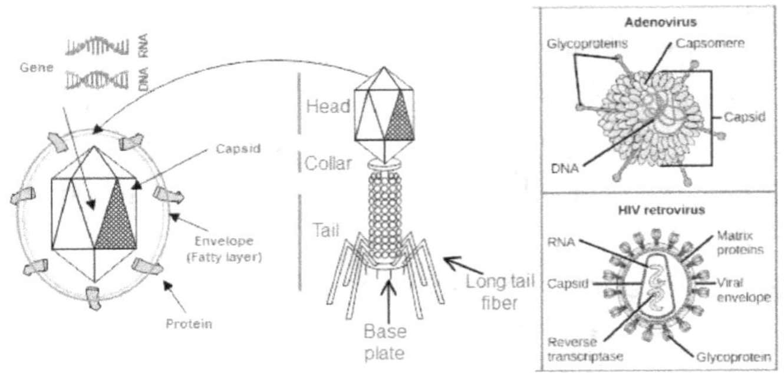

Fig. 3.36 Schematic diagram of Viruses (source:wiki).

Sizes: Viruses come in a variety of sizes (10-200 nm). They are only visible with an electron microscope and cannot be seen with a regular microscope.

Detection: Antigenic responses to viral proteins are frequently used to detect viral infection.

Types of viruses:

1. **DNA-containing viruses**-Examples: adenoviruses, papoviruses, and poxviruses; diseases causing DNA viruses: upper respiratory infections, herpes simplex, herpes zoster, chickenpox, and smallpox

2. **RNA-containing viruses**-Examples: arboviruses, myxoviruses, picornaviruses, and rhinoviruses; disease-causing RNA viruses: these viruses are the root cause of several diseases, including encephalitis, gastroenteritis, influenza, measles, meningitis, mumps, poliomyelitis, and rabies.

3. The human immunodeficiency virus (HIV) or retrovirus (RNA viruses), which causes AIDS.

The Life cycle of Viruses:

1. A virus (Fig. 3.37) enters a host cell and reproduces its nucleic acid to cause an infection of the host cell. The virus attaches itself to the host cell's surface first.

2. When an undamaged virion connects to a specific "receptor" site, the replication cycle begins.

3. The attachment phase occurs between the virion's outer structure and the host cell's cell surface structure (Example. HIV interacts with the CD4 receptor on immune system cells. Rhinoviruses bind to ICAM-1, and Epstein-Barr virus binds to the CD 21 receptors on B cells). At the site of attachment, enzymic digestion of the host plasma membrane may occur. In some situations, the complete viral particle or its infectious nucleic acid reaches the cell.

4. After acquiring attachment, the virion begins the penetration phase. In this phase, the virus can enter the host cell. In some cases, receptor-mediated endocytosis, a fusion of the viral envelope with the cell membrane, or direct penetration of the membrane can complete the penetration phase.

5. Viruses must be uncoated after entering the cell. A stripped nucleic acid or nucleocapsid form of the virus within the host cell usually contains polymerase enzymes. When an uncoated form of the virus is within the host cell, it is no longer infectious.

6. Once the virus has invaded the host cell and uncoated itself, it begins a phase of its life cycle known as "the eclipse period", which varies in length depending on the virus. During this stage, the virus takes advantage of host resources to replicate and manufacture viral proteins.

7. In retroviruses, the virus carries reverse transcriptase enzyme activity that generates a DNA template. The DNA template is then integrated into the host genome, referred to as a provirus at this point, and transcribed into both genomic RNA and mRNA for translation into viral proteins, resulting in the formation of new virus particles.

8. Host cells that can support viral reproduction are said to be in permissive (nonrestrictive) phases. In this phase, the infection is referred to as "the production of additional viral particles" (the viral DNA or RNA becomes uncoated and replicates). When fresh infectious viral particles are generated, the host cell's metabolism may be devoted to the formation of viral products. The new viruses combine and escape the cell, which is destroyed, invading new cells, which causes the host cell to die.

9. In some other circumstances, the presence of viral particles does not significantly affect the host cell's metabolism, and the infected cell can survive.

10. During viral reproduction, about 100,000 new virions can be generated within the host cell. The replication cycle of the virus can last anywhere from a few hours to more than three days.

11. In a normal acute viral infection, the infected cell usually dies 10 to 48 hrs after infection. Some viruses, such as the herpes simplex virus, can lie dormant for months until they are triggered into an infectious form by stress factors such as sunburn, fever, or cold exposure.

12. The reproduction of an infective virion within the nonpermissive cells is unable to complete, resulting in an unsuccessful infection.

13. When a virus is nonfunctional within the host cell, it may also result in an unsuccessful infection.

14. In either case, the viral genome may remain in a surviving host cell, resulting in a dormant infection for many years. An infection can cause a cell to convert from normal to malignant.

15. Each virus can only infect a specific type of cell. Such viruses are classified into three types: those that target plants, those that affect animals (including humans), and those that affect single-cell organisms (microbes and bacteria).

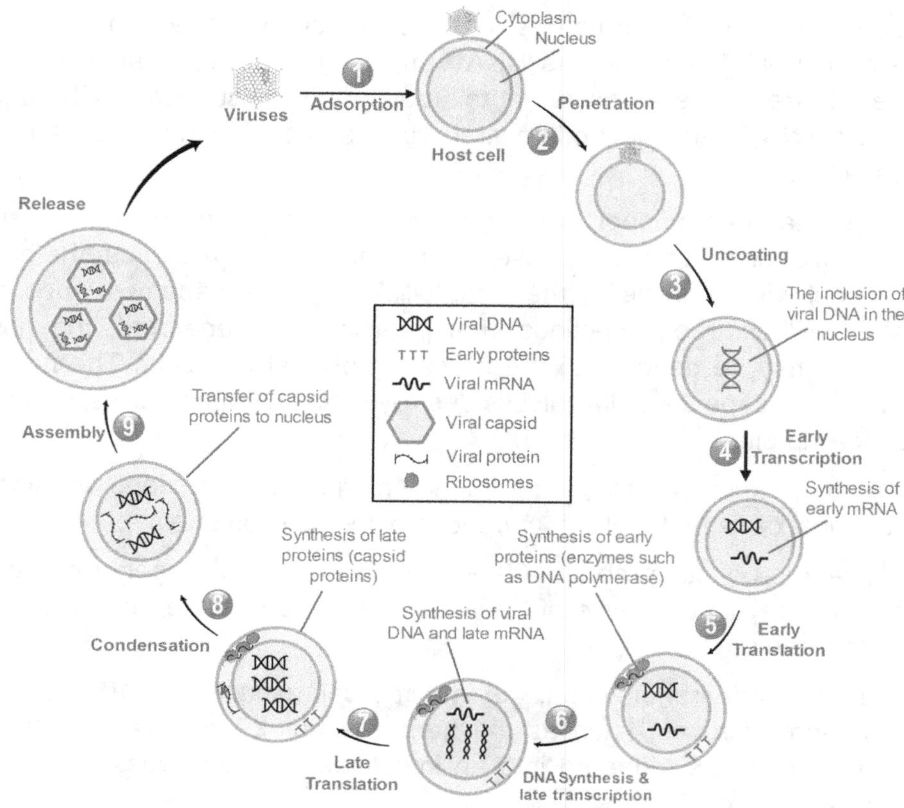

Fig. 3.37 The stages of the viral life cycle.

Summary of Viral Infection

Each type of virus has a unique mechanism of infection. The basic scheme of infection can be illustrated as follows: A virus is absorbed onto the surface of a host cell by electrostatic or hydrophilic interaction. Virus-specific receptors are likely to be found in many viruses. The virus then penetrates the host cell's membrane, allowing the nucleic acid to be freed from its protein-protected state. Therefore, it loses its virus identity. The viral nucleic acid then begins to function as if it were a member of the "host" cell. When the viral genome begins to replicate, it is transcribed either in the cytoplasm or in the nucleus of the host cell. As a result of these events, a substantial amount of viral nucleic acid and protein is produced, which is used to create new virions. During this step, the host cell's replication mechanism is shut off, and the described cycle is repeated indefinitely until the death or medication process.

Antiviral Agents

Antiviral agents are chemical substances used to treat viral infections. Specific antiviral drugs are used for specific viruses' infections, just like antibiotics.

The challenge of the development of antiviral agents is distinct from that of antibacterial agents. However, while great progress has been made in the treatment of bacterial infections, progress in the treatment of viral disorders has been slow. The antibacterial agents could be developed by choosing certain metabolic pathways and enzyme systems in bacterial cells. It is necessary to develop antiviral drugs that selectively block virally encoded or produced enzymes while ignoring host cell enzymes involved in related biochemical processes. The problem lies with antiviral agents' development, which is somewhat complicated. Antiviral agents can inhibit a far smaller number of viral-specific enzymes than antibacterial agents. Only a small number of drugs are available for treating a small number of viral infections. Currently, the progress of the antiviral agent has been made through studying metabolic analogues, random testing, and antiviral lead compounds.

Approaches for Development of Antiviral Drugs

Antiviral drugs for the treatment of viral infections are developed using three different approaches: The first step is immunization as a preventive measure. Second, the use of endogenous antiviral substances such as interferon, which is considered to bind to certain receptors on the cellular membrane's surface and trigger RNA and protein synthesis inside the cell, resulting in an antiviral effect. The third point is the use of antiviral drugs. Interfering with a virus's capacity to enter a target cell is one strategy for developing antiviral drugs. Currently, several "entry-inhibiting" or "entry-blocking" drugs are being developed.

Development of Antiviral Drugs

Two entry-blockers, such as amantadine and rimantidine, have been used as antiviral agents.

A second strategy could be adopted when a virus infects a cell. This method creates "nucleotide or nucleoside analogues," which resemble the building blocks of the RNA or DNA of the virus and stop the enzymes from synthesizing the RNA or DNA of the virus once the analogue is integrated.

Acyclovir, the first successful antiviral, is a nucleoside analogue that works against herpes virus infections. Zidovudine (AZT), the first antiviral drug approved for HIV treatment, is also a nucleoside analogue.

Idoxuridine, cytarabine, and vidarabine, the first-generation antiviral drugs, were the first commercial products used as antiviral drugs. Because of their limited therapeutic index, they are only used for a few clinical purposes. These drugs have a direct influence on viral replication and get involved in host cell functions.

Amantadine, acyclovir, ribavirin, and zidovudine were later available as treatments for viral infection. Ribavirin, ampligen, dideoxycytidine, and foscarnet are the novel drugs being considered for the treatment of acquired immunodeficiency syndrome (AIDS).

Classification:

1. Agents Inhibiting Virus Attachment, Penetration, and Early Viral Replication - Ex. amantadine, rimantadine, interferon

2. Neuraminidase Inhibitors – Ex. zanamivir, oseltamivir

3. Entry (Fusion) Inhibitors - Ex. enfuvirtide

4. Acyclic Nucleoside Analogs – Ex. acyclovir, valacyclovir, ganciclovir

    (a) Conventional Nucleoside Analogs –Ex. idoxuridine, ribavirin, vidarabine,

    (b) Nonnucleoside Analogs – Ex. fomivirsen, foscarnet

    (c) Agents Affecting Translation by the Ribosome – Ex. methisazone

5. Antiretroviral (Anti-HIV) Agents Including Protease Inhibitors

    (a) Nucleoside Reverse Transcriptase Inhibitors – Ex. zidovudine, didanosine, stavudine, zalcitabine, lamivudine

    (b) Nonnucleoside Reverse Transcriptase Inhibitors – Ex. nevirapine, delavirdine, loviride

    (c) HIV Protease Inhibitors – Ex. saquinavir, indinavir, ritonavir

    (d) HIV Integrase Inhibitors – Ex. raltegravir

3.7.1 Amantadine Hydrochloride

Historical Background

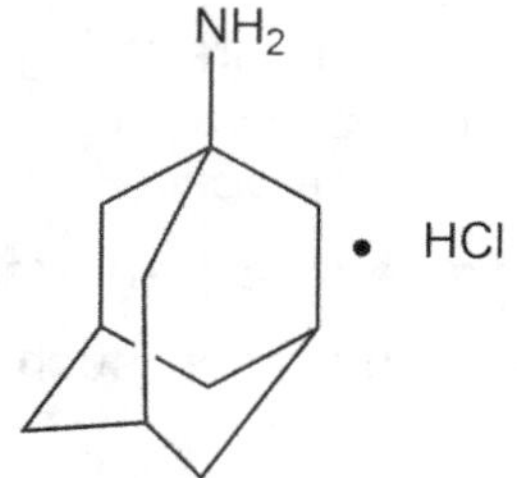

Fig.3.38 Chemical structure of Amantadine hydrochloride.

✓ Amantadine was approved in 1976 for the treatment of influenza virus A and was first used in West Germany in 1966. In 1976, the USFDA approved amantadine as a prophylactic drug against influenza A.

✓ Amantadine is an antiviral drug that also has anti-Parkinson's properties.

Chemical Structure: (Fig. 3.38)

Chemical Name:

1-adamantylamine hydrochloride; adamantan-1-amine hydrochloride

Mechanism of Action

The actual mechanism of amantadine's antiviral effect is unknown. It's thought to be an ion channel blocker. It has also been hypothesized that asymmetrical tricyclic primary amines prevent RNA virus particles from penetrating the host cell. It also prevents the viral DNA from being uncoated in the early stages of replication. According to recent research, amantadine blocks the influenza A virus' M2 proton-selective ion channel, which slows viral replication.

Uses

✓ Amantadine hydrochloride is effective against influenza A but not influenza B virus infection in the respiratory system.

✓ It has a relatively narrow therapeutic range and is exclusively used to treat and prevent influenza A infections. It's also used to treat Parkinson's disease.

3.7.2 Rimantadine Hydrochloride

Historical Background

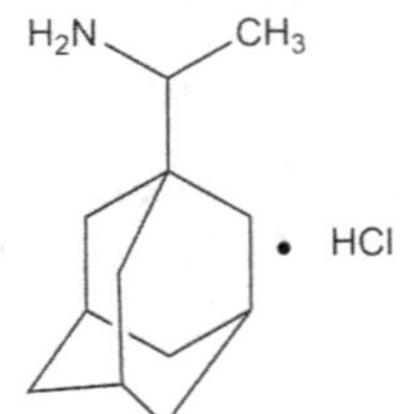

Fig.3.39 Chemical structure of Rimantadine hydrochloride.

- ✓ **William W. Prichard** of Du Pont & Co. developed rimantadine in 1963 and received a patent in 1965. Rimantadine was approved for medicinal use in 1993.

- ✓ Rimantadine is an antiviral agent that is derived from amantadine. It is made of adamantane, which is an alicyclic molecule with a methyl group ($-CH_3$) bonded to an amine ($-NH_2$). It has a higher level of action than amantadine against influenza type A.

Chemical structure: (Fig. 3.39)

Chemical name: α-methyl-1-adamantanmethylamine hydrochloride; 1- (adamantan-1-yl) ethan-1-amine hydrochloride

Structure-Activity Relationship

1. Amantadine and rimantadine are the hydrochlorides of 1-aminoadamantane and its α-methyl derivatives, respectively.
2. Both chemical compounds are cyclic amines.
3. They prevent influenza A viral RNA from getting uncoated and hence multiplying within the infected host cell.
4. In high-risk patients, they are effective in both preventing and treating influenza A infections.

Mechanism of Action

Rimantadine acts by interacting with the M2 viral protein, which transports acid ions through the influenza virion shell. The acid ions aid in the disintegration of the virion coat, allowing the viral RNA to be released into the infected cell's cytoplasm. Rimantadine prevents viral uncoating and stops the cycle of viral replication and infection by inhibiting M2. Additionally, rimantadine, like amantadine, can disrupt influenza virus assembly during viral replication.

It's a pharmacologically and structurally related synthetic adamantane derivative of amantadine. It appears to be more efficient against the influenza A virus than amantadine hydrochloride, with fewer CNS adverse effects. Rimantadine hydrochloride is hypothesized to obstruct virus uncoating by preventing virus-specific proteins from being released. It may block the production of viral-specific RNA, but it does not affect virus adsorption or penetration. It seems to have a virustatic (stopping the growth of viruses) effect early in the viral replication process.

Uses

Rimantadine has been used to treat and prevent influenza A virus infections. It is also used in the treatment of Parkinson's disease.

3.7.3 Idoxuridine

Historical Background

William H. Prusoff of Yale University synthesized it in the late 1950s. It was initially used as an antiviral agent in 1962 after being developed as an anticancer drug.

Chemical Structure: (Fig. 3.40)

Chemical Name:

1-(4-hydroxy-5-(hydroxymethyl)tetrahydrofuran-2-yl)-5 -iodopy- rimidine-2,4(1*H*,3*H*) -dione

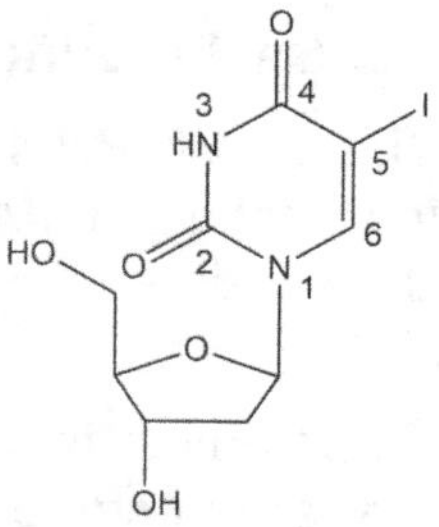

Fig. 3.40 Chemical structure of Idoxuridine.

Mechanism of Action

Idoxuridine is a halogenated pyrimidine compound. The chemical compound is an analogue of thymidine nucleoside. It acts as an antiviral agent against DNA viruses by inhibiting their replication through a competitive inhibition mechanism. It is converted to an active triphosphate form by the thymidine kinase enzyme. The phosphorylated compound inhibits cellular DNA polymerase, which is required for viral DNA synthesis. The drug's triphosphate form is subsequently integrated into viral nucleic acid synthesis via a false pairing system that replaces thymidine. When transcription takes place, incorrect viral proteins are produced, resulting in incorrect viral particles.

Idoxuridine affects viral DNA but does not affect viral RNA. Idoxuridine's principal activity is to prevent viral DNA replication by integrating directly into the DNA. Thymidine kinase phosphorylates idoxuridine to form an active triphosphorylated complex. The resulting complex inhibits viral and cellular DNA synthesis.

Uses

- ✓ Idoxuridine eye drops are used to treat herpes simplex keratitis (inflammation of the cornea).

- ✓ It is used topically to treat cutaneous herpes simplex and herpes zoster.

3.7.4 Trifluridine

Historical Background

Trifluridine is a thymidine analogue as well. Its chemical name is 5-trifluoromethyl-2-deoxyuridine. **Charles Heidelberger** and his colleagues developed the drug in 1964.

Chemical Structure: (Fig. 3.41)

Chemical Name:

1-(4-hydroxy-5-(hydroxymethyl)tetrahydrofuran-2-yl)-5-(trifluoromethyl)pyrimidine-2,4(1*H*,3*H*)-dione; 5-trifluoromethyl -1-(2-deoxyribofu-ranosyl) pyrimidin-2, 4-(1*H*.3*H*)-dione

Structure Activity Relationship

1. Fluorinated nucleoside analogues are drugs that interact with DNA and RNA. They were developed mainly for the treatment of cancer and viral infections.

2. Fluorine atoms can be found in both the base and the sugar moiety. The fluorination of nucleosides is a popular research topic.

3. The fluorine atom can mimic the hydrogen or hydroxyl function, converting the substrate to a key enzyme inhibitor (for example, 5-fluorouracil).

4. It can protect the nucleoside bond from hydrolysis (2'-fluoronucleoside) and increase drug stability.

5. It can also be directly involved in enzymatic reactions. Among the enzymes that fluoro nucleosides and fluoronucleobases could potentially target are thymidylate synthase, ribonucleotide diphosphate reductase, DNA polymerases, and viral reverse transcriptases.

Fig. 3.41 Chemical structure of Trifluridine.

Mechanism of Action

The antiviral mechanism of action of trifluridine involves the suppression of viral DNA synthesis. Trifluridine monophosphate inhibits thymidylate synthetase irreversibly, and its triphosphate inhibits DNA polymerases competitively compared to thymidine triphosphate. At low concentrations, trifluridine is incorporated into cellular DNA and inhibits cellular DNA production.

Uses
✓ Trifluridine is commonly used as a 1% ophthalmic solution for topical Herpes simplex virus (HSV) keratitis treatment.
✓ Topical trifluridine has also been used to treat aciclovir-resistant HSV infections on the skin.
✓ It's used to treat herpes infections in the eyes.

3.7.5 Acyclovir

Historical Background

Howard Schaeffer discovered acyclovir (aciclovir) in 1974 as part of a screening effort for antiviral drugs that began in the 1960s at Burroughs Wellcome in the United States. In 1982, the first topical formulation of the drug was made available to physicians. The new era of antiviral drugs began with the discovery of aciclovir.

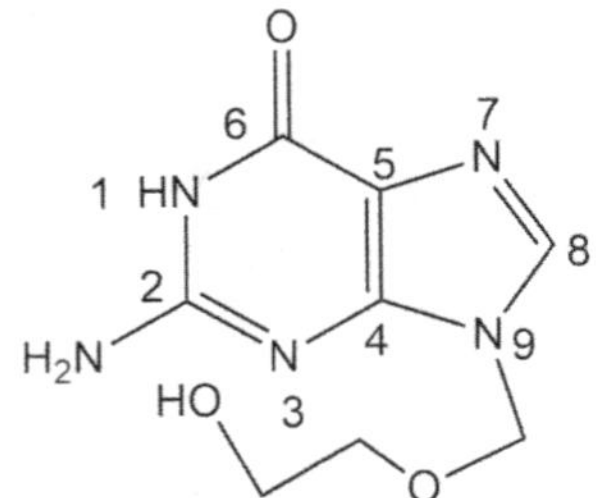

Fig. 3.42 Chemical structure of Acyclovir.

Aciclovir is highly selective and has low cytotoxicity. The synthesis of aciclovir was based on nucleosides obtained from *Cryptotethya crypta*, a Caribbean sponge.

Chemical Structure: (Fig. 3.42)

Chemical Name:

2-amino-9-((2-hydroxyethoxy)methyl)-1,9-dihydro-6H-purin-6-one;
9-(2-Hydroxyethoxymethyl)guanine

Structure Activity Relationship

1. Antiviral action is dependent on the length of the acyclic side chain connected at N-9.

2. Inactive analogues are produced when the hydroxy methylene group on the acyclic side chain is substituted with other substituents. As a result, the $-CH_2OH$ group is required for antiviral action.

3. When the acyl side chain was slightly modified, the 9-alkoxy derivative was developed, which is extremely active against herpes simplex and varicella zoster viruses.

4. Acyclovir has undergone several structural changes in order to produce high-potency medicines.

Synthesis: (Fig. 3.43)

1. It's prepared by alkylating guanine in triethylamine with 1-benzoyloxy-2-chloromethoxyethane.

2. Guanines had their hydroxyl and amino groups protected by a trimethylsilyl group before being treated with hexamethyldisilazane.

3. The subsequent product, 9-(2-benzoyloxymethoxymethyl) guanine, is extracted after hydrolysis.

4. The benzoyl protecting group from the hydroxyethoxymethyl fragment is removed by treating it with a methanol solution of ammonia, yielding acyclovir.

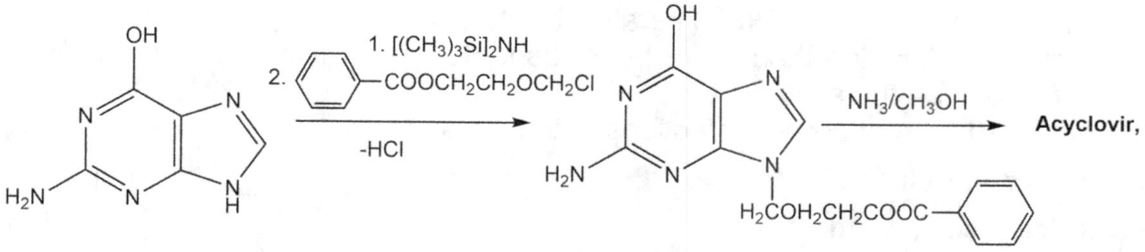

Fig. 3.43 Synthesis of Acyclovir.

Mechanism of Action

Acyclovir is not an antiviral agent itself. It only acts as an antiviral agent when phosphorylated within infected cells. Acyclovir is phosphorylated to its monophosphate form mainly by viral-induced thymidine kinase, which does so much more efficiently than cellular thymidine kinases. Acyclovir monophosphate is phosphorylated to diphosphate and triphosphate in the infected host cell, mostly via cellular enzymes. The drug is activated and concentrated increasingly in the infected cell as phosphorylation occurs, adding another selective component to the drug's activity. In comparison to biological DNA polymerases, acyclovir triphosphate competes with viral DNA polymerases. Acyclovir triphosphate binds very firmly to viral DNA polymerase, effectively inactivating it; also, acyclovir inserted into the developing DNA viral chain causes DNA chain termination due to the absence of 2'- or 3'-carbons from the guanosine analogue. As a result, multiple phases in the antiviral process target viral replication while having little influence on normal, uninfected cell functions and DNA replication.

The transformation of pyruvate to triphosphate and later inhibition of viral DNA synthesis are the mechanisms of antiviral activity. It acts in a very selective manner. Acyclovir diffuses into a virus-infected cell and phosphorylates herpes simplex thymidine kinase to a monophosphate. Acyclovir is not used as a substrate by uninfected cells. The monophosphate is then converted to a diphosphate and then to a triphosphate, which inhibits viral DNA polymerase as well as viral DNA, where it acts to break the chain, preventing further elongation of the DNA chains.

Uses

- ✓ It is used to treat viral infections caused by the herpes simplex virus (types I and 2) as well as the varicella-zoster virus (zoster and chickenpox).
- ✓ It's also used to treat herpes simplex infections in the eyes and genetilia (female reproductive system).

3.7.6 Ganciclovir

Historical Background

The USFDA approved an oral capsule form of ganciclovir in 1994 and an oral prodrug form of ganciclovir in 2001.

It differs from acyclovir by possessing a hydroxymethyl group at the 3' position of the acyclic side chain. It has 8–20 times the *in vitro* activity of acyclovir against CMV and is as active against HSV-1 and HSV-2.

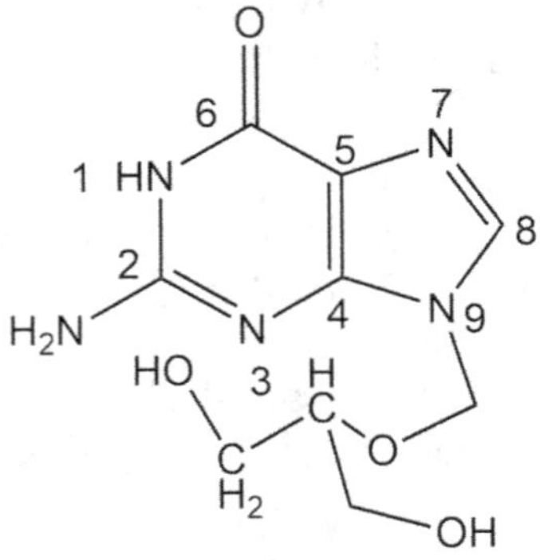

Fig. 3.44 Chemical structure of Ganciclovir.

Chemical Structure: (Fig. 3.44)

Chemical Name:

2-amino-9-(((1,3-dihydroxypropan-2-yl)oxy)methyl)-1,9-dihydro-6H-purin-6-one;[9-(1,3-dihydroxy-2-propoxymethyl) guanine]

Mechanism of Action

It blocks viral DNA synthesis. During HSV infection, a virus-induced enzyme, the viral thymidine kinase, which phosphorylates intracellular ganciclovir to the monophosphate derivative. During CMV infection, a viral protein kinase phosphorylates intracellular ganciclovir into the monophosphate derivative. Cellular enzymes produce the diphosphate and triphosphate forms of ganciclovir. In CMV-infected cells, ganciclovir triphosphate concentrations are at least 10-fold higher than in uninfected cells. Ganciclovir triphosphate concentrations in CMV-infected cells are also more than 10-fold higher than acyclovir triphosphate concentrations, and the intracellular release of ganciclovir triphosphate is prolonged (16.5 to >24 hours). Ganciclovir triphosphate is a competitive inhibitor of deoxyguanosine triphosphate incorporation into DNA. It inhibits viral DNA polymerases more effectively than host cellular DNA polymerases. When ganciclovir triphosphate is incorporated into viral DNA, viral DNA chain elongation slows and eventually stops.

Uses

✓ Ganciclovir is used to treat cytomegaloviral (CMV) infections in AIDS patients and other immunocompromised individuals.

✓ It is also commonly used in the treatment of retinitis (inflammation of the retina of the eye), colitis (inflammatory bowel disease), and esophagitis (inflammation that may damage the tissues of the esophagus), as well as to prevent and cure CMV illness in transplant patients.

3.7.7 Zidovudine

Historical Background

Zidovudine (ZDV) is a nucleoside (a compound consisting of a purine or pyrimidine base) with a thymidine-like structure. It was the first drug to show promise in extending the lives of patients with an AllDS or AIDS-related complex.

Researchers in the United States first developed zidovudine (azidothymidine) as an anticancer agent in the 1960s. Two decades later, the pharmaceutical company Burroughs Wellcome, USA, undertook its antiviral test, specifically anti-HIV activity. On March 19, 1987, the company got FDA approval for the first AIDS drug.

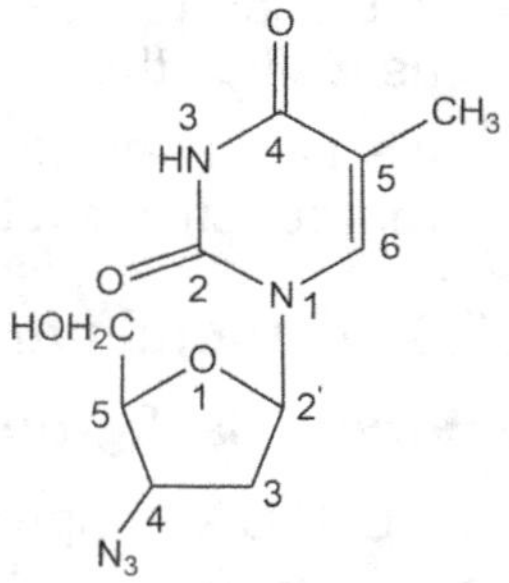

Fig. 3.45 Chemical structure of Zidovudine.

It is a thymidine analogue in which the azido (N_3) group is replaced by the 3-carbon atoms of the dideoxyribose moiety.

Chemical Structure: (Fig. 3.45)

Chemical Name:

1-(4-azido-5-(hydroxymethyl)tetrahydrofuran-2-yl)-5-methylpyrimidine-2,4(1H,3H)-dione; 3-azido-3-deoxytimidine

Mechanism of Action

It inhibits the replication of RNA tumour viruses (retroviruses), which are the causative factors of AIDS and T-cell leukemia. Retroviruses guide the synthesis of a provirus via reverse transcriptase (a DNA copy of a viral RNA genome). HIV infection is caused by proviral DNA integrating into normal cell DNA. The cellular thymidine kinase converts

ZDV to 5'-mono-, di-, and triphosphates. Because reverse transcriptase uses ZDV-triphosphate as a substrate, these phosphates are then integrated into proviral DNA. Due to the presence of an azido group in ZDV, this mechanism prevents normal 5',3'-phosphodiester bonding. This results in the end of DNA chain elongation. ZDV-triphosphate, which selectively inhibits reverse transcriptase and consequently viral DNA polymerase at the appropriate dose concentration, prevents the growth of HIV. ZDV is an effective HIV-1 inhibitor that also suppresses HIV-2 types.

Uses

- ✓ It is used to treat HIV infection and AIDS.
- ✓ It was previously used alone, but it has proven to be more effective when combined with other antiretroviral drugs.

3.7.8 Didanosine

Historical Background

On October 9, 1991, the USFDA approved didanosine as the second drug for the treatment of HIV infection after zidovudine. **Morris J. Robins** (Professor of Organic Chemistry at Brigham Young University) and **R.K. Robins** were the first to synthesize it in 1964.

It contains inhibitors of nucleoside reverse transcriptase. Inosine (a nucleoside compound) and didanosine are structurally similar compounds.

It is 2', 3'-dideoxyinosine chemically, and it differs from inosine by having hydrogen atoms on the ribose ring instead of the 2'-and 3'-hydroxyl groups. It's a prodrug that's bioactivated into dideoxyadenosine triphosphate by metabolism.

Chemical structure: (Fig. 3.46)

Chemical Name:

9-(5-(hydroxymethyl)tetrahydrofuran-2-yl)-1,9-dihydro-6H-purin-6-one

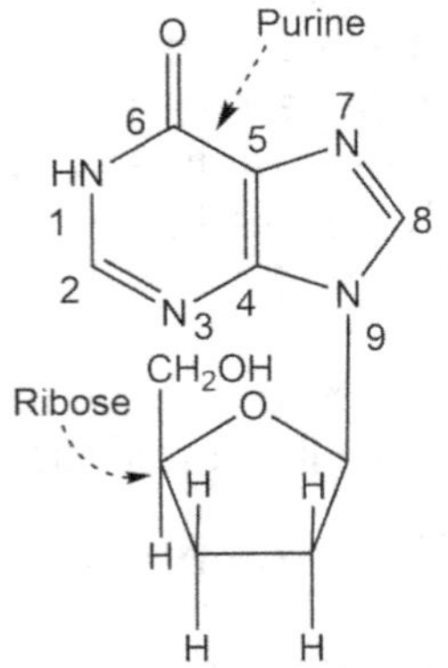

Mechanism of Action

It is a prodrug that is metabolized into dideoxyadenosine triphosphate. Dideoxyadenosine triphosphate is a competitive inhibitor of viral reverse transcriptase. It is inserted into the growing viral DNA in place of deoxyadenosine triphosphate. As a result, the absence of a 3'-hydroxyl group in this agent breaks the chain elongation of the virus. It has a virustatic effect on retroviruses. The antiretroviral activity of didanosine is enhanced when combined with ZDV.

Fig. 3.46 Chemical structure of Didanosine.

Zalcitabine is a synthetic pyrimidine nucleoside analogue that can be used as an alternative to ZDV. It inhibits nucleoside reverse transcriptase. Zalcitabine has a cytosine-like chemical structure. The 3'-hydroxyl group of the 2'-deoxyribose molecule of cytosine is substituted with a hydrogen atom, which makes it different from 2'-deoxycytidine.

Uses

It is used to treat HIV infection in combination with other antiretroviral drugs.

3.7.9 Zalcitabine

Historical Background

Jerome Horwitz initially synthesized zalcitabine in the 1960s, and Samuel Broder, Hiroaki Mitsuya, and Robert Yarchoan at the National Cancer Institute, USA, went on to develop it as an anti-HIV drug. The USFDA approved zalcitabine as the third antiretroviral for the treatment of HIV/AIDS. It was first approved as monotherapy on June 19, 1992 and then again in 1996, with a combination of zidovudine.

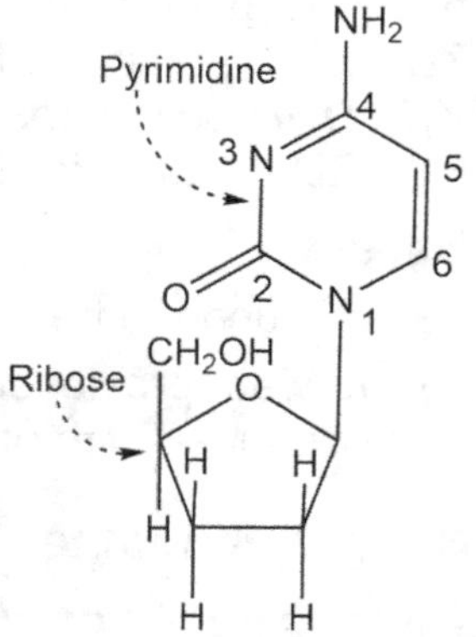

Chemical Structure: (Fig. 3.47)

Chemical Name:

4-amino-1-(5-(hydroxymethyl)tetrahydrofuran-2-yl)pyrimidin-2(1H)-one

Fig. 3.47 Chemical structure of Zalcitabine.

Mechanism of Action

Zalcitabine is a synthetic nucleoside analogue of the naturally occurring nucleoside deoxycytidine, with hydrogen replacing the 3'-hydroxyl group. By cellular enzymes, zalcitabine is transformed into the active metabolite, dideoxycytidine 5'-triphosphate, within cells. Dideoxycytidine 5'-triphosphate suppresses HIV reverse transcriptase activity by competing with deoxycytidine 5'-triphosphate as a natural substrate and incorporating itself into viral DNA. The absence of a 3'-OH group in the integrated nucleoside analogue inhibits the synthesis of the 5' to 3' phosphodiester linkage. This linkage is required for DNA chain elongation. As a result, viral DNA growth is stopped. Dideoxycytidine 5'-triphosphate, the active metabolite, is also a cellular DNA polymerase inhibitor.

Uses

It is an oral drug used to treat infections caused by the human immunodeficiency virus (HIV).

3.7.10 Lamivudine

Historical Background

Lamivudine (2'-deoxy-3'-thiacytidine) is a first-generation nucleoside reverse transcriptase inhibitor that was approved for the treatment of HIV-1 infection in 1995 and hepatitis B virus (HBV) infection in 1998.

Lamivudine is an L-enantiomeric analogue of cytosine. It inhibits viral reverse transcriptase enzymes and inhibits HIV replication at dosages that are safe for human polymerases.

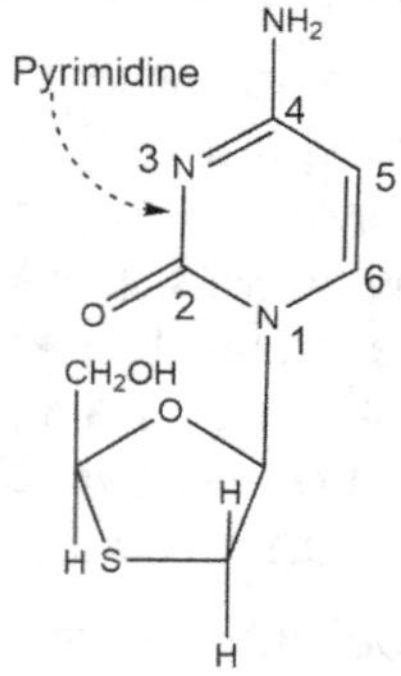

Fig. 3.48 Chemical structure of Lamivudine.

Chemical Structure: (Fig. 3.48)

Chemical Name:

4-amino-1-(2-(hydroxymethyl)-1,3-oxathiolan-5-yl) pyrimidin-2(1H)-one;
1-[2-(hydroxymethyl)-1,3-oxathiolan-5-yl] cytosine

Mechanism of Action

Lamivudine is a nucleoside analogue of 2'-deoxycytosine. It exerts its effect as a DNA chain terminator to inhibit further viral DNA replication. Lamivudine 5'-triphosphate is the active metabolite of lamivudine. The intracellular kinases that produce the metabolite compete with the virus's naturally occurring cytidine triphosphate. The metabolite is incorporated into DNA and stops DNA chain elongation. Lamivudine is a highly effective inhibitor of HIV-1 reverse transcriptase enzymes.

Uses

✓ It is used in the prevention and treatment of HIV/AIDS.

✓ It is also used to treat chronic hepatitis B infections when other treatments are ineffective.

✓ It is effective against both HIV-1 and HIV-2 types of infection.

✓ It is often used in conjunction with other antiretrovirals, such as zidovudine and abacavir, to treat HIV infection.

3.7.11 Loviride

Historical Background

The Janssen antiviral drug loveride, also known as loviride, demonstrated effectiveness against HIV. Loviride is an inhibitor of non-nucleoside reverse transcriptase.

Chemical Structure: (Fig. 3.49)

Chemical Name:

2-((2-acetyl-5-methylphenyl)amino)
-2-(2,6-dichlorophenyl)- acetamide

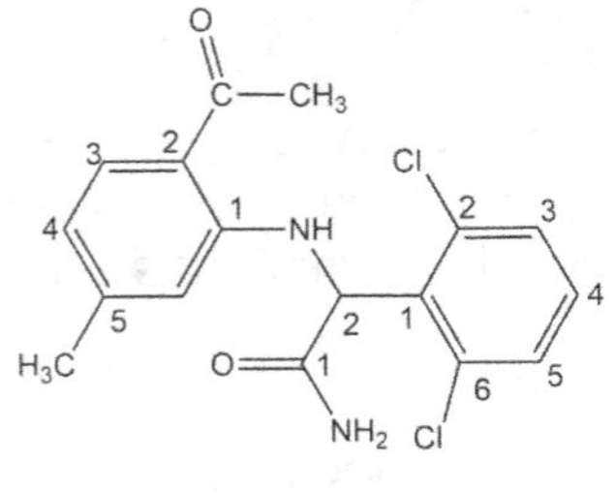

Mechanism of Action

It's reverse transcriptase (RNA-directed DNA polymerase) inhibitors, which prevent DNA from being synthesized on an RNA template.

Fig. 3.49 Chemical structure of Loviride.

It is thought to interfere with viral replication. It binds to certain cell surface receptors, preventing viral entry or the uncoating of DNA. As a result, it blocks the late stages of virus assembly or inhibits viral protein synthesis. Additionally, it interferes with viral DNA polymerase.

Uses

It is used in the treatment of HIV-1 & HIV-2 types of infections.

3.7.12 Delavirdine

Historical Background

Delavirdine is an inhibitor of non-nucleoside reverse transcriptase with specific activity against HIV-1. It has no activity against the reverse transcriptase of HIV-2. In 1997, the US FDA gave it approval.

Chemical Structure: (Fig. 3.50)

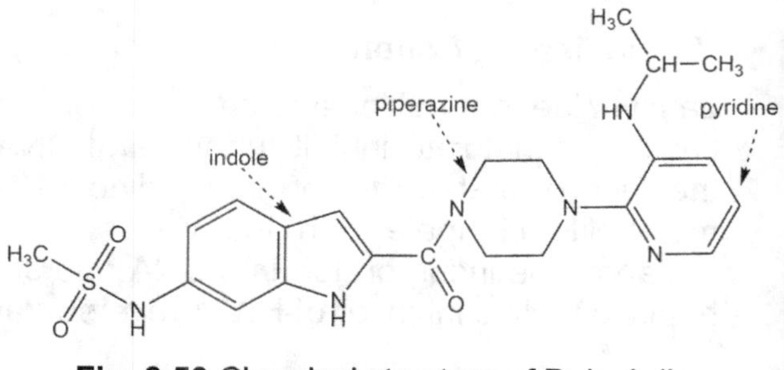

Fig. 3.50 Chemical structure of Delavirdine.

Chemical Name:

N-(2-(4-(3-(isopropylamino)pyridin-2-yl) piperazine-1-carbonyl)-1H-indol-6-yl)methane sulfonamide

Mechanism of Action

Delavirdine inhibits the activity of reverse transcriptase and DNA-directed DNA polymerase. The process leads to chain termination in HIV-1 after the enzyme-substrate complexes are formed.

Nonnucleoside reverse transcriptase inhibitors (NNRTIs) have a different mechanism of action than nucleoside/tide analogues. N(t)RTIs (nucleoside reverse transcriptase inhibitors) suppress HIV replication by incorporating into the elongating strand of viral DNA, resulting in chain termination. NNRTIs, on the other hand, are not integrated into viral DNA and instead directly suppress HIV-1 replication by binding non-competitively to HIV-1 reverse transcriptase. The drugs bind to a hydrophobic region adjacent to the active site catalytic residues in the enzyme-DNA complex. This leads to a slower reverse transcription process. NNRTIs do not affect nucleotide-binding sites. NNRTIs do not inhibit human DNA polymerases, unlike nucleoside/tide analogues. The drugs have unique specificity for HIV-1, except for etravirine, which has antiviral efficacy against HIV-2.

Uses

- ✓ It is used in the treatment of HIV-1 infection.
- ✓ It is given in combination with zidovudine in the treatment of HIV.

3.7.13 Ribavirin

Historical Background

Researchers from the International Chemical & Nuclear Corporation (ICN), which is now known as Valeant

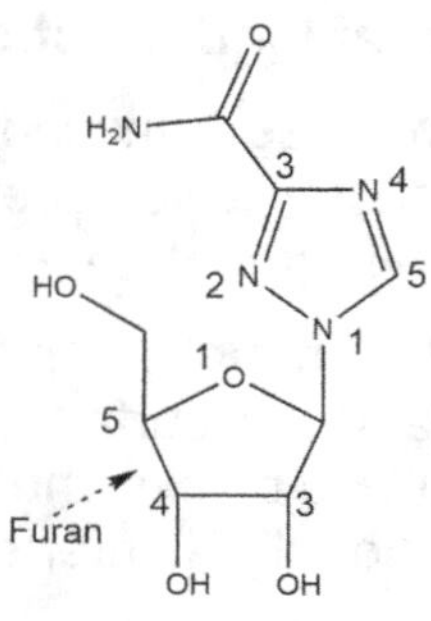

Fig. 3.51 Chemical structure of Ribavirin.

Pharmaceuticals Canada, initially discovered and manufactured ribavirin in 1970. **Joseph T. Witkovski** and **Ronald K. Robins**, two chemists, developed this compound.

Chemical Structure: (Fig. 3.51)

Chemical Name:

1-(3,4-dihydroxy-5-(hydroxymethyl)tetrahydrofuran-2-yl)-1H-1,2,4-triazole-3-carboxami de

Structure Activity Relationship

1. The 1,2,4-triazole ring, carboxamide group, and β-D-ribofuranosyl moiety are all important for this drug's antiviral activity.

2. Ribavirin's base moiety is similar to nicotinamide's monocyclic base. It is also particularly active in RNA-related metabolism due to its sugar component (ribose with a hydroxy group at the 2' carbon position).

3. Following absorption, cellular enzymes break down the molecule into monophosphates, diphosphates, and triphosphate metabolites. As a result, these compounds inhibit viral nucleic acid synthesis, primarily by changing messenger RNA synthesis.

4. A variety of ribavirin analogues, particularly 3-carboxamide derivatives (found to be comparable to ribavirin) and thiocarboxamides, have been produced which are only active against DNA viruses.

Mechanism of Action

Ribavirin is a guanosine analogue compound. It acts as an antiviral agent that is effective against both DNA and RNA viruses. It undergoes phosphorylation to form a triphosphate metabolite by the adenosine kinase enzyme. As a result, it inhibits viral-specific RNA polymerase and disrupts messenger RNA and nucleic acid synthesis.

Uses

✓ In infants and children, ribavirin is used to treat respiratory syncytial virus infections.

✓ It has also been used in the treatment of various illnesses, such as measles, hepatitis, and influenza.

✓ The combination of oral ribavirin and interferon α-2b is beneficial in the treatment of chronic hepatitis C.

3.7.14 Saquinavir

Historical Background

Saquinavir was the first approved protease inhibitor for AIDS patients to treat HIV.

The pharmaceutical company Roche developed saquinavir. The USFDA approved saquinavir as the sixth antiretroviral and the first protease inhibitor in 1995. In combination with other antiretroviral medications, it is still routinely used to prevent and treat HIV infection in adults and children.

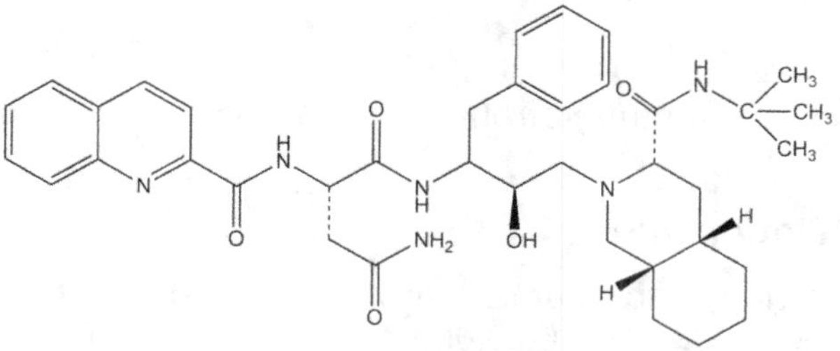

Fig. 3.52 Chemical structure of Saquinavir.

Chemical Structure: (Fig.3.52)

Chemical Name:

(2S)-N1-((3R)-4-((3S,4aS,8aS)-3-(tert-butylcarbamoyl)octahydroisoquinolin-2(1H)-yl)-3-hydroxy-1-phenylbutan-2-yl)-2-(quinoline-2-carboxamido)succinamide

Mechanism of Action

Saquinavir acts as a protease inhibitor. Proteases are enzymes that break down proteins into smaller components. The HIV protease is required for both intracellular viral replication and the release of mature viral particles from infected cells. It binds to the active site of the viral protease. Thus, blocking viral polyprotein fragmentation and thereby preventing virus development. It also inhibits both the HIV-1 and HIV-2 types of viruses.

Uses

- ✓ It is used to treat and prevent HIV infection and acquired immunodeficiency syndrome (AIDS).

- ✓ It is used to treat HIV infection in conjunction with nucleoside reverse transcriptase inhibitors.

3.7.15 Indinavir

Historical Background

Indinavir is an HIV protease inhibitor that is derived from a pentanoic acid amide compound. Merck developed the chemical compound in 1994. In March 1996, the USFDA approved it as the 8th antiretroviral drug for the treatment of HIV.

Chemical Structure: (Fig. 3.53)

Chemical Name:

(*S*)-1-((2*S*,4*R*) -4-benzyl-2-hydroxy -5-(((1*S*,2*R*)-2-hydroxy-2,3-dihydro-1*H* -inden-1-yl)- amino)-5-oxopentyl) -N-(tert-butyl) -4-(pyridin-3-ylmethyl) piperazine -2-carbo-xamide;N-[2 (*R*)-hydroxy-1(*S*)-indanyl] -5-[2(*S*) -(1,1-dimethylethlaminocarbonyl) -4-(pyridin-3-yl) me- thylpiperazin-1-yl] -4[*S*] -hydroxy-2[*R*] -phenylmethylpentanamide

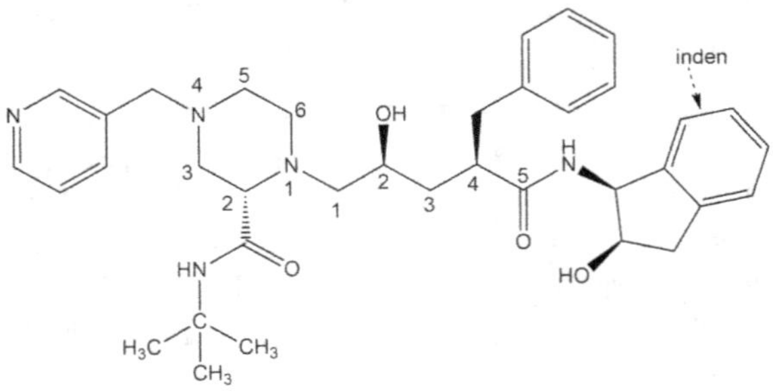

Fig. 3.53 Chemical structure of Indinavir.

Mechanism of Action

Indinavir's mode of action is competitive inhibition. The drug binds to HIV protease's active catalytic site, preventing the enzyme from breaking down polypeptides into active, infectious proteins. This inhibition lowers the number of fragmented polypeptides in the blood, which helps lower the amount of active HIV RNA in the body.

Uses

It is used to treat HIV & AIDS in combination with other nucleoside reverse transcriptase inhibitors.

3.7.16 Ritonavir

Historical Background

Ritonavir is manufactured by AbbVie, Inc. (Abbott, USA). It was approved by the USFDA on March 1, 1996. After saquinavir, it was the second protease inhibitor to be approved in the United States.

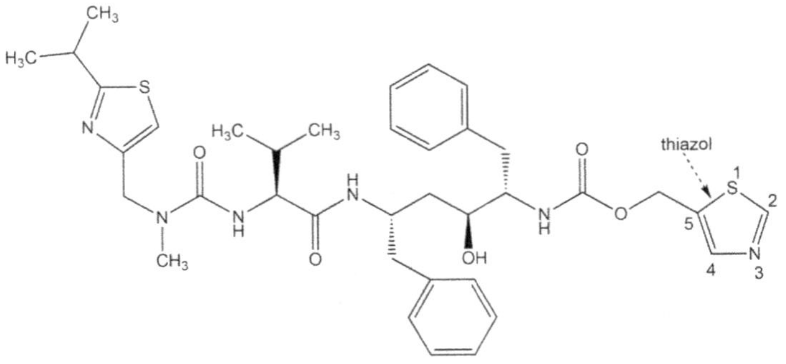

Fig. 3.54 Chemical structure of Ritonavir.

Chemical Structure: (Fig. 3.54)

Chemical Name:

Thiazol-5-ylmethyl ((2S,3S,5S)-3-hydroxy-5-((S)-2-(3-((2-isopropylthiazol-4-yl)methyl)-3-methylureido)-3-methylbutanamido)-1,6-diphenylhexan-2-yl)carbamate

Mechanism of Action

It is an antiretroviral drug that acts by binding to the HIV-1 protease enzyme. The HIV-1 protease catalyzes the breakdown of protein precursors, resulting in the formation of new viral particles. Protease inhibitors interfere with this breakdown process, preventing the formation of new virus particles.

It is a protease inhibitor that inhibits the replication of the Human Immunodeficiency Virus Type 1. HIV-1 protease is a proteolytic enzyme. The enzyme converts viral polyprotein precursors into individual functional proteins. Ritonavir binds to the protease active site and reduces the enzyme's activity. This inhibitor blocks viral polyprotein fragmentation, resulting in the generation of immature, non-infectious viral particles. Protease inhibitors are typically taken with at least two additional anti-HIV drugs.

Uses

It is given in combination with other antiretroviral agents for the treatment of HIV-1 infection.

CHAPTER 4

ANTIFUNGAL AGENTS
ANTI-PROTOZOAL AGENTS
ANTHELMINTICS
SULPHONAMIDES AND SULFONES

4.1 Antifungal Agents

Fungi are one of the most varied groups of organisms on Earth. In contrast to bacteria, fungi have eukaryotic cellular processes that make them closer to humans than bacteria. Out of over two million fungus species, around 600 are recognized as human fungal pathogens, with only 3-4% of these species accounting for >99% of invasive fungal infections. In comparison to superficial fungal infections, which are prevalent in humans, these infections are often life-threatening and have a higher fatality rate.

Fungi are more complicated organisms when compared to bacteria or viruses. They have ribosomes, components of the cellular membrane, and a nuclear membrane. As a result, antibacterial agents are typically ineffective against pathogenic fungi.

Mycoses (fungal infections) are less common than bacterial or viral infections. Several fungus species are harmful to humans. Some fungal infections can migrate to the skin's surface and cause localized symptoms, while others can be systemic and life-threatening. Some of these organisms (for example, *Candida*) can move from the skin to the internal organs, causing systemic infections with life-threatening effects. *Candida* (candidiasis or candidosis) and dermatophyte fungi such as *Epidermophyton*, *Microsporum*, and *Trichophyton* (tinea; ringworm) are some of the fungi that can cause infections of the hair, mucous membranes, nails, or skin. *Aspergillus*, *Blastomyces*, *Candida*, *Coccidioides*, *Cryptococcus*, *Histoplasma*, and *Paracoccidioides* are the fungi that cause systemic infections in humans.

In most cases, fungal (mycotic) infections are difficult to treat. Dermatophylic, mucocutaneous, and systemic fungal infections are the three types of fungal infections that are commonly observed in humans.

Natural antibiotics or synthetic antifungal agents related to imidazole and triazole heterocycles make up the majority of antifungal drugs used in clinical practice.

Dermatophytic fungal infections are most prevalent, causing infections of the skin, hair, and nails. Tolnaftate, undecylenic acid, haloprogin, clotrimazole, and miconazole are all topical antifungal agents used to treat fungal infections. Griseofulvin is taken orally and is used to treat deep infections, particularly infections of the nail bed.

Currently, ketoconazole is commonly used to treat severe dermatophytes.

Candida albicans infections, which affect wet skin and mucous membranes, are the most common type of mucocutaneous infection (i.e., gastrointestinal tract, perianal (the area around the anus), and vulvovaginal (female) areas. To treat such infections, amphotericin B, miconazole, clotrimazole, and nystatin are applied topically. Ketoconazole is given orally for systemic infections.

Systemic fungal infections are extremely rare, but they can be quite dangerous since they are chronic and difficult to diagnose and cure. So, athlete's foot, ringworm, and candidiasis (thrush), as well as systemic infections (*cryptococcal meningitis*) could be cured by using antifungal drugs. These drugs kill the fungal organism without affecting the host by using distinctions between mammalian and fungal cells.

Antifungal drugs can be classified chemically as polyenes, imidazole and triazole derivatives, allylamines, and others. Polyenes (nystatin, amphotericin B, and natamycin) bind to sterols in the fungus cell wall, most notably ergosterol. The contents of the cell leak out, and the cell dies as a result. Because human (and other animal) cells possess cholesterol instead of ergosterol, they are less vulnerable. Antifungal drugs in the imidazole and triazole groups inhibit the enzyme cytochrome P_{450} 14α-demethylase (imidazoles: miconazole, ketoconazole, clotrimazole, econazole, mebendazole, butoconazole, and fluconazole). This enzyme converts lanosterol to ergosterol and is necessary for the formation of fungal cell walls. In humans, these drugs also prevent steroid production. The allylamines (naftifine, terbinalfine, butenafine, and amorolfine) inhibit squalene epoxidase, another enzyme necessary for the synthesis of ergosterol. Griseofulvin suppresses fungal mitosis via binding to polymerized microtubules. An antimetabolite is flucytosine. Antifungal drugs are classified as dermatophytic, mucocutaneous, and systemic.

Definition

Antifungals are drugs that treat fungal infections by inhibiting the synthesis of the fungal cell membrane, cell wall components, membrane permeability, nucleic acid synthesis, and the fungus' mitotic spindle function during cell division.

History of antifungal agents

1. In 1958, the first broad-spectrum antifungal, amphotericin B deoxycholate, was introduced. It has significant antifungal efficacy but is linked to renal damage.

2. Flucytosine, a pyrimidine analogue first discovered in 1973, is effective against *Candida* and *Cryptococcus*. Drug resistance and toxicity limit its use.

3. Fluconazole and itraconazole were among the first-generation azoles introduced in the 1990s.

4. Amphotericin B was introduced in the 1990s and has broad-spectrum activity with less toxicity.

5. Echinocandin drugs were introduced in the 2000s and have strong anti-Candida properties. They are only available in parenteral form.

6. The second generation of azole compounds, such as voriconazole, posaconazole, and isavuconazole, entered the market in the early 2000s. The broad spectrum of activity against filamentous fungus is a major advantage of these drugs.

Classification

1. Naturally occurring:

   (a) Polyene antibiotics Ex. amphotericin B, nystatin, natamycin,

   (b) A spiro system antibiotic: Ex. griseofulvin

2. Synthetic Agents:

   (a) Azoles

      (i) Imidazoles: Ex. clotrimazole, econazole, miconazole, oxiconazole, ketoconazole, butoconazole, tioconazole, miconazole, ketoconazole

      (ii) Triazoles: Ex. fluconazole, itraconazole, voriconazole, terconazole,

   (b) Allylamine: Ex. terbinafine

   (c) Thiocarbamate: Ex. tolnaftate

   (d) Miscellaneous: Ex. naftifine hydrochloride, butenafine

4.2 Antifungal Antibiotics

Polyene antifungal antibiotics

This unique family of antifungal drugs and the first successful therapy against deep-seated fungal infections emerged from the polyene antifungal discovery. Polyenes are macrocyclic lactone rings that have hydrophilic and lipophilic regions. The hydrophilic area is composed of multiple alcohols, carboxylic acids, and, in most cases, sugar. The lipophilic area holds a chromophore (a molecule responsible for its color) with four to seven conjugated double bonds. The number of conjugated double bonds is directly proportional to antifungal activity *in vitro* and inversely proportional to mammalian cell toxicity. Amphotericin B, for example, has seven conjugated double bonds and is approximately ten times more toxic to fungi.

4.2.1 Amphotericin-B

Historical Background

  ✓ **Donovick R., Gold W., Pagano JF.,** and **Stout HA** identified the drug in 1956 following fermentation of the actinomycete *Streptomyces nodosus*. The organism was recovered from a soil sample taken in Venezuela's Orinoco River region. It was approved as a therapeutic treatment in 1959 and made commercially available in 1960.

  ✓ Amphotericin is a combination of two closely related compounds known as amphotericins A and B. Amphotericin B is more active and is used to treat fungal infections both systemically and locally.

✓ One of the most significant scientific achievements of the twentieth century was the discovery of amphotericin B and its therapeutic applications.

✓ Despite the discovery of many novel antifungal drugs, including second generation triazoles and echinocandins, amphotericin B remains the most extensively used antifungal drug.

✓ Amphotericin B is a member of the polyene macrolide class. This class also includes amphotericin A and nystatin. The latter compound is said to be the first antifungal drug for the treatment of mycoses.

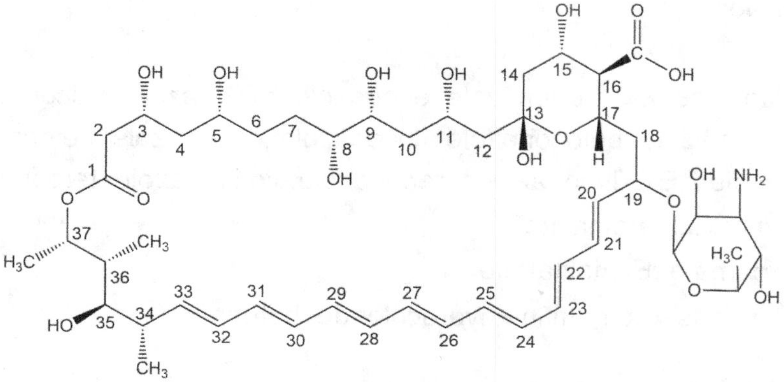

Fig. 4.1 Chemical structure of Amphotericin-B.

Chemical Structure: (Fig. 4.1)

Chemical Name:

3*R*,5*R*,8*R*,9*R*,11*S*,13*R*,15*S*,16*R*,17*S*,19*R*,34*S*,35*R*.36*R*,37*S*)-19-(3-amino-3,6-dideoxy-β-D-mannopyranosyloxy)-16-carboxy-3,5,8,9,11,13,15,35-octahydroxy-34,36-dimethyl-13,17-epoxyoctatriaconta-20,22,24,26,28,30,32-heptaen-37-olide

Structure-Activity Relationship

1. The drug's antifungal activity is primarily dependent on four positions of the chemical structure. They are (1) the formation of a hydroxyl group at C-13; (2) the absence of a negative charge in the acid group; (3) the polyene itself; and (4) ionizable nitrogen.

2. Ergosterol is a protein that is an important part of the membrane of fungal cells. The mycosamine and C-35-OH groups in the drug are very important in binding the ergosterol.

Chemistry

1. It has seven double bonds in trans disposition.

2. Amino sugar mycosamine is glycosidically linked through position 19 of the aglycone macrolide.

3. The molecule has a primary amino group in the sugar part and a carboxylic group at position C-16.

4. It forms a soluble salt in both acidic and basic environments.
5. It is amphoteric. As such, it is named amphotericin.

Mechanism of Action

The polyenes act by directly interacting with the sterols in the fungal membrane and disrupting their integrity. This interaction arises due to the drug's high affinity for fungal ergosterol. This complex then creates pores in the fungal membrane, which leak ions out of the cells, causing them to die. Despite this, the drug has a lower affinity for human cholesterol, which explains why it has a stronger effect on pathogens than on host cells.

Depending on the dose, it has both fungistatic and fungicidal effects. Amphotericin B has an antifungal effect because it binds to sterols, specifically ergosterol, in the cellular membranes of susceptible fungi. This reaction creates gaps in the membrane and increases membrane permeability to simple molecules, diminishing the membrane's function as an osmotic barrier and rendering the cells more vulnerable to destruction. Amphotericin B is active against both developing and dormant cells. However, this drug does not react very selectively to host mammalian cells.

The polyenes bind to the sterol-containing membranes of fungi, with the drugs inserting themselves into the membranes and disrupting their functions. The lipophilic portion of the drug penetrates the lipid bilayer of the cell membrane, generating a pore. Polyene-treated cells' membranes become leaky, and the cells eventually die. As a result of the loss of important cell constituents, including ions and relatively small organic compounds. Polyenes have a stronger affinity for ergosterol-containing membranes than cholesterol-containing membranes. This explains why they are more harmful to fungal cells.

Uses

1. It is still the first-line treatment for severe, acute systemic fungal infections.
2. It is used to treat common fungal infections such as candidomycosis, aspergillosis, histoplasmosis, cryptococcosis, coccidioidomycosis, blastomycosis, and pulmonary mycoses.
3. It is taken orally for intestinal candidiasis.

4.2.2 Nystatin

Historical Background

Nystatin is derived from bacteria. Two women scientists at the Division of Laboratories and Research of the New York State Department of Health, **Elizabeth Lee Hazen** and **Rachel Fuller Brown**, discovered it in *Streptomyces noursei* in 1950. Hazen found a promising microorganism in the soil of a friend's dairy farm. **Jessie Nourse**, the farm's owner's wife, was the inspiration for the microorganism's name. In 1954, Hazen and Brown named the compound Nystatin after the New York State Health Department.

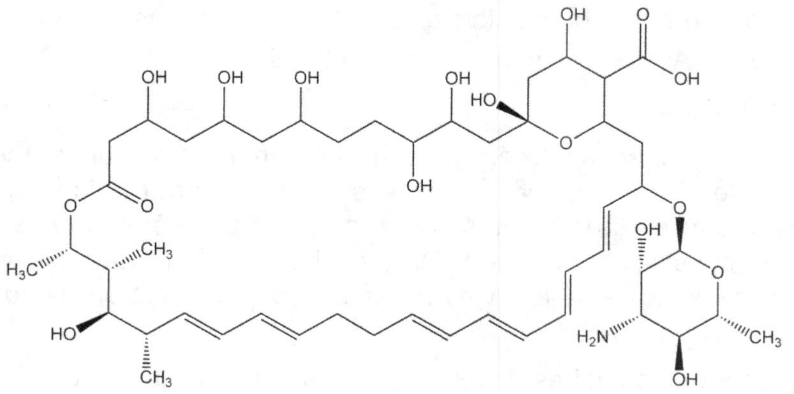

Fig. 4.2 Chemical structure of Nystatin.

Chemical Structure: (Fig. 4.2)

Chemical Name:

(1*S*,15*S*,16*R*,17*R*,18*S*,19*E*,21*E*,25*E*,27*E*,29*E*,31*E*)-33-(((2*S*,3*S*,4*S*,5*S*,6*R*)-4-amino-3,5-dihydroxy-6-methyltetrahydro-2*H*-pyran-2-yl)oxy)-1,3,4,7,9,11,17,37-octahydroxy-15,16,18-trimethyl-13-oxo-14,39-dioxabicyclo[33.3.1]nonatriaconta-19,21,25,27,29,31-hexaene-36-carboxylic acid

Chemistry

1. A1, A2, and A3 are the biologically active components of Nystatin. The primary active principle in the official product is nystatin A1.

2. The structure is similar to that of amphotericin. In this ring, the macrolide ring contains separate tetraene and diene chromophores. A methylene bridge separates the two chromophores. The macrolide ring is linked glycosidically to mycosamine.

3. Its primary target is *Candida spp.* Nystatin is more toxic and is not used systemically.

Mechanism of Action

The mechanism of action of Nystatin for antifungal activity is similar to that of amphotericin B. It is a polyene antifungal drug. It binds to the ergosterol in the fungal cell membrane, causing permeability alterations of the cell membrane and, finally, cell lysis.

Nystatin is an antifungal polyene that binds to sterols in both fungal and human cell membranes. It is normally fungistatic *in vivo*, but at high concentrations, it can be fungicidal. It has a stronger affinity for ergosterol, a sterol found in fungal cell membranes, than cholesterol, a sterol found in human cell membranes. Yet, it is too toxic to be used systemically. The membrane integrity of both fungal and human cells is compromised as a result of this binding, resulting in the loss of intracellular potassium and other cellular contents.

Uses

1. It is used solely to treat candidiasis of the skin, mucous membranes, GI tract, and vaginal candidiasis.
2. It is used to prevent the development of candidomycosis after long-term treatment with penicillin.
3. In immunocompromised patients, it has also been used as a preventative measure. It is used to treat oral candidiasis.

4.2.3 Natamycin

Historical Background

In a *Streptomycetes* culture filtrate, **Jacques Waisvisz** discovered natamycin in 1955. The organism was identified in a South African soil sample. Its name comes from the Natal region of South Africa, where it was initially discovered. *S. natalensis* fermentation is used to make commercial preparations.

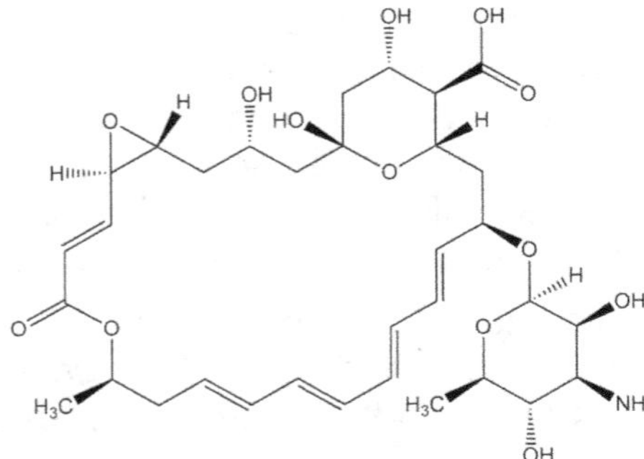

Fig. 4.3 Chemical structure of Natamycin.

It is also produced by some streptomyces species: *S. lydicus*, *S. chattanoogensis* and *S. gilvosporeus*.

It was originally named pimaricin to honor Pietermaritzburg (a city in South Africa).

The spectrum of its activity is somewhat narrower than that of amphotericin and nystatin, but at the same time, it is less toxic.

Chemical Structure: (Fig.4.3)

Chemical Name:

(1*R*,3*S*,5*R*,7*R*,8*E*,12*R*,14*E*,16*E*,18*E*,20*E*,22*R*,24*S*,25*R*,26*S*)-22-(((2*R*,3*S*,4*S*,5*S*,6*R*)-4-amino-3,5-dihydroxy-6-methyltetrahydro-2*H*-pyran-2-yl)oxy)-1,3,26-trihydroxy-12-methyl-10-oxo-6,11,28-trioxatricyclo[22.3.1.0^{5,7}]octacosa-8,14,16,18,20-pentaene-25-carboxylic acid

Mechanism of Action

Natamycin is a polyene amphoteric macrolide antibiotic. It works by disrupting the fungal cell membrane by binding to ergosterol, the major sterol in the cell membrane. As a result, pores form within the cell membrane. This complex leads to cellular cations and anions draining out, resulting in fungal cell death.

Uses

1. It is used to treat superficial fungal infections and in ophthalmology.
2. This drug is used to treat fungal infections around the eyes, such as eyelid, conjunctiva, and cornea infections. It comes in the form of eye drops or lozenges (for oral infections).

3. It's also used as a preservative in the food sector (to prevent fungus growth in dairy products and other foods).

4.2.4 Griseofulvin

Historical Background

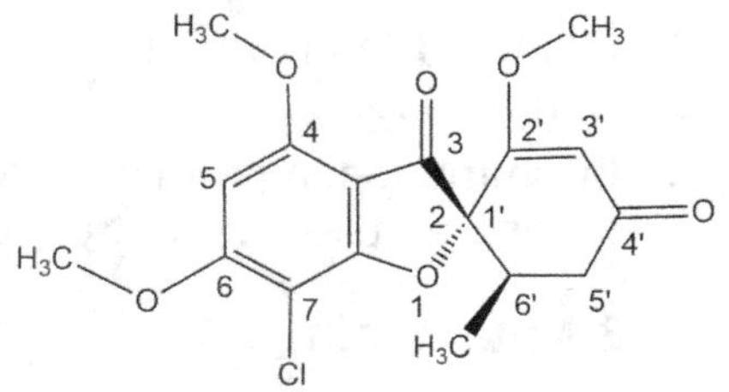

Griseofulvin is an antifungal antibiotic that is used to treat a variety of fungal infections in the skin. It is produced by a certain fungal species called *Penicillium*. It was isolated in 1939 as a soil fungus called *Penicillium griseofulvum* (developed by **A. E. Oxford** and coworkers). This was used to cure ringworm in cattle and was later used to fight bacterial infections in humans. The first human studies with griseofulvin were conducted in 1958. In 1959, the FDA gave its official approval.

Fig. 4.4 Chemical structure of Griseofulvin.

The name "griseofulvin" was suggested for this novel compound because the parent mould was called *Penicillium griseofulvum*. Other organisms, such as *P. janczewskii*, *P. patulum*, and *P. raistriki*, have been used to make griseofulvin.

Chemical Structure: (Fig. 4.4)

Chemical Name:

(2*S*,6'*R*)-7-chloro-2',4,6-trimethoxy-6'-methyl-3*H*-spiro[benzofuran-2,1'-cyclohexan]-2'-ene-3,4'-dione

Structure-Activity Relationship

1. The structure of griseofulvin is unique. It has two chiral centers and a spiro system (a twisted structure in which two or more rings are linked together by one common atom).

2. X-ray diffraction was used to identify the configuration.

3. Even though griseofulvin has been prepared in all four geometric isomers. Only one, which corresponds to a natural antibiotic, has antifungal activity.

4. If the 7-chloro substituent is substituted with a fluoro group, the antibiotic retains its action.

5. The 2'-propoxy or 2'-butoxy analogues show higher *in vitro* activity when used in place of the natural 2'-methoxy group.

Mechanism of Action

Griseofulvin is fungistatic rather than fungicidal, even at significant concentrations. The interruption of the formation of chitin, a substance found in fungal cell walls, was at first thought to be griseofulvin's mode of action. Although the exact mechanism of action is uncertain, several possibilities have been suggested. The potential of griseofulvin to damage the mitotic spindle structure, halting fungal cell growth in the M-phase of its life cycle, is one possibility. Another theory is that griseofulvin causes fungal cells to produce faulty DNA, preventing them from replicating.

Uses

1. Griseofulvin is an oral antifungal drug for treating dermatophyte infections of the skin, scalp, hair, and nails.
2. It's taken orally to treat superficial fungal diseases like fingernail and toenail infections, but when applied topically, it doesn't penetrate the skin or nails.

4.3 Synthetic Antifungal Agents

Before the advent of antibiotics, the most effective antifungal drugs were chemical substances such as powerful fungicides and surface antiseptics that inactivated essential enzymes with heavy metals. Bacteria, protozoa, fungi, mammals, and plants were all extremely poisonous to these substances.

Organic chemicals with more specific antifungal activity, such as sulfur compounds, fatty acids, benzoic acid, phenol derivatives, and quaternary ammonium compounds, have been used topically to treat superficial mycoses.

Potassium iodide: In 1903, **de Beurmann** and **Gougerot** reported the favorable benefits of the first oral chemotherapeutic treatment, potassium iodide. It acts on sporotrichosis, the only mycosis that reacts to this drug. Iodine acts as a direct antifungal agent in the therapeutic effect of potassium iodide.

Sulfonamides: In the next 40 years, antifungal chemotherapeutic drugs were employed as sulfonamides and aromatic diamidines.

Flucytosine: It is an antimetabolite from the fluoropyrimidine class. **Grunberg E., Titsworth E.,** and **Bennett M.** reported the compound's antifungal activity in 1963.

Azoles: Imidazoles Antifungal imidazoles have a pivotal role in mycosis therapy. In 1944, **Wooley D. W.,** reported that benzimidazole inhibits bacterial and fungal growth. As such, several antifungal imidazole compounds have been developed, including thiabendazole, mebendazole, and chlorimidazole.

The first oral azole was **clotrimazole**, a tritylimidazole. It is efficacious in both human and experimental mycoses. Miconazole, ketoconazole, and other imidazoles (tioconazole, sulconazole, and isoconazole) have been used successfully in superficial mycoses treatments.

Triazoles: Terconazole, a topical agent; itraconazole; and fluconazole, a systemic drug, are three novel triazoles that have shown promise as antifungal agents.

Allylamines: Allylamine derivatives are a novel class of synthetic antifungal agents. Tolnaftate is the most potent of almost 4,000 compounds generated from naphthiomate and is mostly active against dermatophytes *in vitro*. It is still used as a reference agent in the development of novel antifungal drugs.

Classification

(a) Azoles derivatives
   (i) Imidazole derivatives: clotrimazole, econazole. butoconazole. oxiconazole, tioconazole, miconazole, ketoconazole
   (ii) Triazole derivative: terconazole, itraconazole, fluconazole

(b)   Fluorinated pyrimidine: flucytosine

(c)   Allylamines: naftifine, amorolfine, butenafine, tolnaftate

(d)   Chitin synthetase inhibitors: nikomycin Z

(e)   Peptides/proteins inhibitors: cispentacin

(f)   Fatty and other acids: propionic acid, undecylenic acid. resorcinol. benzoic acid

4.3.1 Clotrimazole

Historical Background

Karl Hienz Buchel (Bayer) first developed clotrimazole as an antifungal drug in the late 1960s. Bayer obtained a patent on it in 1972, and in 1973 it was available on German markets under the brand name Canesten. It was the first of a family of azole derivatives. Because of its mild side effects and uncomplicated metabolic profile, this drug has gained widespread acceptance for the treatment of vaginal yeast infections and athlete's foot.

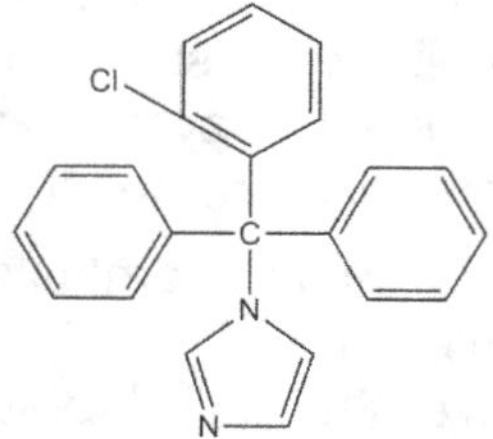

Fig. 4.5 Chemical structure of Clotrimazole.

It has been added to the list of essential medications by the World Health Organization.

Chemical Structure: (Fig. 4.5)

Chemical Name: 1-((2-chlorophenyl)diphenylmethyl)-1*H*-imidazole

Mechanism of Action

The interactions of azole compounds with membrane components may explain the antibacterial activity, as well as the subsequent activity against non-proliferating fungal cells. It's been proposed that the plasma membrane's unsaturated fatty acid components could be the target of imidazole activity. On the other hand, there is significant experimental evidence that sterol biosynthesis inhibition is the primary antifungal mechanism. The manufacture of ergosterol, which is an essential and integral element of the fungal cytoplasmic membrane, is depicted schematically (**Fig. 4.6**). Clotrimazole and other azoles have mainly caused the demethylation of 24-methyleneedihydrolanosterol, which then causes another systemic reaction. The gradual depletion of ergosterol in the cytoplasmic membrane is thought to cause changes in the membrane structure, eventually leading to a fatal efflux of ions and cytoplasmic material.

Clotrimazole acts by disrupting the fungal cytoplasmic membrane's permeability barrier. Clotrimazole suppresses ergosterol production in a concentration-dependent manner by blocking 14α-lanosterol demethylation. The cell can no longer build an intact and functional cell membrane when ergosterol synthesis is suppressed. Ergosterol also stimulates the growth of fungal cells in a hormone-like manner, resulting in a dose-dependent suppression of fungal growth.

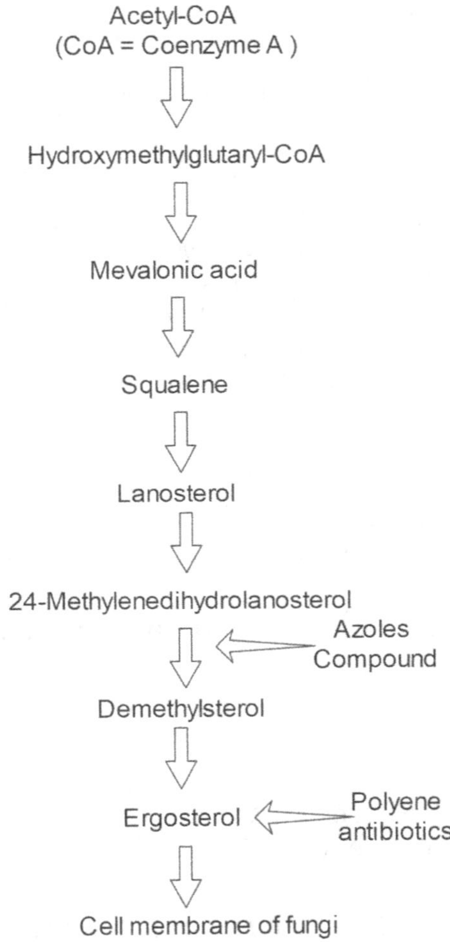

Fig. 4.6 Mechanism of action of antifungal drugs.

Uses

1. Clotrimazole is used topically to treat superficial candidiasis, as well as pityriasis versicolor (skin rash) and dermatophytoses.

2. It's also utilized in the treatment of vaginal candidiasis, and ringworm including athlete's foot.

3. It can be taken as throat lozenge by mouth for oropharyngeal candidiasis or applied as a cream, or ointment to the skin or in the vagina.

4.3.2 Econazole

Historical Background

It was discovered in 1969 by Janssen Pharmaceutica Ltd., Belgium, and used for medical purposes in 1974.

Chemical Structure: (Fig. 4.7)

Chemical Name:

1-(2-((4-chlorobenzyl)oxy)-2-(2,4-dichlorophenyl)eth yl)-1*H*-imidazole

Mechanism of Action

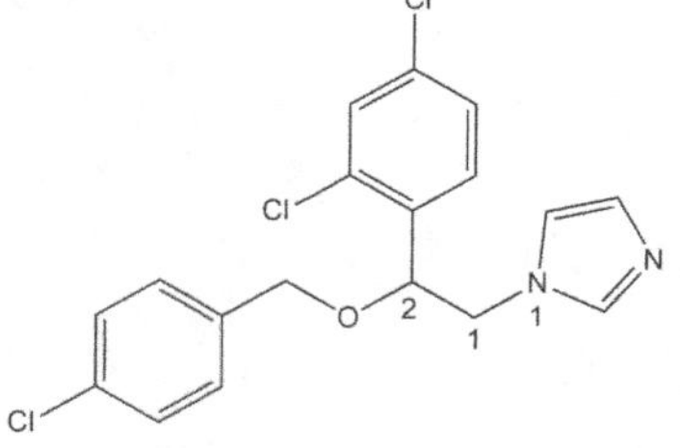

Fig. 4.7 Chemical structure of Econazole.

Econazole nitrate, an azole antifungal drug. It inhibits the 14α-lanosterol demethylase enzymes, which are mediated by cytochrome P_{450} in fungi. This enzyme is responsible for the conversion of lanosterol to ergosterol. The increase in 14α-methyl sterols is linked to the loss of ergosterol in the fungal cell wall. This process could explain econazole's fungistatic properties. Demethylation in mammalian cells is less responsive to econazole inhibition.

Uses

1. Econazole nitrate is applied topically as creams, lotions, and powder in the treatment of fungal infections including candidiasis, dermatophytosis, and pityriasis versicolor.

2. This is also used to treat *tinea versicolor* (a fungus that discolors the skin), and yeast infections of the skin.

4.3.3 Butoconazole

Historical Background

Butoconazole nitrate, an imidazole class compound, was developed by Syntex Research in Mexico. It is active as an antifungal drug both *in vitro* and *in vivo* in animal models.

It was granted a patent in 1975 and approved for medicinal usage in 1983.

Chemical Structure: (Fig. 4.8)

Chemical Name:

1-(4-(4-chlorophenyl)-2-((2,6-dichlorophenyl)thio)but yl)-1H-imidazole

Mechanism of Action

It is a synthetic imidazole derivative compound with fungistatic characteristics. It disrupts the steroid synthesis of fungi by preventing the conversion of lanosterol to ergosterol, altering the lipid composition of fungal cell membranes. This further causes a change in cell permeability, which inhibits the growth of fungi. Many dermatophytes and yeasts are susceptible to butoconazole nitrate. It also has antibacterial properties against gram-+ve bacteria.

Fig.4.8 Chemical structure of Butoconazole.

Uses

1. It is useful for treating dermatophytoses and pityriasis versicolor-related skin conditions.
2. In the treatment of vaginal candidiasis, butoconazole nitrate is used as a 2% vaginal cream. It relieves the vaginal burning, itching, and discharge that can occur with this illness.

4.3.4 Oxiconazole

Historical Background

In 1989, oxiconazole nitrate (1%) cream was approved in the USA for the treatment of *tinea pedis*, *tinea cruris*, and *tinea corporis* on a once-daily basis.

Chemical Structure: (Fig. 4.9)

Chemical Name:

(*Z*)-1-(2,4-dichlorophenyl)-2-(1*H*-imidazol-1-yl)ethan-1-one O-(2,4-dichlorobenzyl)oxime

Mechanism of Action

It inhibits ergosterol biosynthesis. Ergosterol is essential for fungi to maintain the integrity of their cytoplasmic membranes. It acts by disrupting the enzyme cytochrome P_{450} in fungi (also known as lanosterol 14α-demethylase). It is crucial for the fungal cell membrane structure. Fungal cell death occurs when this enzyme is inhibited. It has also been shown to reduce intracellular ATP concentrations and impair DNA synthesis. Oxiconazole, like other imidazole antifungals, can increase zinc permeability in the membrane, increasing its cytotoxicity.

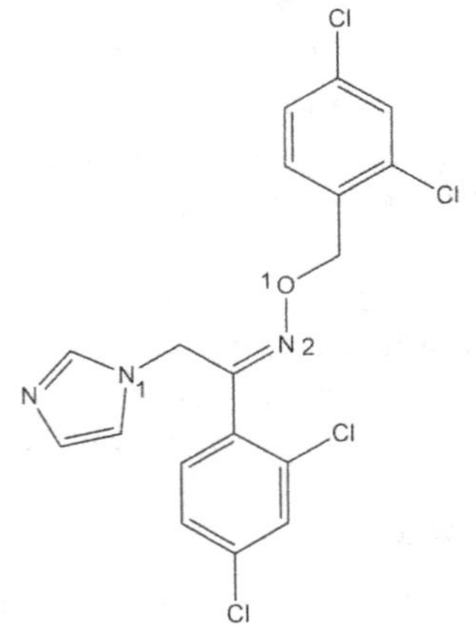

Fig.4.9 Chemical structure of Oxiconazole.

Uses

1. It is applied topically as a cream or lotion to treat skin infections such as athlete's foot, jock itch, or ringworm.
2. It is used to treat a skin rash caused by *Candida spp.* (tinea versicolor: this is characterized by lightening or darkening of the skin of the neck, chest, arms, or legs).
3. It's used to treat common pathogenic dermatophytes in the form of creams and lotions.

4.3.5 Tioconazole

Historical Background

Tioconazole, like miconazole and clotrimazole, is a novel imidazole antifungal drug. It has a broad spectrum of activity and is more effective against *Candida albicans* in *in vitro* than other imidazoles.

It was granted a patent in 1975 and approved for therapeutic purposes in 1982.

Chemical Structure: (Fig. 4.10)

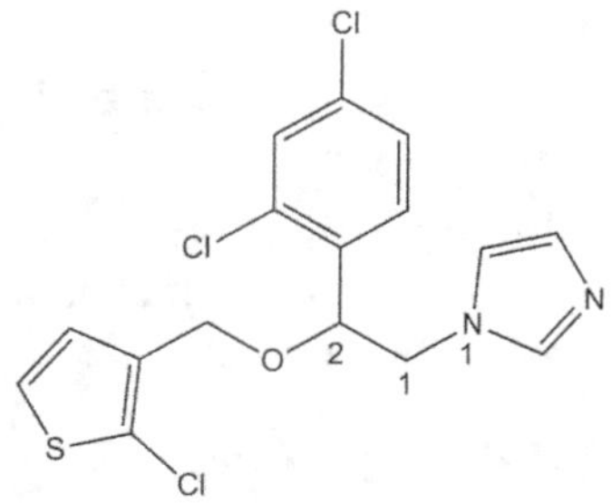

Chemical Name:

1-(2-((2-chlorothiophen-3-yl)methoxy)-2-(2,4-dichloroph enyl)ethyl)-1*H*-imidazole; 1-[2-[(2-chloro-3- thienyl) methoxy]-2-(2,4-dichlorophenyl)ethyl]-1*H*- imidazole

Mechanism of Action

It inhibits fungal oxidative enzymes, resulting in harmful hydrogen peroxide accumulation; it also inhibits the synthesis of ergosterol, a vital part of the fungal cell wall, which becomes permeable to intracellular contents. A lack of selectivity leads to significant adverse effects from these actions.

Tioconazole works by altering the permeability of the fungal cell membrane. Ergosterol is a constituent of the fungal cell membrane. The constituent is necessary for the survival of the fungi. It interacts with the 14α-demethylase enzyme (also known as the cytochrome P_{450} enzyme) of the fungi. The enzyme takes part in converting lanosterol to ergosterol. Hence, it inhibits ergosterol synthesis. When ergosterol synthesis is inhibited, cellular permeability is altered. This event is causing leakage of cellular contents such as phosphorus-containing substances and potassium. As a result, lysis of the cell causes.

Uses

1. It is applied topically to treat oral, skin, and vaginal infections.

2. It is useful in treating vulvovaginal candidiasis.

3. Tioconazole nitrate is used topically to treat superficial candidiasis, dermatophytosis, and pityriasis versicolor.

4. Tioconazole ointments are used to treat vaginal yeast infections in women.

5. It's utilized in ringworm therapy as a topical (skin) preparation.

4.3.6 Miconazole

Historical Background

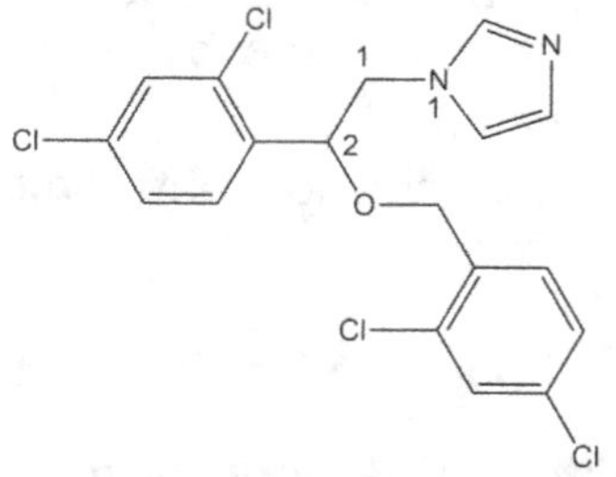

Antifungal drugs such as miconazole and econazole were both developed by Janssen Pharmaceutica (Belgium). Miconazole, a phenethyl imidazole synthesized in 1969, was the first azole to be used parentally. It was approved for medicinal use in 1971.

It is effective against a wide range of yeasts and dermatophytes when applied topically.

Fig. 4.10 Chemical structure of Tioconazole.

Fig.4.11 Chemical structure of Miconazole.

Chemical structure: (Fig. 4.11)

Chemical Name:

1-(2-((2,4-dichlorobenzyl)oxy)-2-(2,4-dichlorophenyl)ethyl)-1*H*-imidazole

Synthesis

1. It is synthesized from 2,4-dichloracetophenone with a bromination process. Under this process, it is obtained as 2,4-dichlorophenacylbromide.

2. When combined with imidazole, 2,4-dichlorophenacylbromide to form 1-(2,4-dichlorophenyl)-2-(1*H*-imidazol-1-yl) ethan-1-one.

3. Reducing the carbonyl group of the subsequent molecule with sodium borohydride gives 1-(2,4-dichlorophenyl)-2-(1*H*-imidazol-1-yl)ethan-1-ol.

4. The hydroxyl group of the intermediate is alkylated by 2,4-dichlorobenzylbromide using a powerful base such as sodium hydride to make the final product miconazole (Fig.4.12).

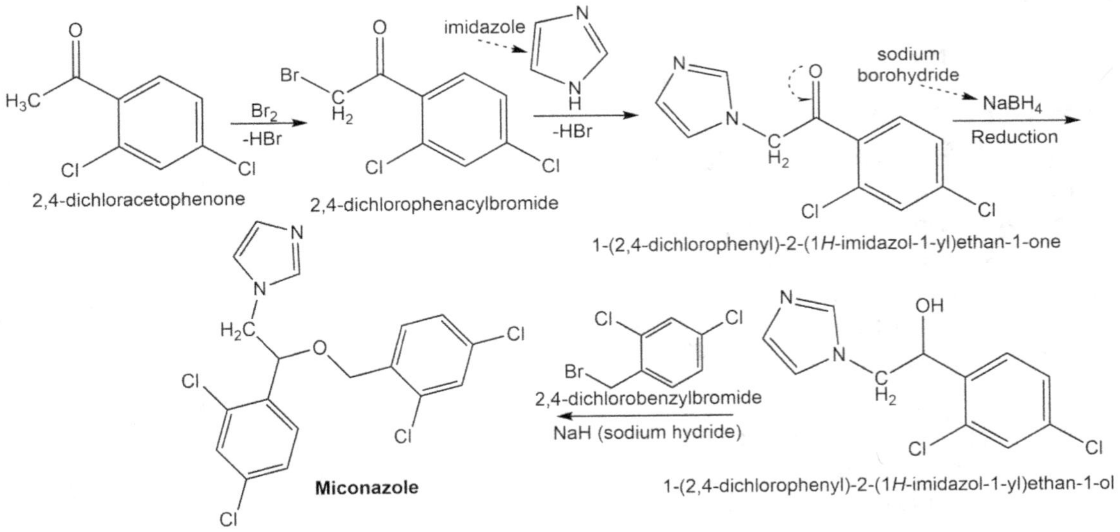

Fig.4.12 Synthesis of miconazole.

Mechanism of Action

It inhibits the synthesis of ergosterol by fungi. Ergosterol is the main sterol component of fungal plasma membranes, and inhibits the fungal cytochrome P_{450} dependent enzyme lanosterol 14α–demethylase. The lack of ergosterol and the accumulation of 14-methylated precursors make it difficult for ergosterol to perform its primary function in fungal membranes. As a result, altered membrane fluidity and the activity of numerous membrane-bound enzymes (e.g., chitin synthase). Fungal growth and replication are slowed as a result of this treatment. Several other effects have also been seen, such as stopping the transformation of yeast mycelia into fungi, making it harder for fungi to stick to surfaces, and having direct toxic effects on membrane phospholipids.

These agents interfere with the enzyme system responsible for the demethylation of lanosterol and its conversion to ergosterol. The N-3 atom of the azole ring binds to the ferric ion atom in the heme prosthetic. The heme prosthetic is a tightly bound, specific non-polypeptide unit that some proteins need to do their job in the body. The prosthetic group may be organic (such as a vitamin, sugar, or lipid) or inorganic (such as a metal ion), but not composed of amino acids) to prevent the activation of the oxygen for insertion into lanosterol. Cytochrome P_{450} is more sensitive to azole containing compounds. They are analogues of enzymes in mammalian cells. Ergosterol is the main sterol of the fungal cell membrane.

Uses

1. Miconazole nitrate and econazole nitrate are applied topically in the form of creams, lotions, and powders to treat fungal infections such as candidiasis, dermatophytosis, and pityriasis versicdor.

2. It can be taken orally and used to treat oropharyngeal and intestinal candidiasis.

3. It has been used to treat fungal infections intravenously.

4.3.7 Ketoconazole

Historical Background

Janssen Pharmaceutica in Belgium synthesizes and produces ketoconazole, an imidazole derivative. It was FDA approved in 1981. It was started as a prototype antifungal therapy of the imidazole class. It was the first oral therapy for systemic fungal infections.

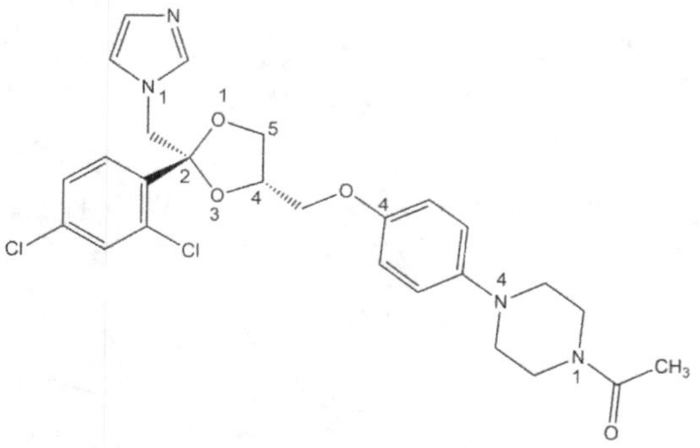

Fig. 4.13 Chemical structre of Ketoconazole.

For almost a decade after its release, it was the only systemic antifungal available. Oral itraconazole has taken the place of oral ketoconazole for several mycoses.

It is fungistatic; however, it didn't work as well in immunocompromised patients.

Chemical Structure: (Fig. 4.13)

Chemical Name:

1-(4-(4-(((2R,4S)-2-((1H-imidazol-1-yl)methyl)-2-(2,4-dichlorophenyl)-1,3-dioxolan-4-yl) methoxy)phenyl)piperazin-1-yl)ethan-1-one;1-Acetyl-4-(4-((2RS,4SR)-2-(2.4-dichloroph -enyl)-2-(1H)-imidazol-1ylmethyl)-1,3-dioxolan-4-yl)meth-oxy)phenyl)piperazine.

Mechanism of Action

Ketoconazole is an antifungal drug that acts by blocking the enzyme cytochrome P_{450} 14α-demethylase. This enzyme prevents the fungus from producing triglycerides and phospholipids. Ketoconazole, in particular, suppresses the formation of lanosterol, a precursor to ergosterol biosynthesis. Fungi require ergosterol to preserve their membrane integrity. The fluidity of the membrane increases without ergosterol, which limits fungal development.

Ketoconazole is an antifungal drug that is structurally related to imidazole. It inhibits the fungal synthesis of ergosterol, a component of fungal cell membranes. It works by blocking the enzyme cytochrome P_{450} 14α-demethylase (CYP51A1). This enzyme is involved in the sterol biosynthesis pathway's conversion of lanosterol to ergosterol. When compared to ketoconazole, fluconazole, and itraconazole, they require lower doses to kill fungi because they have a higher affinity for fungal cell membranes.

Uses

✓ It was the first orally active azole antifungal drug, and it proved effective for both superficial and systemic infections.

✓ It is active against numerous fungi that can cause human disease, including *candida*, *histoplasma*, *coccidioides*, *blastomyces* (but not *aspergillus*), *chrornomycosis*, and *paracoccidioidomycosis*.

✓ It's used topically to treat fungal infections of the skin and mucous membranes, such as athlete's foot, ringworm, candidiasis (yeast infection or thrush), and fingernails.

✓ Topically applied cream for candidal or dermatophyte infection

✓ It's also used as a shampoo to treat dandruff (seborrheic dermatitis of the scalp) and other skin conditions, potentially by lowering Malassezia furfur levels on the skin.

✓ Other azole antifungal drugs, such as itraconazole, have largely replaced it as a first-line systemic antifungal drug. Because ketoconazole is more toxic, has a lower absorption rate, and has a narrower spectrum of activity.

4.3.8 Terconazole

Historical Background

It is a topical triazole antifungal drug that has structural similarities to ketoconazole.

Triazole-based drugs soon gained popularity and rapidly grew due to their broad range of antifungal activity and lower toxicity. It was the first triazole-based antifungal drug to be developed specifically for human use. Janssen Pharmaceutica developed it in 1983. Previously, all triazole-based drugs were used to treat Candida-related fungal infections.

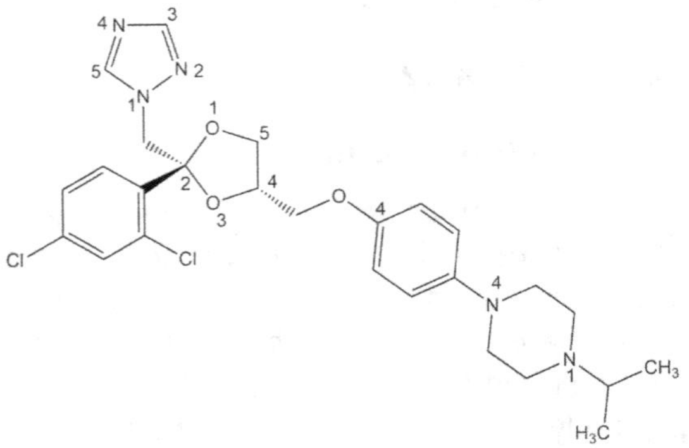

Fig. 4.14 Chemical structure of Terconazole.

Chemical Structure: (Fig. 4.14)

Chemical Name:

1-(4-(((2R,4S)-2-((1H-1,2,4-triazol-1-yl)methyl)-2-(2,4-dichlorophenyl)-1,3-di-oxolan-4-yl) methoxy)phenyl)-4-isopropyl piperazine

Mechanism of Action

Terconazole binds to the heme iron component of the fungus lanosterol cytochrome P_{450} enzyme, also known as CYP3A4. ERG11 is a gene that regulates the production of lanosterol. Fungi have lanosterol in their plasma membrane. It is a member of the methylsterol family. In a fungal cell, lanosterol is demethylated through 14-demethylation. This method results in the formation of zymosterol, a crucial component of the ergosterol biosynthesis pathway in fungi that leads to cell membrane components. This design provides membrane fluidity. This occurs when lanosterol is transformed into 4,4'-dimethyl cholesta-8,14,24-triene-3-ol. This affects the integrity of the cell membrane, as well as transport and catabolism. Membrane fluidity and the activity of membrane-bound enzymes eventually diminish. It has also been proven to prevent fungal morphologic change and cell attachment. Because humans do not utilise lanosterol in this pathway, terconazole is only effective against fungi.

It inhibits the enzyme lanosterol 14α-demethylase in sensitive fungi. As a result, there was a decrease in the quantity of ergosterol. Ergosterol is required for organisms to form membranes and maintain proper permeability.

Uses

✓ It is used to treat vaginal yeast infections and to prevent chronic *vulvovaginal candidiasis*.

✓ It comes in the form of a lotion or a suppository. It acts by interfering with the formation of lipids in yeast cells. It possesses a broad range of spectrum of activity when compared to azole compounds, but not when compared to triazole compounds.

✓ It is recommended to use vaginal cream or suppositories.

4.3.9 Itraconazole

Historical Background

The US FDA approved itraconazole, a broad-spectrum triazole from Janssen Pharmaceutica, in 1992. It was found to be less toxic than ketoconazole and to have a broad spectrum of activity against *Candida spp.*, *Aspergillus spp.*, *Cryptococcus neoformans*, *Coccidioides immitis*, *Histoplasma capsulatum*, *Blastomyces dermatitidis*, *Paracoccidioides brasiliensis*, *Sporothrix schenckii*, and some *phaeohyphomyce*. It has gradually replaced ketoconazole as the therapy of choice for nonmeningeal, non-life-threatening cases of *histoplasmosis*, *blastomycosis*, and *paracoccidioi-domycosis*. In terms of spectrum activity, it performs better than fluconazole. It has potent activity against *aspergillosis* and *sporotrichosis* species. Fluconazole, on the other hand, has a better pharmacological and toxicological profile. Itraconazole was only available in capsule form. Fluconazole and itraconazole are both significant advancements in the treatment of systemic fungal infections.

Chemical Structure: (Fig. 4.15)

Chemical Name:

4-(4-(4-(4-(((2R,4S)-2-((1H-1,2,4-tri-azol-1-yl)methyl)-2-(2,4-dichlorophenyl)-1,3-dioxolan-4-yl)methoxy)phenyl)piperazin-1-yl)phenyl)-2-(sec-butyl)-2,4-dihydro-3H-1,2,4-triazol-3-one

Stereochemistry

1. There are three chiral centres in the molecule. The triazolomethy-lene and aryloxymethylene dioxo-lane-ring substituents are always *cis* to one another, and the two chiral centers in the dioxolan centres are fixed to one another.

2. A combination of four stereoi-somers is used in the therapeutic formulation (two enantiomeric pairs).

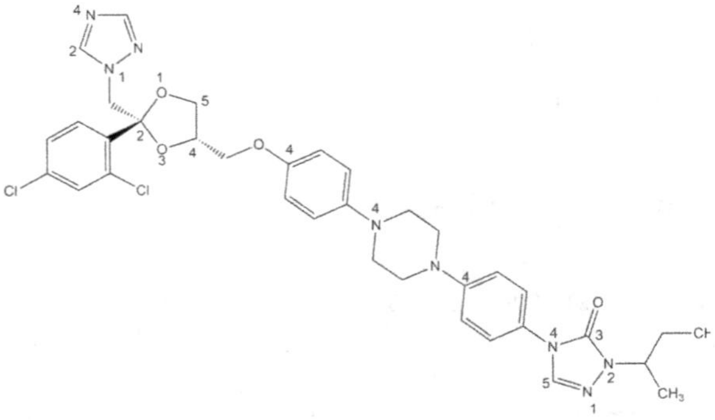

Fig. 4.15 Chemical structure of Itraconazole.

3. *In vitro* studies suggest that stereoisomers with a (2S,4R) configuration in the dioxolane ring are 4-fold more powerful than those with a (2R,4S) structure.

Mechanism of Action

Itraconazole acts by preventing lanosterol 14α–demethylase, a fungal cytochrome P_{450} dependent enzyme. When this enzyme is blocked, it prevents the conversion of lanosterol to ergosterol, which disrupts the formation of fungal cell membranes. It has fungistatic and fungicidal activity against yeast-like fungi and *Aspergillus* spp.

Uses

✓ It is used to treat a variety of fungal illnesses, including aspergillosis, blastomycosis, coccidioidomycosis, histoplasmosis, and paracoccidioidomycosis. It can be administered orally or intravenously.

✓ It is taken orally to treat oropharyngeal and vulvovaginal candidiasis, pityriasis Versicolor, and dermatophytosis that is not responding to topical treatment.

✓ It is used to treat fungal infections in those who have a poor immune system.

✓ Recently, the anticancer properties of itraconazole have also been investigated.

4.3.10 Fluconazole

Historical Background

- ✓ Pfizer in the USA developed the broad-spectrum triazole antifungal drug known as fluconazole. It was approved in early 1990 and addresses many of the imidazole-containing compound's drawbacks.

- ✓ Fluconazole and itraconazole exhibited a broader spectrum of antifungal action than the imidazole-containing compounds. It has a significantly better safety profile when compared to amphotericin B and ketoconazole.

Chemical Structure: (Fig. 4.16)

Chemical Name:

2-(2,4-difluorophenyl)-1,3-di(1*H*-1,2,4-triazol-1-yl)propan -2-ol

Mechanism of Action

Fluconazole interferes with the conversion of lanosterol to ergosterol. Ergosterol, the prime sterol constituent, is present in yeast and fungal cell membranes. This interaction is caused by the azole attached to fungal cytochrome P_{450}. This enzyme is responsible for the demethylation step required for 14α-methylsterol conversion to ergosterols. The accumulation of 14-methylsterols and reduced membrane fluidity is

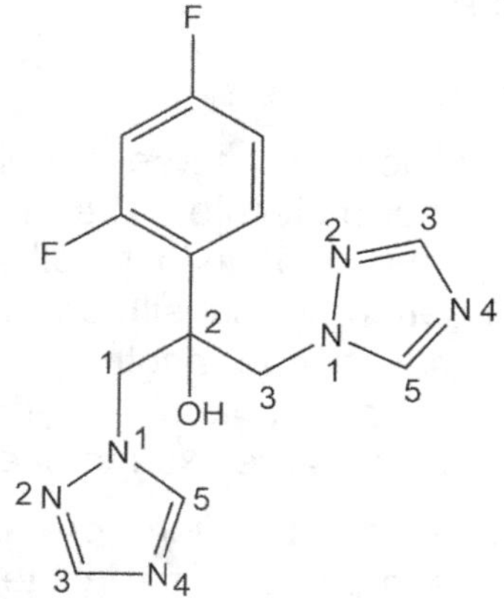

Fig. 4.16 Chemical structure of Fluconazole.

believed to produce a decrease in membrane-bound key enzyme activity with subsequent increases in free fatty acids. The permeability of the fungal membrane is disrupted as a result of this.

Fluconazole interacts with 14α-demethylase, a cytochrome P_{450} enzyme that catalyzes the conversion of lanosterol to ergosterol. It inhibits the formation of ergosterol, which is an important component of the fungal cell membrane, by increasing cellular permeability. Other activities of the drug include preventing endogenous respiration and fungal growth. It's also crucial to remember that fungi produce more methyl sterols in tandem with the loss of sterols. These sterols are the primary source of fluconazole's fungistatic activity.

Uses

1. It is used to treat a variety of fungal illnesses, including candidiasis, blastomycosis, coccidiodomycosis, histoplasmosis, dermatophytosis, and pityriasis versicolor.

2. It is employed to prevent candidiasis in those individuals at high risk, such as those who have undergone an organ transplant, premature neonates, or people with low blood neutrophil levels.

3. It is given either orally or intravenously.

4.3.11 Naftifine hydrochloride

Historical Background

Naftin (naftifine hydrochloride) is an allylamine antifungal that is used to treat tinea infections on the skin. The US FDA approved naftifine cream, 1%, for the first time on February 29, 1988.

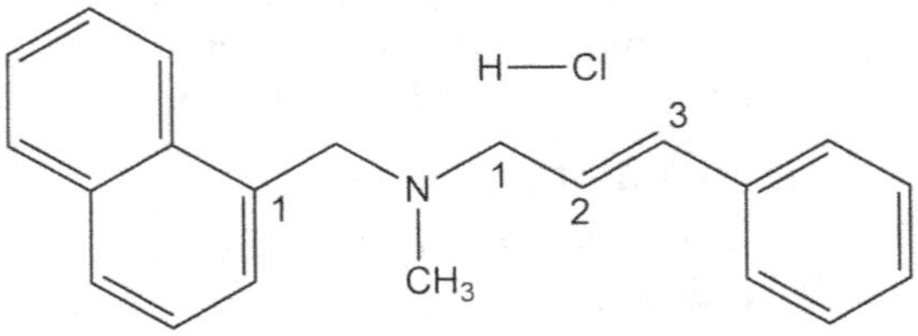

Fig. 4.17 Chemical Structure of Naftifine hydrochloride.

It has been demonstrated to have high *in vitro* antifungal activity against dermatophytes and to be an effective topical drug for the treatment of *tinea cruris*, *tinea corporis*, and *tinea pedis*.

Chemical Structure: (Fig. 4.17)

Chemical Name:

(*E*)-N-methyl-*N*-(naphthalen-1-ylmethyl)-3-phenylprop-2-en-1-amine hydrochloride

Structure-Activity Relationship

A. Changes to the Naphthalene System

1. Substituents in position 4 of the naphthalene nucleus, such as $-CH_3$, $-Cl$, or $-OCH_3$, produce a slight loss of activity *in vitro* and *in vivo*. The unfavorable effect of a $-CH_3O$ group in position 6 and notably in position 2 is substantially more pronounced. Only a mildly active analogue with $-OH$ in position 2 exists.

2. The replacement of a condensed heterocyclic ring system for naphthyl resulted in *in vitro* active compounds. The benzo[b]furan and chromene rings for naphthyl have reduced activity.

B. Changes at the Amino Group

1. For maximum activity, the amino group must be tertiary. The quaternary compound is inactive. The size of the alkyl group appears to be limited between C^1 and C^2 because the *N*-ethyl derivative is the only such analogue that is still highly active *in vitro* and *in vivo*. The *N*-isopropyl and *N*-allyl compounds exhibit no antifungal action. The analogues of *N*-cyclohexyl, *N*-phenyl, and *N*-benzyl are devoid of action.

2. The insertion of a methyl group between naphthalene's carbon atoms and nitrogen's carbon atoms is tolerated without producing significant activity loss. However, the presence of a methyl group between the double bond and the nitrogen is unfavorable to biological activity.

3. When the amino function was replaced with a thioether, sulfoxide, or sulfone group, antimycotic action was not observed.

C. Changes at the Double Bond

1. The *cis* isomer of the compound is the prime structural alteration at this site that retains significant antimycotic efficacy *in vitro* and *in vivo*. Compounds

containing a triple bond, cyclopropane ring, $-CH_2C=O$, or one less carbon, $-C=O$ or $-CH_2$, exhibit active compounds, although only very weakly. In the absence of the double bond, the analogue with $-CH_2CHOH$ is inactive.

D. Changes at the Phenyl Ring

1. Analogues containing fluorine at positions 2 and 4 of the phenyl rings have antimycotic properties comparable to Naftifine. The 2-Cl and 4-Cl counterparts, as well as the 4-methyl derivative, are slightly less active. In contrast to its efficacy on the naphthalene system, a 4-methoxy substituent in the phenyl ring loses much of its antimycotic activity.

2. The substitution of a monocyclic heteroaromatic ring system for the phenyl ring produces excellent results with the 2- and 3-thiophene analogues, and a lesser effect with the furan derivative. Polar heterocycles, such as N-methyl pyrrole or pyridine, have a significant negative impact on biological function. The use of 1-naphthyl instead of phenyl resulted in an almost complete loss of activity.

3. Cyclohexane compounds and cyclohexenes with the double bond in position 3 are not appropriate phenyl replacements. However, when the cyclohexenyl group is conjugated, a highly active molecule is formed. This molecule is at least as effective as naftifine *in vitro* and on topical treatment in the guinea pig dermatophytosis model.

4. The phenyl ring is rendered inactive by the substitution of -H, $-CH_3$, -CN, $-CH_2OH$, and -COOH. *In vitro*, carboxylic ester analogues are very active, but not *in vivo*.

Mechanism of Action

Naftifine acts as an antifungal by inhibiting squalene 2,3-epoxidase, a crucial enzyme in fungus' ergosterol production. The fungus typically converts squalene to ergosterol. Ergosterol is a sterol found in fungal membranes that is necessary for optimal cell growth and function. Because the enzyme is inhibited, there is a lack of ergosterol and an accumulation of squalene. Due to a decrease in phospholipid and glycoprotein synthesis as well as membrane breakdown, an excess of squalene causes cell death. Naftifine has fungicidal and fungistatic properties against dermatophytes and *Candida* species. It can be fungicidal against *Candida spp.* at higher concentrations. Both gram-+ve and gram-ve bacteria are susceptible to naftifine. It does not inhibit the synthesis of human sterols.

Uses

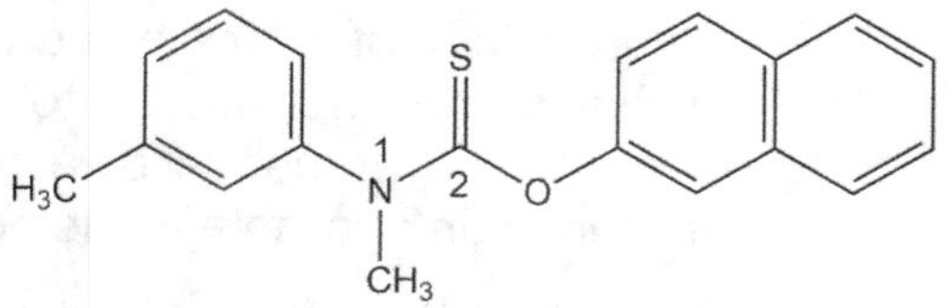

1. It is only allowed to be used externally and superficially as a broad-spectrum anti-dermatophytes and anti-candida infection drug.

Fig. 4.18 Chemical structure of Tolnaftate.

2. The most common application of naftifine is to treat skin tinea infections.

3. It's available in a variety of forms, including cream, powder, spray, and liquid aerosol.

4. It is used in fungal infections like athlete's foot, Pityriasis Versicolor infections, ringworm, and superficial dermatophyte therapy.

4.3.12 Tolnaftate

Historical Background

Tolnaftate is a thiocarbamate. In 1965, Japan's Nippon Soda Company, Ltd., revealed a series of naphthiomates exhibiting antifungal activity. Their research also found that the most promising molecule in the series was O-2-naphthyl m, N-dimethyl-thiocarbanilate (tolnaftate).

It is a topical antifungal drug used to treat a variety of dermatophytes and Microsporum species that can cause infectious illnesses such as *Tinea pedis* (athlete's foot), *Tinea cruris* (jock itch), and *Tinea capitis* (body ringworm).

It does not affect *Candida albicans*, gram-ve, or gram-+ve bacteria. This drug is ineffective in the treatment of fungal infections of the hair and nails when used alone.

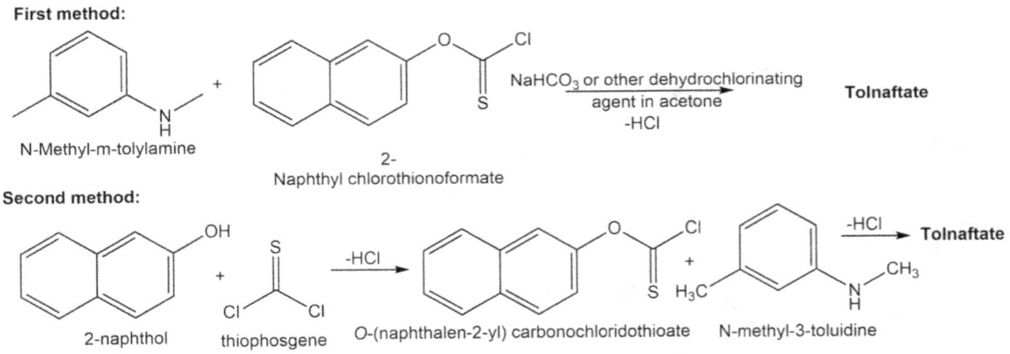

Fig. 4.19 Synthesis of Tolnaftate.

Chemical Structure: (Fig. 4.18)

Chemical Name: O-(naphthalen-2-yl) methyl(m-tolyl)carbamothioate

Synthesis:

First method: (Fig. 4.19)

1. It is prepared by combining N-methyl-m-tolylamine with 2-naphthyl chlorothionoformate in acetone with sodium bicarbonate or another dehydro-chlorinating agent.

2. The finished product is purified by the recrystallization of ethanol.

Second method: (Fig. 4.19)

1. It is prepared by reacting equimolar amounts of 2-naphthol with thiophosgene to get a thiophosgene monosubstituted product.

2. To obtain the desired final product, the intermediate product is treated with N-methyl-3-toluidine.

Mechanism of Action

Tolnaftate acts as a squalene epoxidase inhibitor, preventing squalene from being converted to 2,3-oxidosqualene. As a result, it causes ergosterol deficits and toxic sterol accumulation within the cell membrane. It has been demonstrated that raising squalene levels is harmful, causing cell membrane permeability and, as a result, altering cellular organization. However, this family of antifungal drugs has only a minor effect on the most common *Candida* species and is only effective against dermatophytes.

Uses

It is used to treat or prevent superficial dermatophyte infections and pityriasis versicolor by applying it topically as a solution, powder, or cream.

Structure-activity relationship of the antifungal drug (azole compounds):

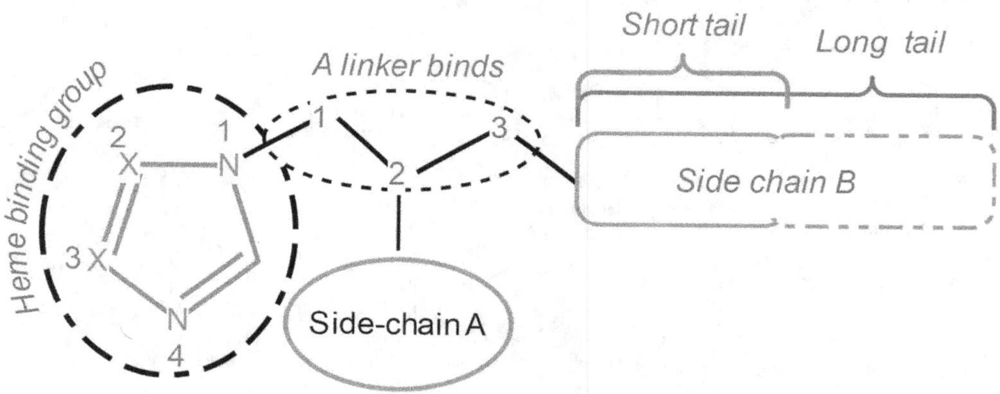

Fig. 4.20 Common structural model of azole.

The structural model of all azole drugs is the same: a heme binding group, a three-atom linker, side-chain A, and side-chain B. (Fig. 4.20)

Heme binding group:

1. This ring is required for the azole group's antifungal activity. In the absence of any substitutions that bind to the linker with N^1 atoms, The active site iron is oriented vertically with respect to the porphyrin (a class of heterocyclic macrocycle organic compounds) plane.

2. The basicity of heteroaromatic nitrogen-containing rings has little bearing on the azole structure's inhibitory efficacy, but it is directly linked to liver damage and drug-drug interactions.

The three-atom linker (1, 2, 3):

1. This three-atom form creates a specific spacing between different arms of structure, resulting in increased potency.

2. Except in topical treatments like clotrimazole analogues and vinyl imidazole derivations, the linker group's first atom number 1 in azole structures is usually carbon and has no modifications.

3. Chirality is critical for the antifungal action of the linker's atoms 2 and 3, which are mainly carbon. The presence of an oxygen atom as a hydroxyl group on C-2 has various advantages, including increased potency due to an indirect H-bond with the active site via water molecules, improved pharmacokinetic characteristics, and water solubility, and more stable metabolism.

4. The addition of a methyl group to C-3 could make it more effective against moulds. The chiral form has a unique conformation in which side-chain B binds to side-chain A and the methyl group fills the lanosterol C-13 binding pocket.

5. Other substitutions with the required activity include CH (double bond with C-3) and two methyl or two F (non-chiral C-3). However, C-3 becomes oxygen, sulfur, or NR_2 (oxime and hydrazine) in some of the first generation structures (miconazole and its derivations), which maintains antifungal activity as well as conformational restriction of structures with a ring on C-2 and C-3, such as dioxalene (itraconazole or ketoconazole). However, they do not enhance potency.

Side chain A:

1. The inhibitory effect of side-chain A in the structure, which is usually a halogenated phenyl, appears to be positioned in the same hydrophobic tunnel as the 17-alkyl chain of lanosterol.

2. Substitutions of the phenyl ring in all carbons are permitted, except groups bigger than chlorine in C-2 and C-6, which have adverse steric conflicts and reduce inhibitor binding affinity at the active site. The fluorine atoms in C-2 and C-4 have a higher potency.

Side chain B:

1. The antifungal activity varies depending on the type of linker in the side chain B to C-3.

2. According to studies, ether, thioether, carbon ($-CH_2-,-CHR,-CR_2$),$-NR_2,-SO_2$, heteroaromatic, or hetroaliphatic (e.g., piperazine, piperidine) rings are well tolerated and effective links. However, amide, ester, and NHR rings reduce antifungal activity.

3. The size of the side chain divides azole drugs into two groups: short-tail and long-tail structures.

(i) For short tail structures

These structures, such as fluconazole, and its derivative compounds, may or may not have minor substitutions in the linker. Hydrophobic, electron-rich, and electron-withdrawing groups (e.g., halogens, –CN, and halogenated heteroaromatic rings) boost potency at the ortho and para positions of phenyl or heteroaromatic rings connected to the linker. Meta-position substitutions reduce antifungal activity.

For Long tail structures

In these structures, like itraconazole and its derivatives, the para-position of a phenyl ring could have a week H-bond acceptor substitution, preferably oxygen (ether, carbonyl) and nitrogen (NR^2), that forms an H-bond with some residue in the active site and also binds to another bulky aromatic group with possible steric and Van der waal's interactions. In the case of itraconazole-like drugs, the addition of a triazole-3-one group may improve pharmacokinetics. This region of the active site has enough room for structural changes to improve the efficacy, physicochemical properties, and pharmacokinetics of targeted antifungal agents.

Classification of azole compounds

There is approximately 40 azole-containing compounds. They are categorized into more than three generations based on what is commercially available.

(i)   First generation azole compounds: Ex. clotrimazole, miconazole, butoconazole, econazole, oxiconazole, tioconazole, luliconazole

(ii) Second generation azole compounds: Ex. ketoconazole, fluconazole, terconazole, Itraconazole,

(iii) Third generation azole compounds: Ex. voriconazole, posaconazole, efinaconazole

(iv) Fourth generation azole compounds: Ex. oteseconazole, quilseconazole

4.4 Anti-protozoal Agents

Diseases related to parasite infections involve a wide range of illnesses, some of which are rather prevalent and others of which are largely unknown to the general community. Some protozoa are parasitic and can cause disease in humans, animals, and plants. Protozoal infections affect an estimated 1.5 billion people worldwide, with malaria (*Plasmodium* spp.) accounting for 500 million clinical cases each year.

Protozoal infections occur around the globe and are a prime cause of morbidity and mortality in several areas, including Africa and the Southeast Asia region.

Other major human infectious diseases caused by protozoans include amebiasis (*Entamoeba histolytica*), giardiasis, babesiosis, Chagas disease (*Trypanosoma cruzi*), leishmaniasis, African sleeping sickness (*Trypanosoma brucei gambiense* and *Trypanosoma brucei rhodesiense*), toxoplasmosis (*Toxoplasma gondii*), trichomoniasis, pneumocystosis (also considered to be fungal infections) and cutaneous leishmaniasis (*Leishmania spp.*) are all classified as parasitic infections. Helminth infections (worms) are parasitic infections. Any one of the three types of helminths—nematodes, cestodes, or trematodes—could be the cause.

Antiprotozoal drugs cure protozoan diseases. They are single-celled eukaryotic parasitic organisms.

4.5 Antiamoebic Drugs

Entamoeba histolytica protozoa, which causes amebiasis, most frequently infects the large intestine and further damages the lungs, liver, brain, and other organs. The gastrointestinal system is susceptible to an attack without causing any clinical symptoms, with moderate symptoms (diarrhea, cramps, meteorism (excess gas)) or signs of acute amoebic dysentery, such as bloody diarrhea, vomiting, fever, and dehydration. The protozoan microorganism *E. histolytica* can cause liver mortality, amoebic hepatitis, and lung abscesses in other organs. There have been reports of heart injury (resulting in pericarditis) and brain damage (resulting in a brain abscess).

The disease affects about 10% of the world's population. In tropical and subtropical areas, it is the most severe. In most cases, the disease is related to poor economic and sanitary conditions.

Occurrence

1. The microbes are spread from person to person via amoebic cysts, a type of amoebic life in which the protozoa have the greatest resistance to external effects.

2. Infection is caused by cysts that are commonly found in contaminated food and drink. Because stomach fluids have a negligible effect on the cysts, they travel into the intestines and mature into trophozoites, which attack the mucous membranes of the intestines, are absorbed, and can spread to other organs.

3. They reproduce, encyst (become enclosed in a cyst), and eventually pass into the environment, completing the cycle. Trophozoites can exist in a host without causing illness or symptoms.

4. Trophozoites can transform into pathogenic forms that penetrate tissues and cause a variety of local and systemic symptoms. Amoebic dysentery can result from trophozoites invading the gut wall and producing ulceration.

5. After a long resting phase, trophozoites may migrate to other tissues, particularly the liver, where they can cause inflammation.

Classification

Amoebicide	Chemical Class	Examples
Luminal	Arsenical compounds	Carbarsone, bismuth glycolylarsanilate
	Hydroxyquinoline derivatives	Chiniofon, clioquinol, iodoquinol
	Dichloroacetamide derivatives	Diloxanide furoate, clefamide, etofamide
	Benzylamine derivatives	Teclozan, chlorbetamide, chlorphenoxamine
	Antibiotic amoebicides	Tetracycline, oxytetracycline, chlortetracycline, erythromycin, paromomycin, and fumagillin
Tissue or systemic	Emetine and its derivatives	Emetine hydrochloride, emetine bismuth iodide, dehydroemetine dihydrochloride
	Aminoquinoline	Chloroquine
	Thiazole derivative	Niridazole
	Nitroimidazoles	Metronidazole, tinidazole, ornidazole secnidazole, nimorazole
	Nithrothiazole	Salicylamide Nitazoxanide
Mixed	Nitroimidazoles	Metronidazole

Antiamoebic drugs (amoebicides) are classified as luminal, systemic, or mixed.

Luminal amoebicides are only effective against amoebae in the gastrointestinal tract. To treat asymptomatic (no symptoms) or mild intestinal amoebiasis, it can be used alone or in combination with a systemic or mixed amoebicide.

Systemic amoebicides are only effective against invasive amoebiasis. They were once commonly used to treat severe amoebic dysentery or hepatic ulcers but are now rarely used.

Mixed amoebicides are effective against both intestinal and systemic amoebiasis.

Trichomoniasis

The flagellated protozoan *Trichomonas vaginalis* is the causative agent of trichomoniasis. Humans are contaminated with this parasite, which causes vaginitis in women and urethritis in men. Sexual contact is the main cause of the infection. Metronidazole or related nitroimidazole drugs are used for trichomonal infections.

In the meantime, many nitroimidazoles were studied for trichomonacidal activity after the discovery of azomycin. Thus, a new chemical compound known as metronidazole was developed. Metronidazole has a wide range of antiprotozoal and antibacterial properties. In the treatment of trichomoniasis and giardiasis, it has become a routine medicine.

Metronidazole's 1-(2-hydroxyethyl) side chain is easily oxidised in the body. Trichomonacides such as tinidazole, nimorazole, and ornidazole have been developed by replacing this side chain. They work similarly to metronidazole in terms of action and use.

4.5.1 Metronidazole

Historical Background

✓ Metronidazole is one of the few antibacterial drugs that was designed to treat a protozoan parasite. Earlier, *Streptomyces spp.* extracts were tested at the Rhone-Poulenc laboratory in France for their ability to inhibit the growth of *Trichomonas vaginalis*, a pathogen that causes vaginal itching.

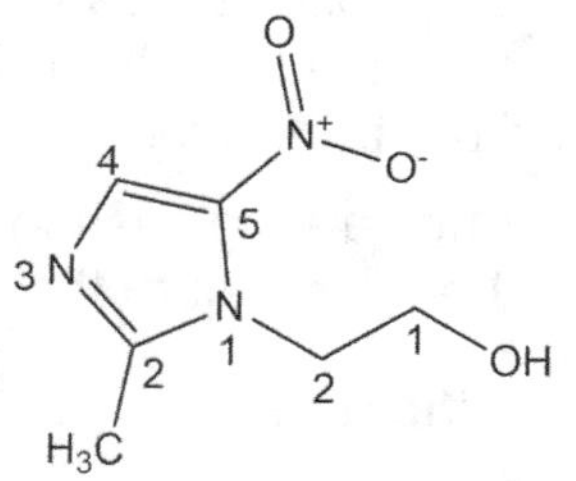

Fig. 4.21 Chemical structure of Metronidazole.

✓ Beginning in 1959, metronidazole, a synthetic derivative of azomycin (a nitroimidazole compound), was used to treat chronic *trichomonad* infections. In 1966, metronidazole was found to be effective against *E. histolytica*, the bacteria that causes amebic dysentery and liver ulcers.

✓ *Giardia lamblia* (also known as *G. duodenalis*) was first identified as a cause of malabsorption and epigastric pain in the 1970s and was treated with metronidazole.

Chemical Structure: (Fig. 4.21)

Chemical Name: 2-(2-methyl-5-nitro-1H-imidazol-1-yl)ethan-1-ol

Synthesis

1. It is synthesised by reacting it with ethane-1,2-diamine and acetone to produce N, N'-(ethane-1,2-diyl)diacetamide.

2. The resulting product is processed with calcium oxide (CaO) to produce 2-methyl-4,5-dihydro-1*H*-imidazole, an intermediate product.

3. After that, the resulting product is reduced with Raney nickel to produce 2-methyl-1*H*-imidazole.

4. Furthermore, the intermediate product is nitrated to produce 2-methyl-5-nitro-1*H*-imidazole.

5. Then, it's treated with 2-chloroethanol or ethylenoxide to produce the desired metronidazole product. (Fig. 4.22)

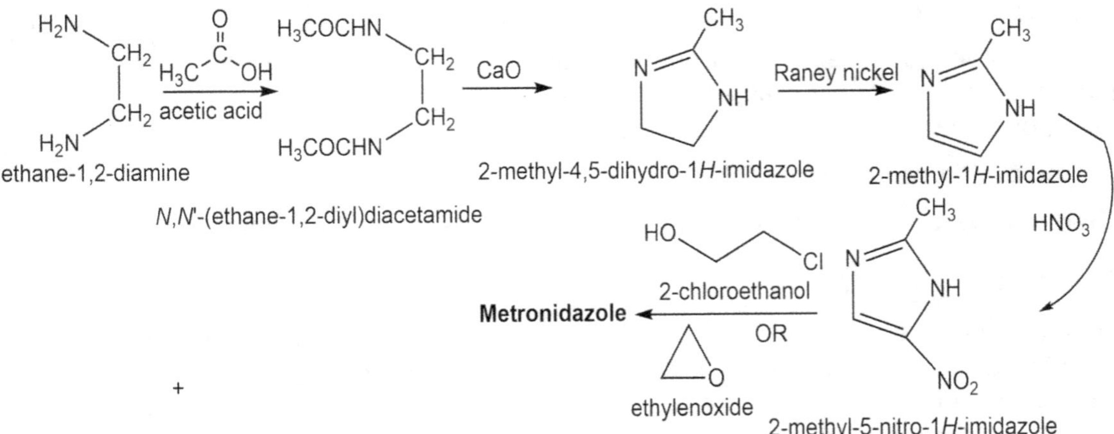

Fig. 4.22 Synthesis of Metronidazole.

Mechanism of Action

Metronidazole enters organisms and inhibits protein synthesis by interacting with DNA, causing the helical structure of DNA to be lost and DNA strands to be broken. As a result, it induces the cell death of sensitive organisms.

Metronidazole's mode of action is a four-step procedure. The first step is for pathogens to enter the organism by diffusing them across cell membranes. The second step includes changing the molecular structure of pyruvate-ferredoxin oxidoreductase by a reduction process. Intracellular transport proteins initiate this process. Metronidazole reduction produces a concentration gradient in the cell, promoting drug uptake and cytotoxic free radical production. Step three involves cytotoxic particles interacting with host cell DNA. This results in DNA strand breaking and DNA helix instability. The breakdown of cytotoxic compounds is the fourth step.

Uses

1. It is the first-line treatment for amebiasis, vaginal trichomoniasis, trichomonad urethritis in males, lambliosis, and amebic dysentery.

2. It is used to treat trichomoniasis, giardiasis, and several infections caused by obligate anaerobic bacteria.

4.5.2 Tinidazole

Historical Background

Tinidazole is a protozoan infection treatment drug. In 1967, it was first used in clinical practice. The US FDA licensed it to treat protozoal illnesses such as trichomoniasis, giardiasis, intestinal amoebiasis, and amoebic liver ulcers.

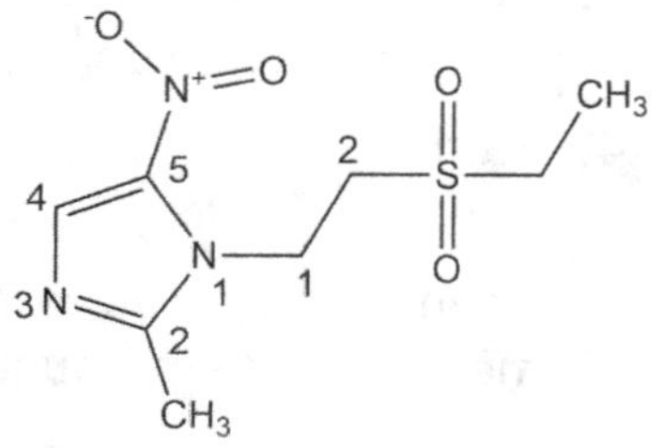

Fig. 4.23 Chemical structure of Tinidazole.

It is commonly used as a treatment for a variety of anaerobic, amoebic, and bacterial illnesses. It belongs to the nitroimidazole class of compounds.

Chemical Structure: (Fig.4.23)

Chemical Name: 1-(2-(ethylsulfonyl)ethyl)-2-methyl-5-nitro-1*H*-imidazole

Mechanism of Action

Tinidazole is an antibacterial and antiprotozoal drug. *Trichomonas* cell extracts reduced the nitro-group of tinidazole. The antiprotozoal activity may be due to the free nitro-radicals formed by this reduction process. An *in vitro* study finds chemically reduced tinidazole. Under the reduction process, it produces nitrites and damages pure bacterial DNA. Furthermore, the drug caused DNA base alterations in bacterial cells and DNA strand breaks in mammalian cells.

It becomes bactericidal only after being transformed into a toxic intermediate metabolite that inhibits bacterial DNA synthesis and breaks existing DNA. The oxidoreductase enzyme of anaerobes and protozoa changes these drugs into harmful derivatives. However, this process does not occur in human cells or aerobic bacteria. These drugs have the same effect on both dividing and nondividing cells.

Uses

✓ It has been used to treat amebic liver ulcerations, trichomoniasis, lambliosis, acute ulcerative gingivitis, and post-operative anaerobic infections.

✓ It is used to treat metronidazole-resistant *Trichomonas spp.* It is given in the treatment of bacterial and trichomonal vaginitis.

✓ It's used to treat almost every protozoan infection.

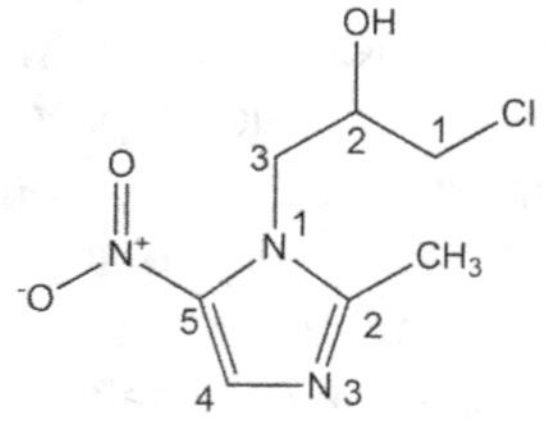

Fig. 4.24 Chemical structure of Ornidazole.

4.5.3 Ornidazole

Historical Background

It was initially developed to treat trichomoniasis before being discovered to have anti-protozoan and anti-anaerobic-bacterial properties.

It is a synthetic nitroimidazole compound. It treats infections caused by anaerobic bacteria and protozoa.

Chemical Structure: (Fig. 4.24)

Chemical Name: 1-chloro-3-(2-methyl-5-nitro-1*H*-imidazol-1-yl) propane-2-ol

Mechanism of Action

During passive absorption into a bacterial cell, the nitro group of ornidazole is converted to an amine group by ferredoxin-type redox mechanisms. The fundamental component responsible for killing bacteria is believed to be the development of redox intermediate intracellular metabolites. Anaerobic bacteria such as *Peplostreptococcus*, *Clostridium*, *Bacteroides fragilis*, *Porphyromonas gingivalis*, and *Fusobacterium*, as well as protozoa such as *Entamoeba histolytica*, *Trichomonas vaginitis*, and *Giardia lamblia*, are all susceptible to the drug.

Uses

1. It treats infections caused by anaerobic bacteria and protozoa.
2. It's used to treat infections of the vaginal, urinary tract, and gastrointestinal tract.
3. It's used to treat amebiasis, giardiasis, and trichomonas infections in the intestine.

Antiamoebic Drugs (Amoebicides)

Classification:

A. Natural product amoebicides: Ex. emetine, dehydroemetine, berberine

B. Synthetic amoebicides: Ex. quiniodochlor (clioquinol), diiodohydroxyquinoline (**iodoquinol**), halquinol, **diloxanide furoate**

C. Antibiotic: Ex. erythromycin, paromomycin, and tetracyclines

4.5.4 Diloxanide Furoate

Historical Background

Diloxanide furoate is a substituted acetanilide that was discovered in 1956. Since its introduction in 1960, this drug has been frequently used to treat asymptomatic or minimally symptomatic people who have *E. histolytica* cysts.

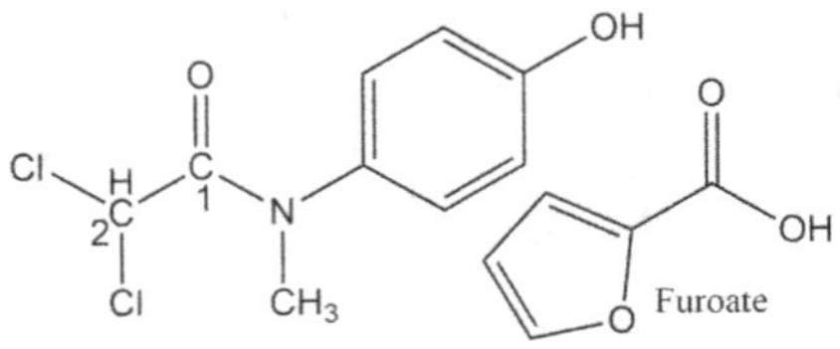

Fig. 4.25 Chemical structure of Diloxanide Furoate.

Diloxanide furoate is a luminal amebicide whose primary manifestation is the clearance of *E. histolytica* cysts. However, paromomycin is the preferred drug for such types of infections. The drug is not effective in either amoebic colitis or extraintestinal infections because it has little or no activity outside the intestinal lumen.

Chemical Structure: (Fig. 4.25)

Chemical Name: 2,2-dichloro-*N*-(4-hydroxyphenyl)-*N*-methylacetamide

Mechanism of Action

Diloxanide inhibits the formation of cysts in *E. histolytica* trophozoites. It shares certain structural similarities with chloramphenicol, implying that it similarly inhibits protein synthesis. The drug is hydrolyzed in the gut by bacterial and gastrointestinal esterases. The drug is converted to diloxanide and furoic acid. After that, it is quickly absorbed, converted to glucuronide, and eliminated in the urine. In the gut lumen, the unabsorbed component of the compound serves as an active antiamebic agent and is excreted in the feces.

Uses

1. It's used to treat *E. histolytica*, the amebiasis carrier. It is given in cases of asymptomatic or mild amebiasis infection.

2. It is used to treat a variety of forms of intestinal amebiasis infections.

3. It is used in invasive amebiasis in conjunction with nitroimidazoles to eradicate luminal cysts.

4. After therapy with metronidazole or tinidazole, it is given to those who are symptomatic. Diloxanide furoate is more effective than diloxanide because it produces higher intestinal concentrations.

4.5.5 Iodoquinol

Historical Background

Iodoquinol, also known as diiodohydroxyquin, is a halogenated oxyquinoline. It is effective against *E. histolytica*, *Dientamoeba fragilis*, *Blastocystis hominis*, and *Balantidium coli*.

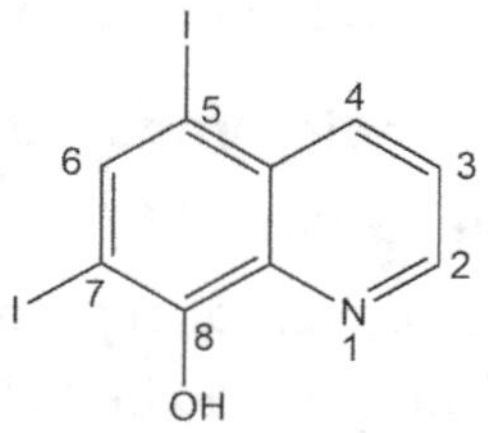

Fig. 4.26 Chemical structure of Iodoquinol.

Chiniofon (8-hydroxy-7-iodoquinoline-5-sulphonic acid) was developed as a result of research into the antibacterial properties of halogenated 8-hydroxyquinolines. Later structural modifications resulted in the production of several related iodinated phenols. Following that, these compounds' amoebic activity was discovered, and several of them (quiniodochlor (clioquinol), diiodohydroxyquinoline (iodoquinol), and halquinol) were proven to be beneficial as luminal amoebicides.

Chemical Structure: (Fig. 4.26)

Chemical Name: 5,7-diiodoquinolin-8-ol

Mechanism of Action

It is amebicidal against *E. histolytica* trophozoites and cysts in the intestinal lumen.

The ability of halogenated 8-hydroxyquinolines to chelate metals from their local surroundings, which may deprive organisms of vital metallic nutrition, is thought to be their mechanism of action. The particular mechanism by which iodoquinol exerts its antibacterial effect remains largely unknown. By chelating essential metal cofactors such as copper, manganese, magnesium, and zinc, they block the RNA-dependent DNA polymerase involved in reverse DNA strand synthesis and RNA synthesis.

Uses

- ✓ It is an amebocide that is effective against *E. histolytica* cysts and trophozoites in the intestinal lumen.

- ✓ II is used to treat intestinal amoebiasis alone or in conjunction with metronidazole.

- ✓ It is used to treat people who have asymptomatic cyst shedding or as an adjunct to existing treatments for invasive diseases.

- ✓ It has also been employed in the treatment of *Blastocystis hominis* and is also effective against *Giardia lamblia* and *T. vaginalis*, but it is usually combined with other drugs.

SAR of Anti-Amoebic Drugs

1. The anti-amoebic activity of (-)-emetine alkaloid is stereospecific. Only one synthetic, (±)-2, 3 dihydroemetine, has anti-amoebic action comparable to natural (-)-emetine.

2. Antiprotozoal activity has been discovered in nitroimidazole (metronidazole) derivative compounds.

3. 8-hydroxyquinolines (clioquinol, iodoquinol) with halogen substitution at C-5 and 7 have amoebic action.

4. Quinoline with an amino group substitution has antimalarial and anti-amoebic properties.

5. 2-phenylthiazolidine-1, 1-dioxides were also observed to be effective against protozoan parasites.

6. The anti-amoebic effect is attributed to the benzyl acetamide derivative group (chlorbetamide).

7. Anti-amoebic action has been established by halogenating acetamide (Diloxanide) and organometallic compounds.

Trypanocides

An antiprotozoal agent that kills trypanosome parasites is known as a trypanocidal agent.

Trypanosomiasis is a term used to describe a range of disorders caused by parasites of the genus *Trypanosoma*. The parasites that cause the two main types of the disease are

(a) African trypanosomiasis: occurs in tropical Africa. Tsetse flies of the genus *Glossinia* spread the disease, caused by the *T. brucei* subspecies.

(b) American trypanosomiasis, or Chagas' disease: occurs in Central and South

America. *T. cruzi* causes the disease, which is spread by blood-sucking triatomid bugs. The heart is the most commonly damaged organ in acute Chagas' illness, but other tissues can also be affected.

Human trypanosomal illness is classified into two types:

(a) Rhodesian: *T. brucei* rhodesiense causes a progressive and usually deadly type of illness with early central nervous system involvement.

(b) Gambian: Sleeping sickness is caused by *T. brucei gambiense*; the disease is more persistent (occurs over a prolonged period) and involves the central nervous system later.

Classification

(i) Dyestuffs and Suramin: Ex. suramin sodium

(ii) Arsenicals: Ex. atoxyl, melarsen

(iii) Diamidines: Ex. stilbamidine, **pentamidine**, propamidine

(iv) Nitrofurans: Ex. nitrofurazone

(v) Nitroimidazoles: Ex. benznidazole

(vi) Miscellaneous: Ex. **eflornithine**

4.5.6 Pentamidine isethionate

Historical Background

Pentamidine was first synthesised in the late 1930s and was only used on a limited basis for the treatment of infections caused by *Trypanosoma gambiense* and *Pneumocystis carinii* between 1967 and 1984.

Pentamidine was first used to treat African trypanosomiasis in 1937 and leishmaniasis in 1940. It was registered as pentamidine mesylate in 1950. It was a reintroduced to the market in isethionate form in 1984. Its efficacy against *Pneumocystis jirovecii* was established in 1987.

Chemical Structure: (Fig. 4.27)

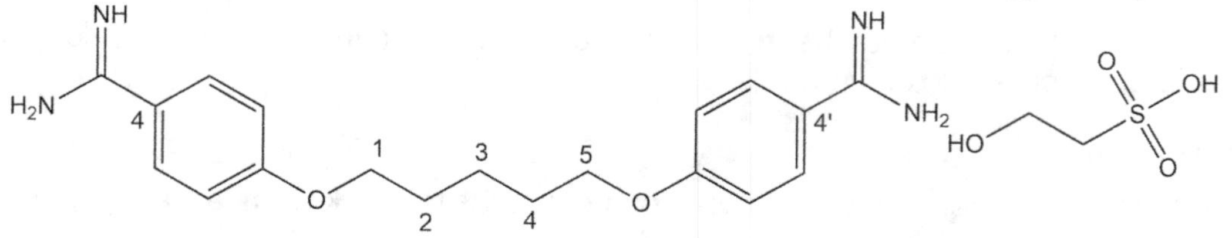

Fig.4.27 Chemical structure of Pentamidine isethionate.

Chemical Name:

4,4'-(pentane-1,5-diylbis(oxy))dibenz -imidamide 2-hydroxyethane-1-sulfonate;
4,4-[pentane-1,5-diylbis-(oxy)]dibenz -amidinedi(2-hydroxyethanesulphonate

Mechanism of Action

Trypanosomes have a defective polyamine synthesis pathway. They are unable to biosynthesize purines from the beginning. They also have the kinetoplast, which is a vast network of mitochondrial DNA. Pentamidine may compete with polyamines for nucleic acid binding. It may bind more selectively to kinetoplast DNA. Kinetoplast DNA has a greater adenosine-thymidine content than nuclear DNA, which could be the site and explanation for preferred kinetoplast DNA binding. Pentamidine inhibits thymidylate synthetase, which is found in a variety of trypanosomatids, raising the possibility of therapeutic action via interfering with DNA biosynthesis.

It specifically binds to the DNA of the *T. cruzi* parasite. It has also been demonstrated to inhibit topoisomerase in *P. jirovecii*. This causes *Trypanosoma* DNA to be split into two strands.

It has been claimed that the mechanism of action of pentamidine varies depending on the organism. It is thought to work by interfering with the essential functions of DNA, RNA, phospholipids, and protein synthesis in various respects. It forms a cross-link between two adenines of adenine-thymine-rich portions of *Trypanosoma* parasite DNA. The drug also inhibits topoisomerase enzymes in the mitochondria of *Pneumocystis jirovecii*. The drug also inhibits type II topoisomerase in the mitochondria of the *Trypanosoma* parasite. This inhibition causes breakage and unfolding of the parasite's circular mitochondrial DNA. The interaction with DNA, or nucleotides, and their derivatives may be responsible for the trypanocidal effect.

Uses

1. The drug has antifungal and antiprotozoal properties. However, it is mostly used to treat *Pneumocystis carinii pneumonia* (PCP).

2. It is used to treat African trypanosomiasis in its early stages.

3. It's also used to treat leishmaniasis (kala-azar), and babesiosis. It's especially useful for people who haven't responded to antimonial therapy.

4. It is also used to prevent and treat infections caused by *Pneumocystis carinii* and PCP in HIV patients.

4.5.7 Eflornithine

Historical Background

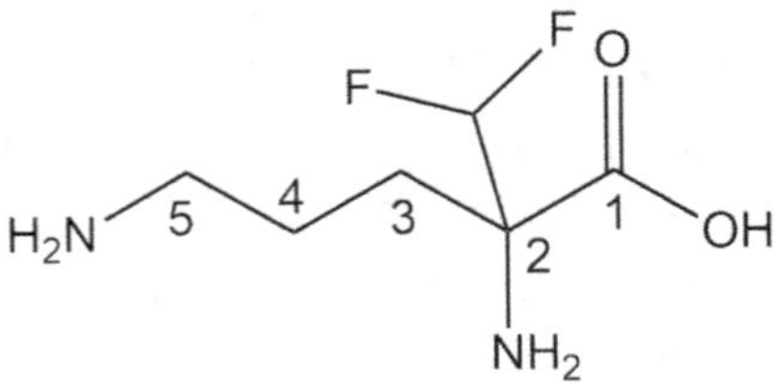

In the late 1970s, the Merrell Dow Research Institute produced eflornithine for cancer treatment. However, it was proven to be unsuccessful in treating cancer. Interestingly, it was discovered in the treatment of African trypanosomiasis (sleeping sickness), specifically the West African strain (*Trypanosoma brucei gambiense*).

Fig.4.28 Chemical structure of Eflornithine.

The compound was identified in 1980 as part of a WHO-sponsored study on polyamine metabolism in trypanosomes by **Cyrus Bacchi**.

Chemical Structure: (Fig. 4.28)

Chemical Name:

2,5-diamino-2-(difluoromethyl)pentanoic acid; 2-(difluoromethyl)-DL-ornithine

Mechanism of Action

Eflornithine irreversibly inhibits ornithine decarboxylase, the first enzyme in the production of the polyamines putrescine and spermidine. The parasite's capacity to maintain its redox state and inhibit reactive oxygen intermediates is impaired when polyamine production is disrupted. Polyamines are required for parasite cell division as well. Although the drug has a comparable effect on humans, it selectively affects trypanosomes. This is because they have a low turnover of ornithine decarboxylase. As a result, eflornithine therapy causes a faster polyamine drop.

Difluoromethyl ornithine inhibits ornithine decarboxylase (ODC), a pyridoxal phosphate-dependent enzyme. Evidence suggests that eflornithine alkylation occurs at cysteine in ODC. The alkylation of ODC prevents putrescine, which is the rate-determining step in the production of polyamines. Eflornithine can also regulate mammalian ODC, but because ODC turnover is so fast in mammals, eflornithine has no major side effects.

Uses

- ✓ It has been used as a trypanocide.

- ✓ African trypanosomiasis (sleeping sickness) and excessive facial hair growth in women, *Pneumocystis carnii pneumonia* (PCP), are treated with this drug.

- ✓ Eflornithine is the drug of choice for treating African sleeping sickness caused by *T. brucei* gambiense. It includes individuals with advanced central nervous system disease, either alone or in combination.

4.5.8 Atovaquone

Historical Background

Atovaquone was initially developed as an antimalarial drug. In 1999, Glaxo Wellcome patented the combination of atovaquone and proguanil for the treatment of malaria.

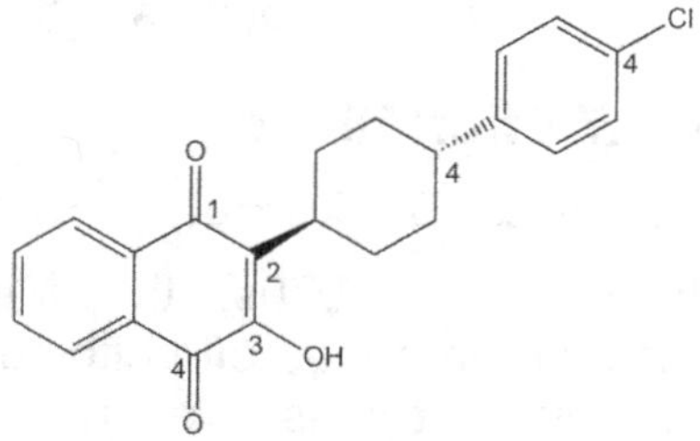

Fig.4.29 Chemical structure of Atovaquone.

Atovaquone is a novel naphthoquinone compound with extensive antiprotozoal activity. It is effective for treating and preventing *Pneumocystis carinii* pneumonia (PCP), as well as for treating and preventing malaria when combined with proguanil. When used with azithromycin, it is also beneficial in the treatment and prevention of babesiosis.

Chemical structure: (Fig. 4.29)

Chemical name:

2-((1r,4r)-4-(4-chlorophenyl)cyclohexyl)-3-hydroxynaphthalene-1,4-dione

Structure Activity Relationship

1. The quinoloid hydroxyl group of atovaquone is shown to be essential for activity. Its replacement with a variety of substituents resulted in a loss of activity.
2. Substitution of the benzenoid ring resulted in a complete or significant loss of activity as well.
3. When the benzenoid ring at C-2 is replaced with an isoalkyl chain, the hydrolapachol compound is produced. The increase in activity was achieved by lengthening the isoalkyl chain at hydrolapachol's C-2 position, but only up to C9.
4. The atovaquone derivative chemical's branched alkyl side chains were twice as potent as their straight-chain or isoalkyl isomers.
5. When the side chain contained an aliphatic or aromatic ring/s at C-2, the maximum number of carbons in the chain associated with optimum activity increased to C10-13.
6. In general, adding double bonds, halogens, or heteroatoms like nitrogen or oxygen to the side chain reduced activity.

Mechanism of Action

Atovaquone is a hydroxynaphthoquinone derivative compound. It specifically inhibits the respiratory chain of protozoan mitochondria at the cytochrome bc1 complex (complex III) by replicating the natural substrate, ubiquinone. The mitochondrial electron transport chain is disrupted, and the mitochondrial membrane potential is disrupted when cytochrome bc1 is inhibited. In humans, atovaquone is effective against all stages of parasites.

Atovaquone's antiparasitic activity is assumed to be due to its ability to block the mitochondrial respiratory chain. It is an inhibitor of ubiquinone reductase, which inhibits the cytochrome bc1 complex. The mitochondrial membrane potential decreases as a result of this process. The *trans* isomer of the chemical is more active than the *cis* isomer, indicating its stereospecific inhibition.

Uses

✓ It is used to treat mild incidences of pneumocystis pneumonia (PCP), but not severe cases.
✓ It's also used to treat *toxoplasmosis*, malaria (when combined with proguanil), and babesiosis (in conjunction with oral azithromycin).

4.6 Anthelmintics

Helminthiasis is the term used for parasitic worm infection. It is one of the most frequent infections and a major public health concern around the world. It affects more than two billion people worldwide. In humans, many worms are parasitic and can cause major health-related problems.

Helminths are distinct from many other parasites in that they multiply outside of the definitive host and can avoid host immune systems. As a result, helminth infections are often chronic, lasting for the duration of the host's life. Helminthiasis is a metazoan infection. The helminths that infect humans are classified into two phyla:

(a) Platyhelminthes (flatworms): Ex. cestode (tapeworms) and trematode (flatworms) are two types of flatworms (flukes or schistosomes)

(b) Aschelminthes (nematodes) (roundworms): Ex. roundworms, hookworms, pinworms, and whipworms

These worms have a cylindrical shape with variations in size, proportion, and structure.

Anthelmintics are drugs that are used to kill parasitic worms or remove them from the affected host. The word "anthelmintic" should not be limited to drugs that work locally to expel worms from the digestive tract. Various forms of worms can infiltrate tissues; therefore, the chemical compounds that are used to treat systemic infections should also be classified as anthelmintics. Anthelmintics are drugs that are used to treat any type of helminthiasis.

Nematode Infections

The zoological organization of nematodes (roundworms) is often higher than that of cestodes or trematodes. Many nematodes are parasitic on humans. The nematodes that mostly infect the intestines may be the first to be considered.

Roundworm (*Ascaris lumbricoides*) affects over a quarter of the world's population. Warm climates are favourable for this parasite. 70-90% of the population in tropical nations may be affected.

Hookworm (*Necator americanus* and *Ancylostoma duodenale*) affects over 20% of the human population. Infection with *N. americanus* is the most common in the United States, whereas infection with *A. duodenale* is seen in other regions of the world.

Whipworm (*Trichuris trichiura*): The infection caused by the parasite can be found all over the world, although it is most common in hot, humid areas. It's common to find it with ascaris and hookworms.

Threadworm, also known as the dwarf threadworm (*Strongyloides stercoralis*), is commonly found in tropical and subtropical areas. They occur with other intestinal helminths.

Pinworm (*Enterobius (Oxyuris) vermicularis*) is most commonly found in school children.

Filarial worms (*Wuchereria bancrofti, Wuchereria (Brugia) malayi,* and *Brugia timori*) are nematodes that primarily infect tissues. Filariasis is a disease caused by this type of parasite. Filariasis is spread primarily by insects. Infection with *W. bancrofti* can be found throughout the tropics, including central Africa, South America, India, China, and Sri Lanka. Other infections caused by filariasis include: *Loa Loa* and *Onchocerca volvulus* are African filarial worm species found in Africa.

Guinea worm (*Dracunculus medinensis*) is a parasite found in Africa and Asia. Infection with *Trichinella spiralis* is common in Europe and the United States. The infection can be contracted by eating raw or undercooked *trichinous* animal flesh.

Pork worm (*Trichinella spiralis*) causes an illness that can affect both the intestine and the whole body. The parasite is the causative agent of the disease trichinosis. It is found in a variety of animals, including rodents, pigs, bears, hyenas, and humans. The worm has long been associated with uncooked pork products.

Classification

A. Chemical

   (i)   Amino-acetonitrile derivatives: Ex. monepantel

   (ii)   Benzimidazoles: Ex. thiabendazole, mebendazole, albendazole, flubendazole

   (iii)   Halogenated salicylanilides: Ex. niclosamide

   (iv)   Imidazothiazoles: Ex. tetramisole

   (v)   Macrocyclic lactones: Ex. ivermectin

   (vi)   Piperazines: Ex. diethylcarbamazine citrate

   (vii)   Pyrazinoisoquinolines: Ex. praziquantel

   (viii)   Spiroindoles: Ex. derquantel

   (ix)   Tetrahydropyrimidines: Ex. pyrantel, morantel

   (x)   Tetrahydroquinolines: Ex. oxamniquine

   (xi)   Miscellaneous: cyclooctadepsipeptides, tribendimidine

B. Based on parasitic infestations:

   (i)   Nematode Infections: antifilarial agents: Ex. diethylcarbamazine citrate, ivermectin

   (ii)   Intestinal nematode infections: Ex. thiabendazole, mebendazole, albendazole

   (iii)   Cestode infection: Ex. niclosamide

   (iv)   Trematode (schistosomiasis) infections: Ex. praziquantel, oxamniquine

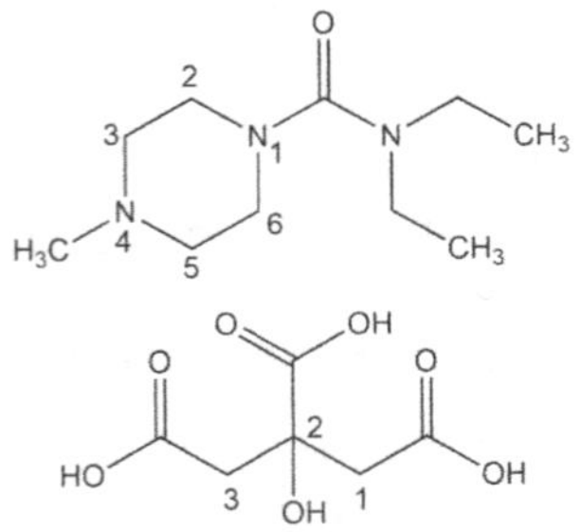

4.6.1 Diethylcarbamazine Citrate

Historical Background

Diethylcarbamazine (DEC) was initially introduced in 1947. It has been found to have high efficacy and safety in the treatment of human lymphatic filariasis. The disease is mostly caused by *Wuchereria bancrofti*.

Fig.4.30 Chemical structure of Diethylcarbamazine citrate.

DEC is remarkably effective as a filaricidal agent. The high prevalence of filariasis among American troops during World War II required the hunt for antifalarial drugs. During the initial tests, piperazine was identified and shown to be effective against nematodes. While the piperazine derivative compound DEC is shown to be effective against microfilaria and filaria.

Chemical Structure: (Fig. 4.30)

Chemical Name:

N,*N*-diethyl-4-methylpiperazine-1-carboxamide   2-hydroxypropane-1,2,3-tricarboxylate; *N*,*N*-Diethyl-4-methylpiperazine-1-carboxamide dihydrogen citrate

Synthesis: (Fig. 4.31)

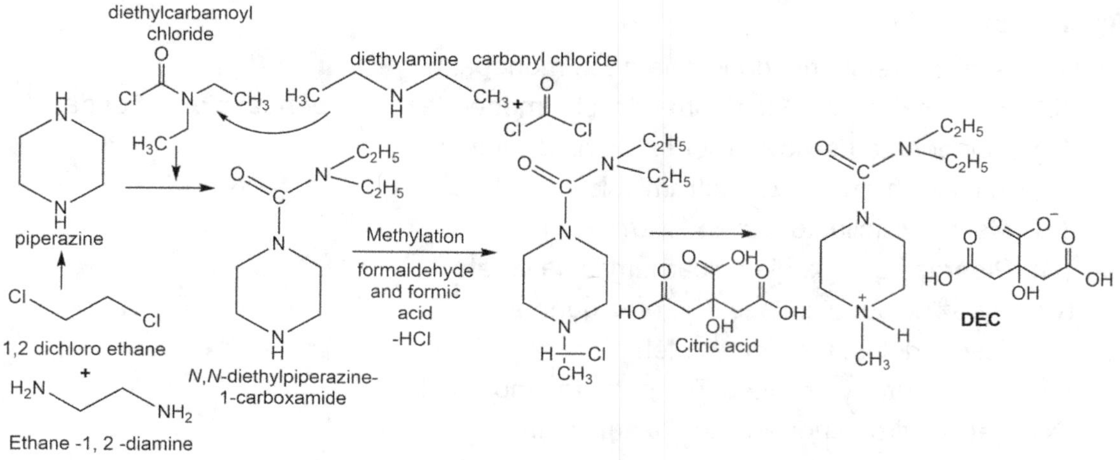

Fig. 4.31 Synthesis of Diethylcarbamazine citrate.

1. Piperazine ring is formed with 1,2 dichloro ethane and Ethane-1, 2 -diamine
2. Condensing piperazine with diethylcarbamoyl chloride yields diethylcarbamazine.
3. Diethylamine and carbonyl chloride can be used to make diethylcarbamoyl chloride.
4. In the presence of formaldehyde and formic acid, the following product (*N*, *N*-diethylpiperazine-1-carboxamide) is methylated to produce *N*, *N*-diethyl-4-methylpiperazine-1-carboxamide.
5. In the presence of citric acid, the base is converted to dihydrogen citrate (DEC).

Structure-Activity Relationship

The piperazine ring of DEC is essential for the drug's activity.

Mechanism of Action

The exact mechanism of DEC's activity is still not fully known. One of the proposed modes of action is platelet-mediated stimulation of microfilariae. This stimulation causes excretory antigens to be released. Another hypothesis suggested that the drug altered prostaglandin metabolism in microfilariae and host endothelial cells. This causes immobilization. The immobilisation results from parasitic cholinergic muscle receptors. Another theory proposes that helminth surface membranes are altered, and microtubule production is disrupted, leading to increased death by the host's immune system. Although DEC's efficacy in filariasis varies, it has not been proven that this is attributable to resistance.

DEC's mechanism of action has been thoroughly explored. However, it is still unknown. DEC appears to be the active form of the drug. Three such methods have been proposed for DEC's mechanism of action. The first is blood platelet involvement, caused by filarial excretory antigens. A more recent investigation revealed that DEC caused morphologic damage to the microfalaria. The removal of the cellular coating exposed antigenic determinants to immune defense mechanisms, resulting in cell damage. Microfalaria organelles were then severely damaged, resulting in death. The second is microtubule polymerization inhibition and preformed microtubule disruption. Interference with arachidonic acid metabolism is the third factor. DEC has anti-inflammatory effects. The anti-inflammatory effect of DEC causes inhibition of cyclooxygenase and leukotriene A4 synthase (leukotriene synthesis). This activity appears to change vascular and cellular binding as well as cell activation.

Uses

✓ It is still the preferred treatment for lymphatic filariasis (*Wuchereria bancrofti*, *Wuchereria (Brugia) malayi*, and *loiasis* (*Loa Loa*)

✓ It's also effective for treating visceral larval migrans & eosinophilia.

✓ It has been used to treat *ascarid* worm infections.

✓ Diethylcarbamazine and oxibendazole are used to treat intestinal helminths.

4.6.2 Ivermectin

Historical Background

Satoshi Mura, a microbiologist at Tokyo's Kitasako Institute, began collecting thousands of soil samples from all across Japan in the late 1960s in search of new antibacterial agents. He sent the soil samples to Merck Research Labs in New Jersey, where his associate, **William Campbell**, tested them against parasitic worms that harm livestock and other animals. A soil sample taken at a golf course southwest of Tokyo proved to be highly effective against worms.

Streptomyces avermictilis was the name given to the bacterium in the culture, which was a new species. In 1981, the novel molecule, ivermectin, was introduced as an animal health treatment. Ivermectin for human use was approved in 1987.

Ivermectin is a potential treatment for *onchocerciasis* (also known as river blindness, a dreadful worm-borne disease spread by flies that blinds millions). In 2015, **Mura** and **Campbell** were awarded the Nobel Prize in Physiology or Medicine.

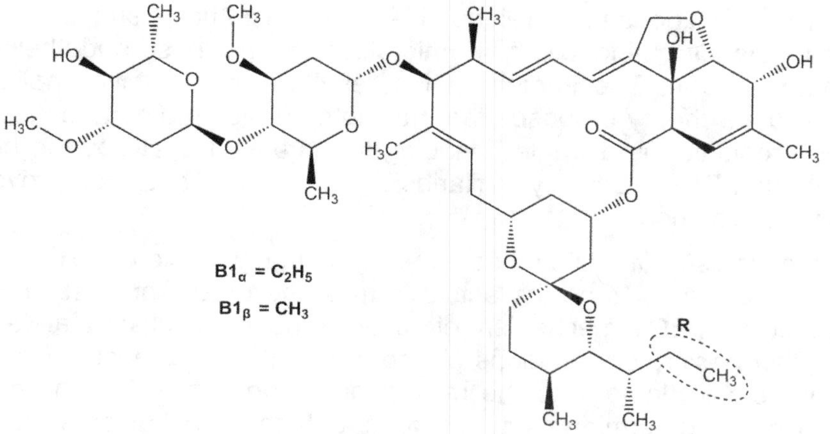

Fig. 4.32 Chemical structure of Ivermectin.

Chemical Structure: (Fig. 4.32)

Chemical Name:

(1*R*,4*S*,5'*S*,6*R*,6'*R*,8*R*,10*E*,12*S*,13*S*,14*E*,16*E*,20*R*,21*R*,24*S*)-6'-[(2*S*)-butan-2-yl]-21,24-dihydroxy-12-[(2*R*,4*S*,5*S*,6*S*)-5-[(2*S*,4*S*,5*S*,6*S*)-5-hydroxy-4-methoxy-6-methyloxan-2-yl]oxy-4-methoxy-6-methyloxan-2-yl]oxy-5',11,13,22-tetramethylspiro[3,7,19-trioxatetr-acy clo[15.6.1.^{14,8}.0^{20,24}]pentacosa-10,14,16,22-tetraene-6,2'-oxane]-2-one

Structure Activity Relationship

1. Natural occurring avermectins (*Streptomyces avermitilis*) are 16-membered macrocyclic lactones that are 80:20 avermectin $B1_\alpha$ and $B1_\beta$. As a result, it's used to control a wide range of insects, mite pests, and fire ants, as well as a veterinary antihelminthic.

2. Ivermectin (IVM) is formed by reducing the C22-23 double bond, which is an 80:20 combination of dihydro avermectin $B1_\alpha$ and $B1_\beta$.

3. Natural avermectins have little biologic activity, but IVM is effective in treating a variety of nematode diseases.

Mechanism of Action

The activity of IVM is hypothesized to involve two mechanisms of action. The first is an indirect action in which microfalaria (an early stage in the life cycle of nematodes) movement is inhibited, allowing cytotoxic cells from the host to attach to the parasite, resulting in parasite eradication. IVM's potential to operate as a γ-aminobutyric acid (GABA) agonist or an inducer of chloride ion influx, resulting in hyperpolarization and muscular paralysis, can cause this effect. The influx of chloride ions appears to be the most likely process. It was recently discovered that IVM binds irreversibly to the glutamate-gated chloride channel of the worm *Haemonchus contortus* when the channel is open. The binding then continues in an open conformation, enabling ions to pass across the membrane and resulting in IVM's paralytic activity. Microfilarial concentrations decrease rapidly as a result of this activity.

IVM's second action causes microfilariae to deteriorate in the uterus. The female worms would discharge fewer microfilariae as a result of this action, and it would take place over a longer period of time. The presence of degraded microfilariae in the uterus prevents continued microfilariae fertilisation and generation.

IVM had antinematodal properties. The antihelmintic action of ivermectin is controlled by glutamate-gated chloride channels in worm neurons and pharyngeal muscle cells. In contrast to endogenous glutamate transmitter-induced channel opening, IVM-activated channels open slowly but irreversibly. This activity causes either hyperpolarized or depolarized neurons or muscle cells of nematode. This leads to parasite paralysis and death. IVM does not readily cross through the mammalian blood-brain barrier to the central nervous system, where glutamate-gated chloride channels are found; hence, the hosts are generally immune to its effects. In onchocerciasis, II has a microfilaricidal effect, while in lymphatic filariasis, it has a microfilaricidal effect.

Uses

- ✓ It exhibits anti-microfilaria activity against *Wuchereria bancrofti*, *Brugia malayi*, *Loa loa*, and *Mansonella ozzardi*, and *Strongyloides stercoralis*.

- ✓ The drug is primarily used to treat onchocerciasis.

4.6.3   Thiabendazole

Historical Background

Thiabendazole is a benzimidazole anthelmintic drug. The chemical structure and mode of action are relevant to albendazole and mebendazole.

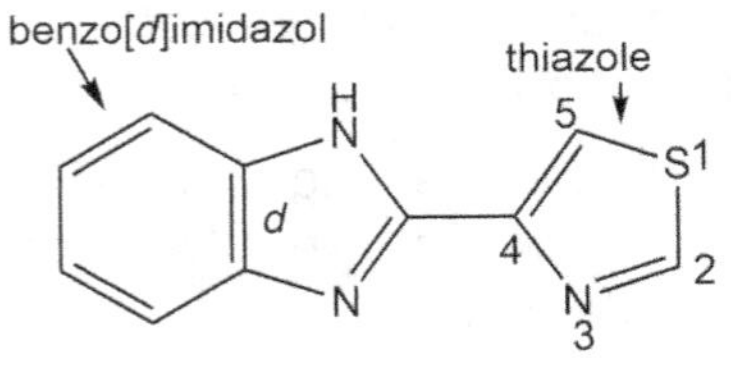

Trichinosis, which is contracted by eating raw or undercooked meat, can cause an elevated temperature, muscle discomfort and swelling, and other threatening symptoms in humans. Dr. **William Campbell**'s research team at Merck discovered the first drug known to kill the *trichinella* parasite in sheep, goats, cattle, and pigs in 1961.

Fig. 4.33 Chemical structure of Thiabendazole.

Thiabendazole was initially registered as a pesticide in the United States in 1969 by Merck and Company, Inc. USA.

Chemical Structure: (Fig. 4.33)

Chemical Name: 4-(1H-benzo[*d*]imidazol-2-yl)thiazole

Mechanism of Action

Thiabendazole is an antihelminthic benzimidazole derivative compound. The exact mechanism of action of thiabendazole is unknown. It inhibits the helminth-specific mitochondrial enzyme fumarate reductase, blocking the citric acid cycle, mitochondrial respiration, and ATP generation, resulting in the helminth's death. Furthermore, it has been reported that thiabendazole inhibits microtubule polymerization. It has a substantial antifertility effect on some trichostrongylids via binding to beta-tubulin.

Uses

✓ It works well on almost all types of intestinal nematodes. It considers as a significant development in the treatment of *Strongyloides stercoralis* infections and cutaneous larva migrans.

✓ It is generally taken orally, although it can also be used topically.

✓ It's been used to treat GI roundworm infections in sheep and goats.

✓ It is also utilized as a preservative and food additive. In the case of bananas, it is used to preserve freshness, and it is a common component in citrus fruit waxes.

4.6.4 Mebendazole

Historical Background

Mebendazole, a broad-spectrum anthelmintic drug, was developed and manufactured by Janssen Pharmaceutica's Research Laboratory in Beerse, Belgium. It is an exceptionally versatile anthelmintic drug that was developed after parbendazole was introduced. The drug was made available in 1972.

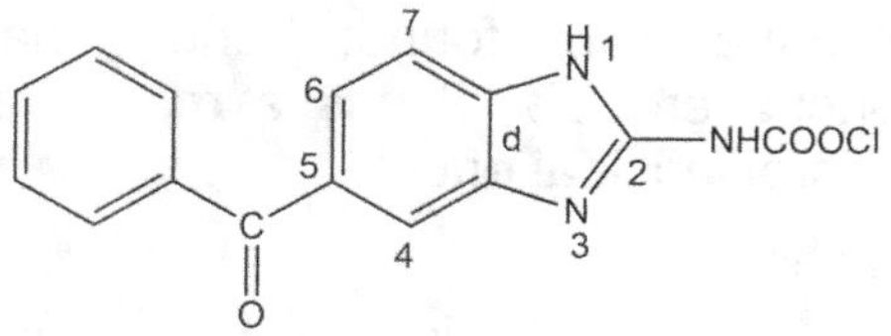

Fig. 4.34 Chemical structure of Mebendazole.

It serves as the model for several benzimidazole derivatives, including albendazole, flubendazole, and flubendazole.

It has a high cure rate for *Ascaris*, threadworms (*Enterobius*), hookworms (*Ancylostoma* and *Necator Spp.*), dwarf tapeworms (*Hymenolepis*), and whipworms (*Trichuris*).

Chemical structure: (Fig. 4.34)

Chemical Name:

Methyl-(5-benzoyl-1*H*-benzo[d]imidazol-2-yl)carbamate;(5-benzoyl-1*H*-benzimidazol-2-yl)-carbamic acid methyl ester

Synthesis

1. It is prepared by reacting fluorobenzene and benzoyl chloride to yield 4-fluorobenzophenone in the presence of AlCl$_3$.

2. When 4-fluorobenzophenone is mixed with nitric acid at a temperature below 5°C, 4-fluoro-3-nitrobenzophenone is formed.

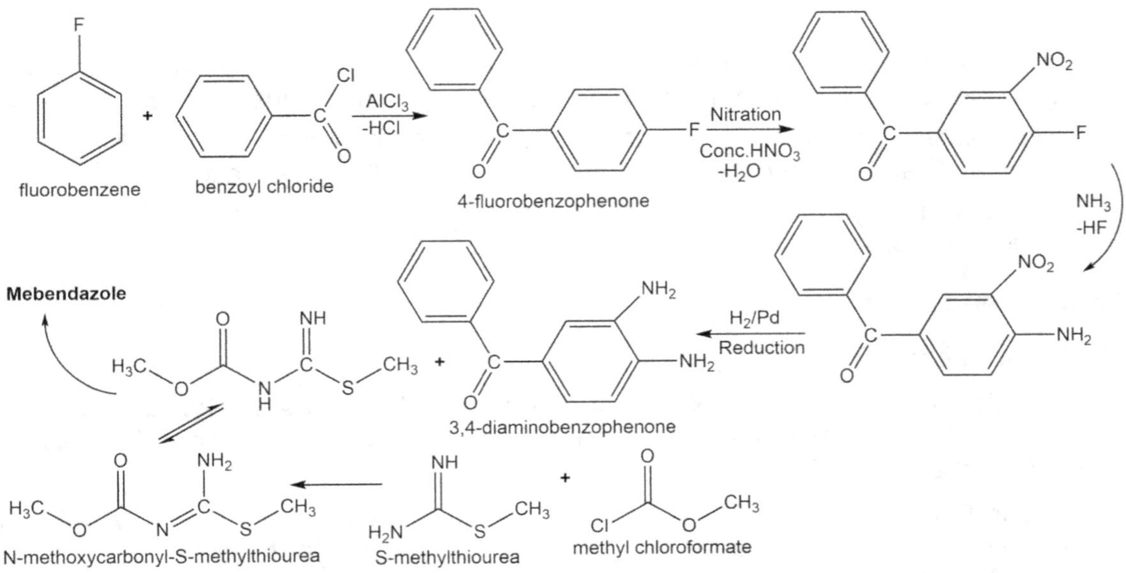

Fig. 4.35 Synthesis of Mebendazole.

3. 4-fluoro-3-nitrobenzophenone is converted to 4-amino-3-nitrobenzophenone by heating it to 125°C in an ammonia solution (nucleophilic aromatic substitution (addition-elimination mechanism)) in methanol.

4. The produced intermediate is now catalyzed by carbon and hydrogen utilizing palladium as a catalyst. The nitro group is changed to an amino group in this case, yielding 3,4-diaminobenzophenone.

5. N-methoxycarbonyl-*S*-methylthiourea, the second reagent, is produced by reacting methyl chloroformate with *S*-methylthiourea.

6. 3,4-diaminobenzophenone reacts with *N*-methoxycarbonyl-*S*-methylthiourea to produce the end product (Fig. 4.35).

Mechanism of Action

Mebendazole binds specifically to β-tubulin in parasite cells, preventing the microtubule chain from extending further. These play a variety of roles in eukaryotic cells, including glucose transport. Because its depolymerization prevents this, the worm progressively depletes its reserves and dies.

It inhibits the formation of microtubules by interacting with the colchicine binding site of β-tubulin. This prevents β-tubulin dimer polymerization in parasitic intestinal cells. Hence, glucose uptake, as well as the digestive and reproductive functions of parasites, are disrupted. It leads to helminth immobility, egg production restriction, and the death of the parasite. It is an excellent drug for treating intestinal helminthic infections with few side effects because it is poorly absorbed in the digestive tract.

It prevents tubulin polymerization. Mitotic spindle formation is interrupted when microtubule assembly is disturbed. Mebendazole also disrupts glucose uptake in the parasite, causing the worms to starve to death.

Uses

- ✓ It can be used to treat pinworm, roundworm, hookworm, and whipworm infections in their intestinal stages, but not larvae that have moved to muscular tissues.

- ✓ *Enterobiasis, ascariasis, ankylostomiasis, strongyloidiasis, trichocephaliasis, trichuriasis,* and mixed helminthiasis are all treated with mebendazole.

- ✓ It works well against intestinal nematode infections and is especially helpful to cure mixed types of infections.

4.6.5 Albendazole

Historical Background

Albendazole was developed by **Robert J. Gyurik** and **Vassilios J. Theodorides** and patented in 1975 by SmithKline Corporation. It was first used as an antihelminthic for sheep in Australia in 1977.

Janssen Pharmaceutical in Belgium (now part of J&J) did a lot of the early work on benzimidazoles as a class, under the guidance of Dr. **Paul Janssen**, an exceptional chemist. Benzimidazoles were first designed as fungicides for plants and then as anthelmintics for animals. Thiabendazole was the first benzimidazole to be invented and approved for human use in 1962.

Parbendazole, fenbendazole, oxfendazole, and cambendazole are examples of veterinary anthelmintics. Mebendazole was the first benzimidazole (BZ) carbamate used in humans, followed by flubendazole (both are Janssen products).

Albendazole was initially employed as an animal anthelminthic in 1977 in the United Kingdom by Smith Kline & French Animal Health. Other benzimidazoles were shown to be significantly less active than albendazole. This was because it was changed to albendazole sulphoxide, an active antihelminthic, whereas almost all other BZs were converted to inert compounds. In 1987, it was finally approved for human use.

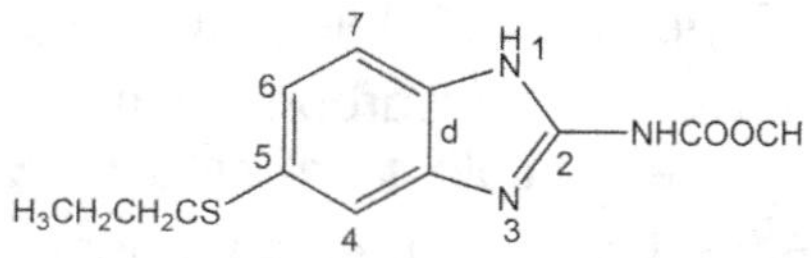

Fig.4.36 Chemical structure of Albendazole.

Chemical Structure: (Fig. 4.36)

Chemical Name:

Methyl(5-(propylthio)-1*H*-benzo[d]imidazol-2-yl)carbamate;(5-(propylthio)-1*H*-benz-imi-dazol- 2-yl)carbamic acid methyl ester

Mechanism of Action

Albendazole prevents parasite tubulin from forming microtubules by inhibiting parasite tubulin polymerization. It has a stronger affinity for the parasite tubulin. Hence, its activity is primarily directed toward the parasite rather than the host. The lack of cytoplasmic microtubules causes the parasites' larval and adult stages to have difficulty absorbing glucose. The worm becomes immobile and eventually dies as a result of its inability to maintain energy production. Albendazole's secondary action could be the suppression of the helminth-specific enzyme fumarate reductase.

It acts as an anthelmintic against sensitive cestodes and nematodes by inhibiting the parasites' glucose intake, resulting in the depletion of glycogen reserves and consequent reduction in adenosine triphosphate levels. As a result, the parasite becomes immobile and eventually dies.

It induces histological changes in the worm's intestinal cells by attaching to the colchicine-sensitive region of β-tubulin. Thus, preventing it from polymerizing or assembling into microtubules (it binds to the parasite β-tubulin much better than mammalian β-tubulin). It impairs the larval and adult stages of the vulnerable parasites' glucose intake and depletes their glycogen stores. It also inhibits the synthesis of spindle fibers, which are required for cell division. As a result, it halts egg production and development and prevents existing eggs from hatching. Cell motility, cell shape maintenance, and intracellular transport are all affected. It alters the helminths' metabolic pathways at higher concentrations by blocking metabolic enzymes such as malate dehydrogenase and fumarate reductase, with the latter resulting in less energy produced by the Kreb's cycle. The parasite becomes immobile and eventually dies due to a decrease in ATP generation.

Uses

1. Albendazole is an excellent treatment for gastrointestinal nematode infections, such as mixed Ascaris, Trichuria, and hookworm infections.

2. It is used to treat *Acaris lumbricoides*, *Ancylostoma duodenale*, *Necator americanus*, *Enterobius vermicularis*, and *Trichuris trichiura* infections.

SAR of Benzimidazole Compounds: (Fig. 4.37)

1. Anthelmintic drugs highlighted the importance of methylcarbamate and thiazole at position 2, phenylthiol, propylthiol, and benzoyl moieties at position 5, and the unsubstituted 1st and 3rd positions of the benzimidazole nucleus for anthelmintic activity.

2. The substitution at C-2 of the benzimidazole ring was used to make many molecules. Thiabendazole was the first broad-spectrum gastrointestinal nematode drug. It is highly active against a wide variety of nematodes.

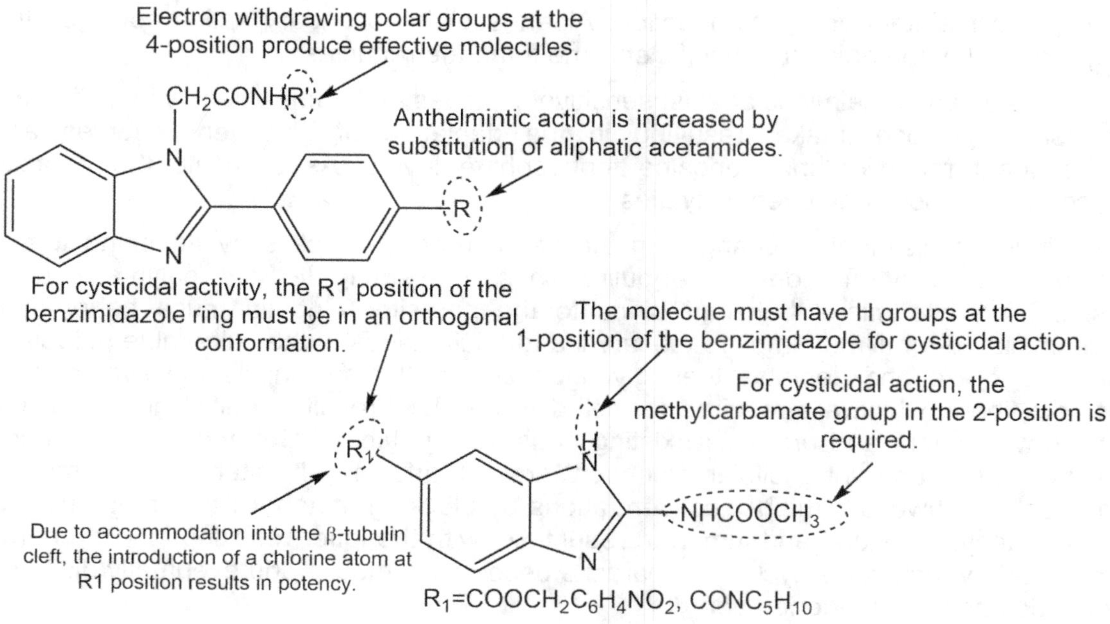

Fig. 4.37 SAR of Benzimidazoles.

3. The C-5 of thiabendazole is hydroxylated, rendering it inactive. As a result, numerous molecules with C-5 substitutions were designed to avoid hydroxylation. The most common compounds are mebendazole and albendazole.

4. Sulfur and fluorine groups at C-5, as well as carbamate substitution at C-2 of the benzimidazole ring, generate a powerful anthelmintic molecule.

5. Anthelmintic action has been found in imidazothiazole-derived compounds.

6. Anthelmintic action is demonstrated by the pyrimidine ring with aromatic and heteroaromatic C-2 substitutions.

7. Certain isothiocyanates have antihelmintic properties.

8. The piperazine ring and its salt exhibit an anthelmintic effect against worms of several species.

9. The 2-phenyl benzimidazole-1-acetamide series was shown to be more active in paralyzing worms in vivo studies. In comparison to standard albendazole, other compounds in the series were more capable of killing worms.

10. For cysticidal efficacy, in *in sillico* investigations demonstrated that the benzimidazole molecule should have an H group at position 1, a methyl carbamate group at position 2, and an orthogonal substituent at position 5.

Mechanism of action

Two processes have been proposed to explain the mechanism of action of benzimidazoles. The first mechanism of the compound explains that the enzyme fumarate reductase appears to be involved in the oxidation of NADH to NAD in helminths. The benzimidazoles can prevent fumarate reductase from functioning. Inhibition of fumarate reductase leads to the separation of oxidative phosphorylation, which is necessary for the synthesis of adenosine triphosphate.

A second mechanism and the principal action of benzimidazoles is their ability to bind to the protein tubulin and block tubulin polymerization into microtubules. Tubulin is a dimeric protein that coexists with polymeric microtubules in a dynamic equilibrium. Binding to tubulin prevents subunits from self-associating and results in a "capping" of the microtubule at the associating end. The microtubule dissociates from the other end, resulting in a net reduction in microtubule length. The unusual selectivity of the benzimidazoles is significant. Although benzimidazole can bind to tubulin in mammals when used as an anthelmintic. It is toxic to the helminth but does not affect the host. It has been suggested that the selectivity of the compound is due to differences in pharmacokinetics between binding to the two distinct tubulin proteins.

Cestode Infections

Cestodes (tapeworms) are worms with flat segments. Fish (*Diphyllobothrium latum*), pig (*Taenia solium*), beef (*Taenia saginata*), and dwarf (*Hymenolepis nana*) tapeworms cause the most dangerous tapeworm infections. Infection with *T. solium* can cause cysticercosis, which is the harboring of cysticerci (larvae) in the human host's tissues. The most commonly infected tissues are the brain, eye, muscles, liver, and lungs. *Hymenolepis nana* infection is more common in children than in adults.

4.6.6 Niclosamide

Historical Background

In 1953, Bayer's chemotherapeutic research laboratories developed niclosamide. It was first sold in 1959 as a molluscicide to kill snails. These are intermediate hosts of *schistosomiasis*. It was shown to be effective against human tapeworm (cestode) infection by Bayer scientists in 1960, and it was sold for human usage in 1962.

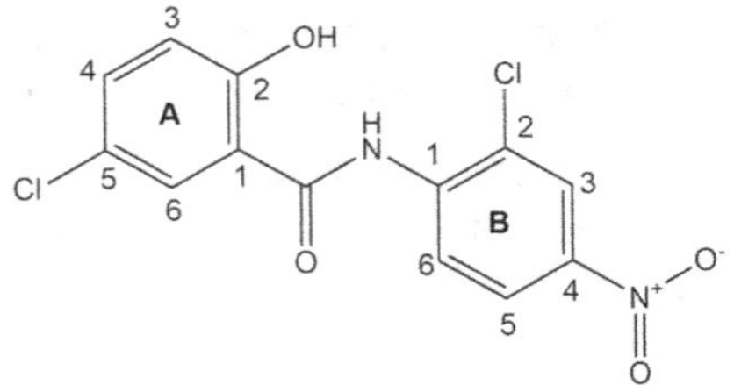

Fig.4.38 Chemical structure of Niclosamide.

It was licenced by the US FDA in 1982 for use in humans to treat tapeworm infection, and it is on the WHO's list of essential medicines.

Chemical Structure: (Fig. 4.38)

Chemical Name:

5-chloro-N-(2-chloro-4-nitrophenyl)-2-hydroxybenzamide:2,5-dichloro-4-nitrosaicylanilide

Structure-Activity Relationship

1. The presence of a hydroxy group at the 2-position in ring A is favourable for tapeworm and fluke activity. This is demonstrated by the fact that removing this OH or replacing it with OCH_3 reduces or eliminates the anthelmintic effect. The replacement of -OH by a cyclic structure, such as 1,3-benzoxazine, results in a reduction of activity.

2. Antihelmintic activity can be retained by having an amide or thioamide bond between aromatic rings A and B (X = CO/CS). However, salicylanilides are more active than thiosalicylanilides. It has been shown that replacing $-CONH_2$ with an amidine, aminomethyl (X = C = NH, $-CH_2$), or ester group reduces the activity.

3. The presence of halogen groups at the 3,5-position in ring A and the 2,4-position in ring B is important for cestodicidal and flukicidal activity. By substituting chlorine at different places of rings A and B, the optimal characteristics of activity are obtained. The use of bromine or iodine instead of chlorine may increase activity while also increasing the toxicity of the resultant compounds. It's also important to note that adding electron-withdrawing groups to ring B, such as nitro or isothiocyanato, ideally at the 4-position, improves anthelmintic action. Similarly, electron-donating groups like amino at ring B's position 4 render the molecule inert or inactive.

4. The activity is retained when rings A or B are substituted with the naphthalene nucleus. However, it has lower inactivity than the parent compound. By substituting heterocycles such as benzothiadiazole or benzimidazole for ring B. The resultant product, N-aryl salicylamides, with weak or no activity, can be developed.

Mechanism of Action

Niclosamide, like other salicylanilides, is a hydrogen ionophore (a chemical species that reversibly binds ions). It transports protons through the inner membrane of mitochondria, causing oxidative phosphorylation to be disconnected from electron transport and inhibiting of ATP synthesis. In isolated mitochondria from helminths and mammals, the same effects have been demonstrated. The combination of low systemic absorption and the protective effect of protein binding reveals selective toxicity.

Its mechanism of action is to block mitochondrial oxidative phosphorylation in mammals and parasites. It prevents the parasite from absorbing glucose and oxygen at the same time.

Uses

1. It removes most tapeworms, including beef, pig, fish, and dwarf tapeworms, but not nematodes.

2. It acts as a molluscicide and is commonly used to get rid of freshwater snails, which are *Schistosoma* spp intermediate's hosts.

3. It is superior to mebendazole and flubendazole in terms of efficacy.

Trematode Infections

Schistosomiasis is a common disease in tropical and subtropical areas, affecting millions of people around the globe. Snails infected with the parasite serve as intermediate hosts. Schistosoma diseases primarily affect the liver, spleen, and gastrointestinal system (*S. mansoni* and *S. japonicum*) or the genitourinary tract (*S. japonicum, S. haematobium*).

Trematodes (flukes) are unbranched, flat, leaf-shaped worms. *S. haematobium*, *S. mansoni*, and *S. japonicum* are the most frequent blood fluke species that cause human schistosomiasis. *S. intercalatum* and *S. mekongi* are less common species.

The pathogenic lung flukes *Paragonimus westermani* and *P. kellicotti* are found in humans. Snails and crabs serve as intermediary hosts for these parasites. *Clonorchis sinensis*, *Opisthorchis viverini*, *O. felineus*, and *Fasciola hepatica* are liver flukes; *C. sinensis* and *Opisthorchis* species exist in man's biliary system. The primary and secondary hosts are snails and fish, respectively. Snails and freshwater plants serve as primary and secondary hosts for *F. hepatica* (the giant liver fluke), which infects the biliary system of humans.

Intestinal flukes include *Fasciolopsis buski*, *Heterophyes heterophyes*, and *Metagonimus yokogawai*. The large intestinal fluke, *F. buski*, is primarily found in Southeast Asia.

4.6.7 Praziquantel

Historical Background

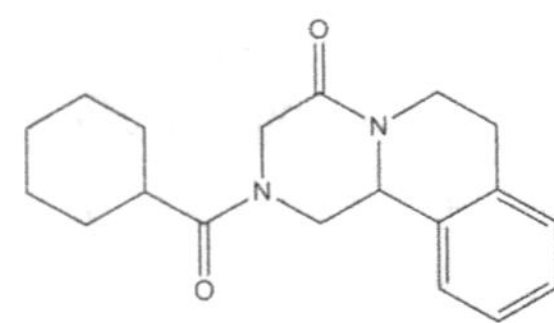

Praziquantel was discovered in the 1970s as a result of a collaboration between the German pharmaceutical companies Bayer AG and E. Merck. It was patented as a veterinary antihelminthic in Germany in December 1973. Bayer collaborated with the World Health Organization to perform clinical trials to prove praziquantel's safety in humans.

Fig.4.39 Chemical structure of Praziquantel.

Its therapeutic activity against a variety of human-pathogenic platyhelminths was verified in tests conducted in the 1970s. Bayer originally marketed it in 1979, following the completion of the required toxicological studies and clinical trials.

It's a pyrazinoisoquinoline derivative, with the *R*- isomer having the majority of the physiological activity. The compound does not influence nematodes, but it is active against cestodes and trematodes.

Chemical Structure:(Fig. 4.39)

Chemical Name:

2-(cyclohexanecarbonyl)-1,2,3,6,7,11b-hexahydro-4*H*-pyrazino[2,1-a]isoquinolin-4-one

Stereochemistry

Since the compound's structure contains an asymmetrical center, it has two distinct absolute configurations: (*R*)- & (*S*)- isomers. The antiparasitic effect is procured from the core isoquinoline pyrazine derivative. It is molecularly intimately related to the (*R*)- isomer. (Fig. 4.40)

Structure-Activity Relationship

A. Substitution of cyclohexane ring

1. The increase in the number of carbon atoms in the ring is encouraging from cyclopropyl to cyclohexyl. The activity will be reduced after the substitution of cycloheptyl.

2. The presence of heteroatoms and/or any substitutions on the ring does not increase activity.

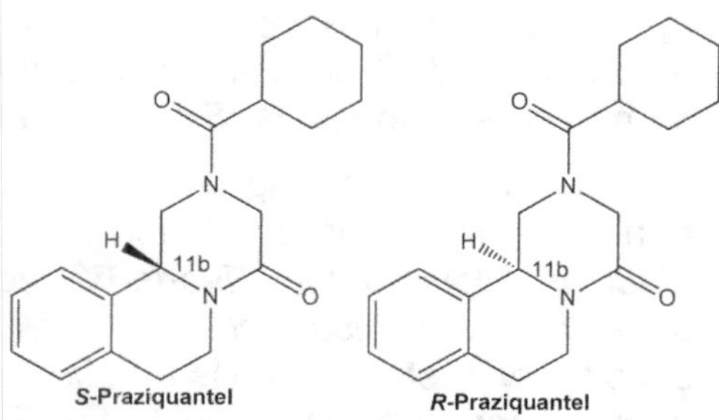

S-Praziquantel   *R-Praziquantel*

Fig. 4.40 Stereochemistry of Praziquantel.

3. For substituted groups, the most active derivatives are those that don't have aromatic rings attached to them. Only by substituting an amine or a fluoride group for the ring can the activity be enhanced.

4. The most active heterocycles found were thiophene and 3-pyridine ring containing compounds.

5. The aliphatic group substitution in the position has resulted in low toxicity of the compound.

B. Substitution at carbonyl group

The presence of a carbonyl or thiocarbonyl group is essential in this position.

C. Substitution at C-4 position

1. The carbonyl group is required for the activity to take place.

2. Only the substitution of thionyl yields identical effects.

D. Configuration in between 11a & 11b position of the ring

The anthelminthic activity is due to the R-isomer.

Fig. 4.41 SAR of Praziquantel.

E. Substitution at C-3 of the ring

Fluorobenzyl and nicotinoyl groups at C-3 enhance the anti-schistosomicidal activity of the derivatives against *S. mansoni*, whereas other groups, such as isobutyryl, reduce the activity at this place (Fig. 4.41).

Mechanism of Action

Praziquantel may have multiple mechanisms of action, which may vary depending on the parasite being treated. Ca^{2+} redistribution appears to be involved in the mechanism of action, either directly or indirectly. When helminths are discovered in the host's lumen (cestode infection), the drug causes muscle contraction and paralysis, which leads to worm removal. It has also been proven to suppress phosphoinositide metabolism, which causes worm paralysis through an unknown mechanism. It causes drug-induced damage to the worm's tissue in intravascular-dwelling schistosomes. As a result, immunological antibodies attack antigens in the helminth. The parasite dies as a result of an antigen-antibody immunologic response. Finally, it regulates the glycogen and energy metabolism of the parasite.

Praziquantel is antihelmintic with a wide range of effects. It appears to affect schistosome cellular membranes by increasing permeability and, as a result, the influx of calcium ions into the cell, resulting in paralysis of the parasite's muscles. As a result, the parasites stop working, and they are expelled from the body.

Uses

1. It is used to treat *schistosomiasis* and is also effective against trematode infections. It works against fluke infections in the intestines, liver, and lungs.

2. In animals and humans, it is clinically efficacious against a wide range of cestode and trematode infections.

4.6.8 Oxamniquine

Historical Background

Richards and **Foster** (Pfizer) discovered oxamniquine in 1969. The chemical compound was derived from lucanthone and hycanthone after hydroxymethylation. The fungus *Aspergillus sclerotiorum* oxidised hycanthone, producing a drug that was later termed oxamniquine by Foster.

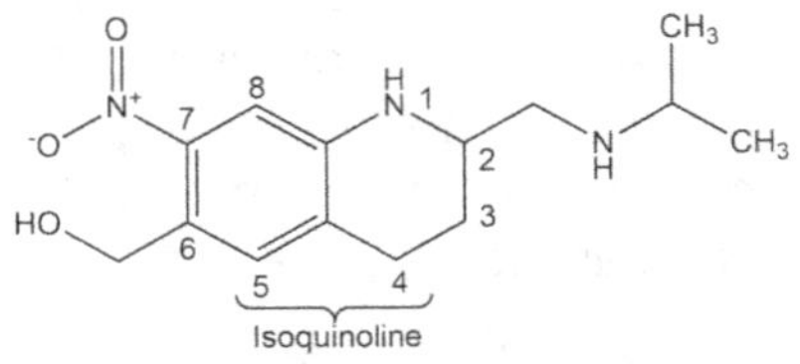

Fig. 4.42 Chemical structure of Oxamniquine.

Pfizer was the first to market it in Brazil. It is less expensive than praziquantel and is effective against *S. mansoni* infections in the intestine and hepatosplenic tract.

Chemical Structure: (Fig. 4.42)

Chemical Name:

(2-((isopropylamino)methyl)-7-nitro-1,2,3,4-tetrah ydro-quinolin-6-yl)methanol; (±)-(7-nitro-2-[(pro-pan-2-yl)amino]methyl-1,2,3,4-tetrahydroquinolin-6-yl)methanol

Stereochemistry

Oxamniquine has an asymmetric carbon and is commercially available in both enantiomers. The S-(+) enantiomer is responsible for the most antischistosomal activity, while the R-(-) enantiomer is only moderately active. (Fig. 4.43)

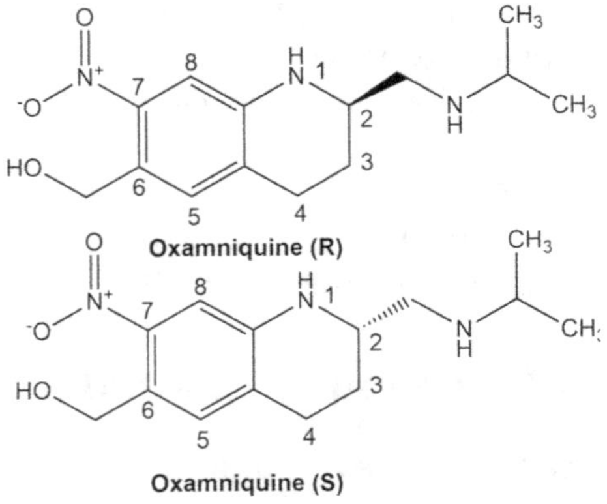

Fig. 4.43 Oxamniquine *R* and *S* enantiomers.

Structure-Activity Relationship

1. Anthelmintic action is derived from the tetrahydroquinoline (Oxamniquine) structure. Anthelmintic action is improved by substituting nitro groups at C-7, isopropyl amino groups at C-2, and hydroxymethyl groups at C-6. If the chlorine group is substituted at C-7, the activity is reduced.

2. *In vivo*, the 6-formyl-oxamniquine derivative molecule retained its efficacy.

3. The modifications to the compound's heterocyclic ring and side chain have shown promise for therapeutic effectiveness. However, the resultant product has shown higher toxicity when compared to oxamniquine. Furthermore, the alkyl side chain can be changed without affecting pharmacological activity, although such changes are linked to an increase in toxicity.

Mechanism of Action

It's a prodrug that's sulfonated by an endogenous sulfotransferase after being taken by the parasite. The enzyme is only found in the parasite when 3-phospho-adenosine-5-phosphosulfate is present. The oxamniquine sulphate ester that results is unstable. The product is spontaneously decomposed into a reactive electrophilic product. The reactive product is capable of alkylating DNA, proteins, and other nucleophilic macromolecules. The parasite could die because of the impairment of cellular metabolic activities.

Oxamniquine is a DNA binding agent with aliphatic amine activity that protonates at physiological pH. This positive charge is thought to contribute to the bioactive form of oxamniquine. It has strong interactions with DNA via an electrostatic connection with the negatively charged phosphodiester group.

The organism converts oxyamniquine to a biological ester. The esterified compound spontaneously dissociates into an electrophilic ionic product. After which it alkylates the helminth DNA, resulting in an irreversible blockage of nucleic acid metabolism. Because resistant helminths do not esterify oxamniquine, the activation does not take place. Oxidative processes lead to inactivation in other metabolic pathways. The metabolites are mostly eliminated in the urine.

Uses

The drug has been shown to be highly effective against *Schistosoma mansoni* from Brazil and useful against *S. mansoni* from West Africa.

4.7 Sulphonamides and Sulfones

Historical Development

✓ Viruses and microbes have infected people since the ancient period. There was little hope for rational treatment of microbial infection until **Antony van Leeuwenhoek** discovered microorganisms in 1676 and then understood their role in infectious illness roughly 150 years later.

✓ Researchers led by **Robert Koch** in the 19th century revealed that specific microbes could always be isolated from the excreta and tissues of people with specific infectious disorders. However, the same microbes were typically absent in healthy people.

✓ **Paul Ehrlich** (1854-1915), a well-known German scientist, discovered a link between dye selective staining and antiprotozoal action. This prompted research into the antibacterial properties of azo dyes.

✓ The discovery of sulfonamides in 1936 in France and Germany marked the start of the contemporary anti-infective era. This discovery was an emergence of Paul Ehrlich's earlier breakthroughs in treating infections with organometallics and his theories of vital staining.

✓ In the late 1920s, **Fritz Mietzsch** and **Joseph Klarer** at Bayer began a systematic effort to synthesize azo dyes for antimicrobials, and **Gerhard Domagk** (1895-1964) researched the mechanism of action of these dyes. Although the dye was proven to be effective in treating streptococcal infections in mice, it was inactive *in vitro*. Clinically, it was found to be beneficial in the treatment of severe staphylococcal septicemias.

✓ **Gerhard Domagk** of Bayer of Germany investigated the antibacterial activity of Prontosil rubrum, a red dye. The dye was detected as effective *in vivo* against *streptococcal* infections in mice. *In vitro*, however, it was inactive.

✓ **Hildegarde Domagk**, the daughter of **Gerhard Domagk**, was the first patient to receive (bright red sulphamoyl azo dye, later named prontosil, in 1932) prontosil for a severe *streptococcal* infection. She was cured with prontosil.

✓ During this time, researchers at the Pasteur Institute, Paris concluded that the azo linkage in prontosil is broken metabolically *in vivo*, resulting in an active entity known as sulphanilamide. At this point, many more researchers began investigating the area of sulphanilamide. Prontosil rubrum is what we call a prodrug nowadays. **Paul Glemo**, a graduate student in Vienna, developed it in 1908.

✓ Domagk's research marked a new age of bacterial infection treatment in humans. He was awarded the Nobel Prize in Medicine in 1939 for the discovery of the antibacterial effects of Prontosil (**Fig.4.44**).

✓ Sulfonamides' antibacterial capabilities were discovered in the mid-1930s. The discovery of sulfanilamide's *in vivo* antibacterial characteristics marked the beginning of the contemporary anti-infective era.

✓ Sulphanilamide, a chemically simple compound that is easy to produce and has no patent constraints, has become widely available for medicinal usage. The use of sulphanilamide in humans, however, was discontinued due to hazardous side effects. It did, however, serve as a model for the development of subsequent sulphanilamides. Many of these have been used in clinical trials, and some of them are still being used today.

✓ More than 5000 molecules of the sulfanilamide class were examined and synthesized within ten years and appeared in 1948. N^1-heterocyclic substituted sulfanilamide, such as sulfapyridine, sulfathiazole, and sulfadiazine, were developed as antibacterial agents.

✓ During 1935–1944, 4,4'-diaminodiphenylsulfone (DDS, dapsone) was reported to have antimycobacterial properties. Though it was not therapeutically useful for human tuberculosis, it was useful for leprosy. The N, N'-diacetyl derivative is also used against resistant *falciparum* malaria strains.

✓ Even though natural and semisynthetic antibiotics have largely replaced sulfonamides in the treatment of systemic bacterial illnesses, sulfonamides remain important antibacterial agents. Co-administering them with dihydrofolate reductase inhibitors has made them more effective, and giving sulfamethoxazole and trimethoprim together is a benefacial to treat a number of bacterial diseases. Sulfonamides were used more frequently with the advent of this combination (co-trimoxazole) in the late 1960s.

✓ Sulfonamides, which were formerly mainstays of antimicrobial chemotherapy, are now considered minor drugs. One of the most likable characteristics of sulfonamides is their low cost, which explains why they have remained on the market for so long.

Chemistry

Sulfa drugs are sulfonamides that are developed from sulfanilamide (*p*-amino-benzene sulfonamide). Sulfonamides have a wide range of pharmacological effects, including hypoglycemics, carbonic anhydrase inhibitors, saluretics, and tubular transport inhibitors. However, antibacterial sulfonamides are termed sulfa drugs. Therapeutically active compounds are often replaced at the N^1 nitrogen, leaving the N^4 position unsubstituted.

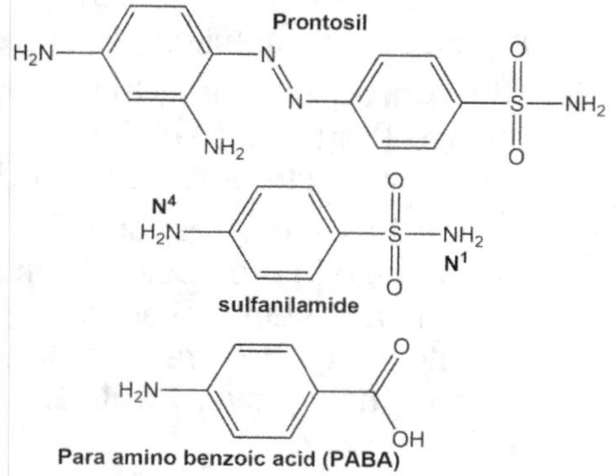

Sulfa drugs are amphoteric. With a pKa range of 4.79 to 8.56, they behave like mild organic acids. Their solubility is improved at an alkaline pH, even though they are only moderately soluble in water. Sodium salts, on the other hand, are easily soluble in water. Sulfacetamide has a neutral pH and is used to treat eye infections.

Fig. 4.44 Chemical structure of sulphanilamide, PABA & Prontosil.

The nitrogen at the para position of an amino group of sulphonamide is labeled as N^4. Whereas, the nitrogen in SO_2NH_2 is designated as N^1. The N^1 position is substituted in systemic sulfa drugs, while the N^4 position is substituted in gut-active sulfa medications. (Fig. 4.44)

About 5000 compounds can be developed by substituting the N^1 and N^4 positions. Thirty of these are clinically significant. Sulfanilamide and its derivatives are more commonly referred to as sulfonamides or sulfa drugs.

Sulphanilamide derivatives with the most effective medical applications feature substituents in place of the sulphonamide group's hydrogen ($-SO_2NH_2$). Substitutions in the amide $-NH_2$ group (the N denoted as N^1) have varying impacts on the molecule's antibacterial activity. Highly powerful compounds have resulted from the substitution of heterocyclic aromatic nuclei at N^1.

Classification

1. Based on chemical structure substitution:

(a) Both N^1 and N^4 substituted sulfonamides Ex. succinyl sulfathiazole, phthalyl sulfathiazole

(b) N^1 substituted sulfonamides Ex. sulfapyridine, sulfathiazole, sulfadimidine (sulfamethazine), sulfamerazine, sulfaphenazole, sulfamethoxazole, sulfadimethoxine, sulfacetamide, sulfaquinoxaline, sulfaethoxypyridazine, sulfamethoxypridazine, sulfasomidine, sulfisoxazole (sulfafurazole), silversulfadiazine, sulfaguanidine

(c) N^4 substituted sulfonamides Ex. prontosil

2. Based on site of action:

(a) Intestinal acting sulfonamides: Ex. succinylsulfathiazole, phthalylsulfathiazole, sulfaguanidine, **sulfasalazine**

(b) Systemic sulfonamides: Ex. sulfadimidine (sulfamethazine), sulfamerazine, sulfaphenazole, sulfamethoxazole, sulfadimethoxine, sulfacetamide, sulfaquinoxaline, sulfaethoxypyridazine

(c) Renal sulfonamides: Ex.sulfisoxazole (sulfafurazole) sulfasomidine

(d) Topical sulfonamides: Ex. sulfamylon, **sulphacetamide** sodium, silver sulphadiazine, **mafenide acetate**

(e) Ophthalmic sulfonamide: Ex. sodiumsulfacetamide

(f) Combination sulfonamide: Ex. trimethoprim

3. Based on duration of action:

(a) Short-acting Suphonamides (half-life less than 20h): Ex. **sulphapyridine, sulphadiazine**, sulphadimidine, **sulfisoxazole**, **sulphamethizole**, sulphasomidlne, sulphathiazole

(b) Intermediate acting Suphonamides (half-life between 10–24h): Ex. **sulphamethoxazol**e, sulphaphenazole

(c) Long-acting Sulphonamides (half-life greater than 24h): Ex. sulphamethoxydiazine, sulphamethoxypyridazine, sulphadimethoxine, **sulfamethazine**

(d) Ultra-long-acting sulphonamides (half-life greater than 50h): Ex. sulfadoxine and sulphalene

4. Based on Chemical structure:

(a) Pyrimidine derivatives: Ex. sulphadiazine, sulphadimidine, sulphasomidine, sulphamethoxydiazine, sulphadimethoxine, sulphadoxine

(b) Pyridazine derivatives: Ex. sulphamethoxypyridazine

(c) Pyrazine derivatives: Ex. sulphalene

(d) Pyridine derivatives: Ex. sulphapyridine

(e) Thiazole derivatives: Ex. sulphathiazole, phthalylsulphathiazole, succinyt-sulphathiazole

(f) Isoxazole derivatives: Ex. sulphamethoxazole, sulphaisoxazole

(g) Pyrazole derivatives: Ex. sulphnphenazole

(h) 1,3,4-thiadiazole derivatives: Ex. sulphamethizole

(i) Aliphatic chain derivatives: Ex. sulphacetamide, sulphugunidine

Structure-Activity Relationship

1. The general structures (Fig. 4.45) describe the fundamental properties of sulfonamides and sulfones for activity.

2. The amino and sulfonyl groups on the benzene ring of sulphanilamide should be in the 1,4 positions. The amino group should be unsubstituted or changed to a free amino *in vivo*.

3. The antibacterial activity is diminished or eliminated when the benzene ring is changed with another ring structure or new substituents are added.

4. The -SO$_2$NH$_2$ is exchanged by -SOC$_6$H$_4$-*p*-NH$_2$, -CONH$_2$, -CONHR, or -COC$_6$H$_4$R, which lowers activity.

5. N^1-monosubstitution can increase activity and can be used with a range of heterocycles; N^1-disubstitution, on the other hand, frequently produces inactive compounds. Because the drug's ionization requires one hydrogen.

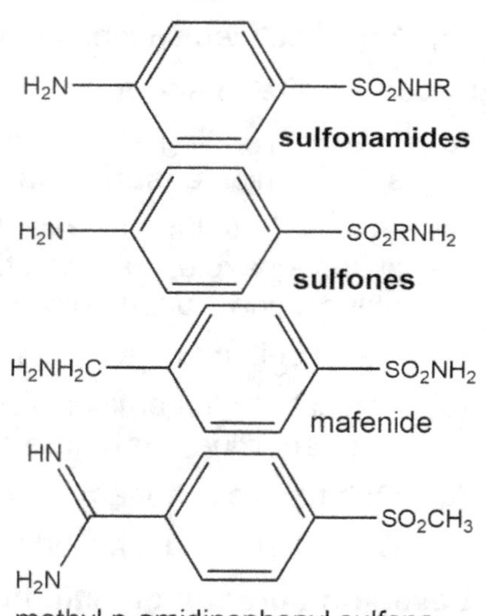

Fig.4.45 Structures of Sulphonamides.

6. The binding to plasmatic proteins is affected by the substituent at N^1 as well as substituents on an N^1 phenyl or heterocyclic ring.

7. The antibacterial activity is influenced by the formal pi charges at the N^1 position. Antibacterial activity increases as these charges increase.

8. Substituting an electron-withdrawing heteroaromatic ring for one of the NH$_2$ hydrogens increased the acidity of the remaining hydrogen and increased its potency. With the right groups in place, the product's antibacterial efficacy rapidly increased, but its water solubility under physiologic conditions increased as well.

9. When R is heterocyclic, sulfonamides have the maximum antibacterial activity.

Although it can also be isocyclic (having just carbon-only rings) or have an acyl group in this position, it can also be isomorphic (having just carbon-only rings) or have an isomer R might be phenylene or a heterocycle in the sulfones; the parent dapsone, where R is phenyl, is the most active.

10. When the amino is replaced with amidino, an active sulfone, methyl p-amidinophenyl sulfone, is formed, even though it is not a sulfonamide. It possesses antibacterial properties, although it is especially effective against *mycobacteria*.

11. Sulphonamides' antibacterial action is linked to the pKa value. Those with a pKa value between 6.0 and 7.5 would have the most activity.

12. The aromatic SO_2 group's strong electron-withdrawing nature renders the nitrogen atom to which it is directly linked somewhat electropositive. As a result, the acidity of the hydrogen atoms linked to the nitrogen increases, resulting in a somewhat acidic functional group (pKa = 10.4).

13. When $-SO_2NH$ is replaced with $-SO_2C_6H_4$ p-NH_2, sulfones are formed, which have lower activities against some bacterial species but are effective against leprosy and some malarial strains.

14. Other structures that are related to this one may be active as well but through a different method. Mafenide, an active sulfonamide, was developed by separating the amino group from the ring with $-CH_2-$.

15. The attachment of unique heterocyclic aromatic substituents to the sulfonamide molecule is the key structural distinction among clinically successful sulfonamides.

16. The sulfonamide binds to the arginine, histidine, and lysine basic sites of the protein. The binding groups are alkyl, alkoxy, and halo groups. The antibacterial activity of sulphonamide is regulated by binding. Protein binding appears to influence the drug's availability and half-life.

17. The pharmacokinetics and antibacterial activity of sulphonamides are both affected by lipid solubility. When lipid solubility increases, the half-life, and antibacterial activity both increase.

Mechanism of Action

Sulfonamides prevent bacterial nucleic acid synthesis by inhibiting the bacterial enzyme dihydropteroate synthetase in the folic acid pathway. Sulfonamides act as a PABA alternative. It inhibits the conversion of PABA to dihydrofolic acid. This activity is bacteriostatic when taken alone. Because the type of activity is a competitive substitution, the tissue concentration of sulfonamide must be kept high enough to prevent bacteria from gaining access to PABA. As a result, sulfonamides are ineffective in pus and necrotic tissue, which offer bacteria additional sources of PABA. The sulfonamides are harmless to mammalian cells because they synthesise dihydrofolic acid from dietary folate rather than PABA. A bactericidal action of sulfonamide could be formed when combined with trimethoprim. Trimethoprim prevents the conversion of dihydrofolic acid to tetrahydrofolic acid by inhibiting dihydrofolate reductase, which inhibits bacterial folic acid synthesis at the next step in the folic acid sequence (Fig. 4.46).

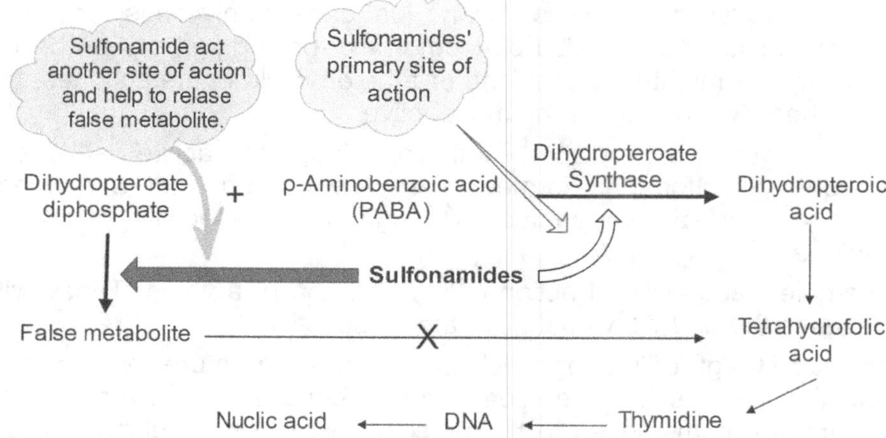

Fig. 4.46 Tetrahydrofolic acid formation via a microbial metabolic route.

Although both bacteria and mammalian cells contain this enzyme, However, far lower quantities of sulphonamides block the bacterial enzyme than the mammalian enzyme. A potentiated sulfonamide combination has lowered antimicrobials' MICs against specific sensitive bacteria. Resistance to the potentiated sulfonamides develops at a slower rate than resistance to the individual drugs; this is a significant benefit because sulfonamide resistance is common and diaminopyrimidine resistance develops quickly when administered alone.

Human dosages of sulfonamides are bacteriostatic. They block the enzyme dihydropteroate synthase, which is essential for the production of folic acid derivatives and, eventually, the thymidine needed for DNA replication. In order to compete with PABA, which is a natural structural component of folic acid derivatives, they bind to the active site. PABA blocks the formation of tetrahydrofolic acid molecules via condensation with 6-hydroxymethyl-7,8-dihydropterin-pyrophosphate to produce 7,8-dihydropteroate and pyrophosphate, which is mediated by enzymes. As a result, sulfonamides can be classified as antimetabolites as well.

Indeed, considerable amounts of PABA can be added to food (in some multivitamin formulations) or to the culture medium to reverse the antibacterial activity of sulfonamides. Most sensitive bacteria are unable to absorb preformed folic acid from their surroundings and convert it to tetrahydrofolic acid. Hence, bacteria synthesise folate at the beginning of the metabolic process. Folates are necessary intermediates in the manufacture of thymidine, which bacteria require for further proliferation. As a result, dihydropteroate synthase inhibition is bacteriostatic.

Humans lack the essential enzymes (including dihydropteroate synthase) to synthesise folates from component parts, so folic acid is supplied in our food. As a result, sulfonamides have no comparably fatal effect on human cell development, and the foundation for sulfonamides' selective toxicity is obvious.

However, the event is a little more complicated for a few bacteria types. In this case, instead of PABA, sulfonamides act on dihydropteroate diphosphate. The resulting metabolite is incapable of undergoing the next required process, glutamic acid condensation, because this false metabolite is also an enzyme inhibitor. Further nucleic acid synthesis is impossible when folic acid levels in bacterial cells decline. As such, the bacteria are unable to proliferate further.

4.7.1 Sulfamethizole

Historical Background

Sulphamethizole is a highly soluble sulphonamide. It is rapidly absorbed and eliminated, making it an effective chemotherapeutic drug for urinary tract infections (UTIs).

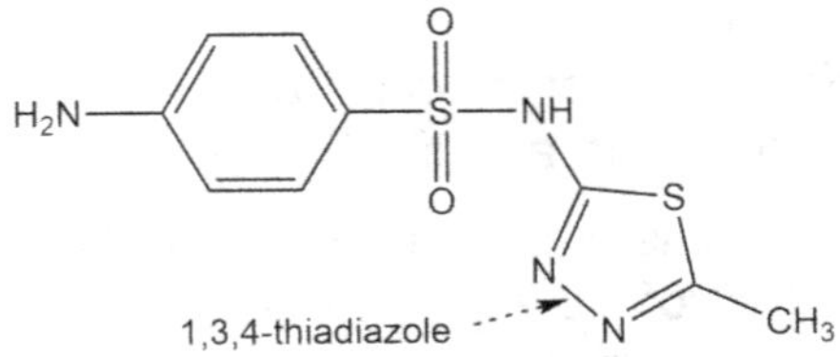

Fig. 4.47 Chemical structure of Sulfamethizole.

It has antibacterial activity against *streptococci*, *pneumococci*, *staphylococci*, *meningococci*, *gonococci*, colon bacilli, and pathogenic dysentery.

Chemical Structure: (Fig. 4.47)

Chemical Name:

4-amino-*N*-(5-methyl-1,3,4-thiadiazol-2-yl)benzenesulfonamide; *N*¹-(5-methyl-1,3,4-thiadiazo1-2-yl) sulphanilamide

Mechanism of Action

Sulfamethizole inhibits bacterial folic acid synthesis by blocking para-aminobenzoic acid (PABA), a dihydropteroate synthetase substrate. As a result, PABA is unable to convert to dihydrofolic acid. PABA is folic acid's immediate precursor. Hence, the cell development of microbes stops and eventually dies. Sulfonamides only inhibit microbes that manufacture their own folic acid. Therefore, other processes influencing the folic acid pathway could also be affected. Sulfonamides do not affect human cells or bacteria that can already utilize folic acid precursors or synthesize folic acid.

Uses

1. It is typically used to treat sensitive organism-caused urinary tract infections that are acute and uncomplicated.

2. If the infection is topical in the urinary system, it is not suitable for treatment.

4.7.2 Sulfisoxazole

It is one of the most extensively used sulpha drugs.

It is commonly used to treat a variety of bacterial diseases, including urinary tract infections.

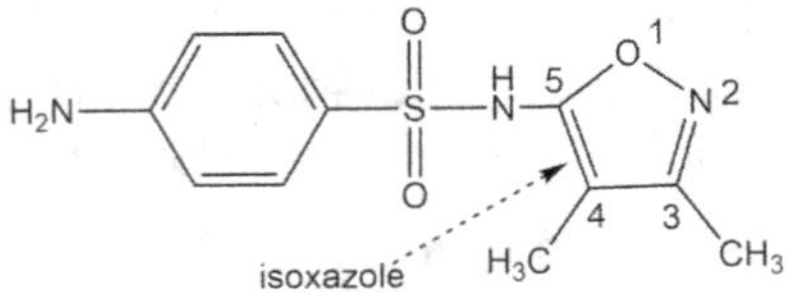

Fig. 4.48 Chemical structure of Sulfisoxazole.

Chemical Structure: (Fig. 4.48)

Chemical Name:

4-amino-*N*-(3,4-dimethylisoxazol-5-yl)benzenesulfonamide; *N*¹-(3,4-Dimethylisoxazol-5-yl) sulphanilamide

Mechanism of Action

Sulfisoxazole is a broad-spectrum sulfanilamide and a synthetic analogue of para-aminobenzoic acid (PABA). It has antibacterial properties. It competes with PABA for the bacterial enzyme dihydropteroate synthase, preventing PABA from being incorporated into dihydrofolic acid, folic acid's immediate precursor. It causes bacterial folic acid production and purine and pyrimidine synthesis inhibition, resulting in slow cell growth and death.

Sulfisoxazole inhibits the enzyme dihydropteroate synthetase. As a result, bacterial dihydrofolic acid synthesis is inhibited. This synthesis occurs when pteridine reacts with para-aminobenzoic acid (PABA). PABA is a substrate of the enzyme dihydropteroate synthetase. The blocked process further prevents the synthesis of folic acid in these organisms.

Uses

This drug is effective against *streptococci, gonococci, pneumococci, staphylococci,* and colon bacillus infections.

4.7.3 Sulfamethazine

Historical Background

Sulfamethazine (also known as sulfadimidine) is a sulfonamide drug. **William T. Caldwell** and co-workers, at Temple University in Philadelphia, USA, were the first to report its synthesis in 1941.

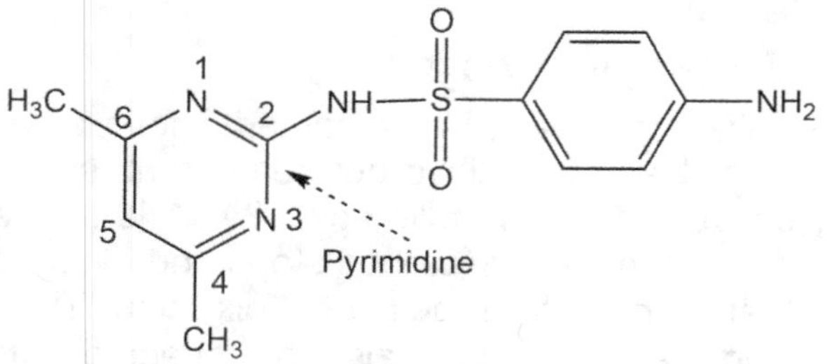

Chemical Structure: (Fig. 4.49)

Fig. 4.49 Chemical structure of sulfamethazine.

Chemical Name:

4-amino-N-(4,6-dimethylpyrimidin-2-yl)benzenesulfonamide; N^1-(4,6-Dimethylpyrimidin-2-yl)sulphanilamide

Mechanism of Action

Sulfamethazine is a sulfonamide drug with a bacteriostatic character. It competes with PABA for binding to dihydropteroate synthase (dihydrofolate synthetase). Hence, it inhibits of bacterial dihydrofolic acid synthesis. The production of DNA and bacterial nucleotides is slow when inhibition of dihydrofolic acid synthesis occurs.

It competes with PABA for binding to dihydrofolate synthetase, an intermediate in tetrahydrofolic acid (THF) synthesis. Thus, its interference with the enzymatic conversion of pteridine and p-aminobenzoic acid (PABA) to dihydropteroic acid. THF is essential for purine synthesis, and inhibiting its synthesis stops bacteria from growing.

Uses

✓ This drug is used to treat pneumococcal, staphylococcal, and streptococcal infections.

✓ It's given in the treatment of sepsis, gonorrhea, and other infectious disorders.

4.7.4 Sulfacetamide

Sulphacetamide sodium is a prescription drug used to treat ocular infections. It has antibacterial properties, and sulfur has mild keratolytic properties.

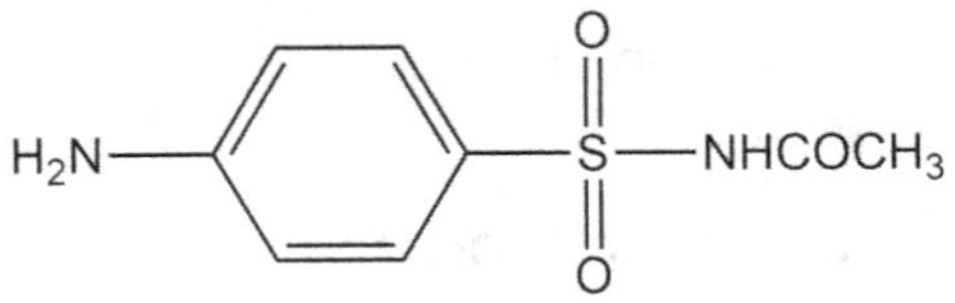

Fig. 4.50 Chemical structure of Sulfacetamide.

Chemical structure: (Fig. 4.50)

Chemical name:

N-((4-aminophenyl)sulfonyl)acetamide; Acetylsulphanilamide

Synthesis

It could be prepared by direct alkylation of acetamide with 4-aminobenzenesulfonyl chloride in the first technique. In the second technique, combining 4-amino-benzenesulfonam- ide with acetic anhydride is the first step. Subsequently, the resulting acetamide is then selectively reductively deacylated with a zinc–sodium hydroxide mixture to get the final product, sulfacetamide. (Fig.4.51)

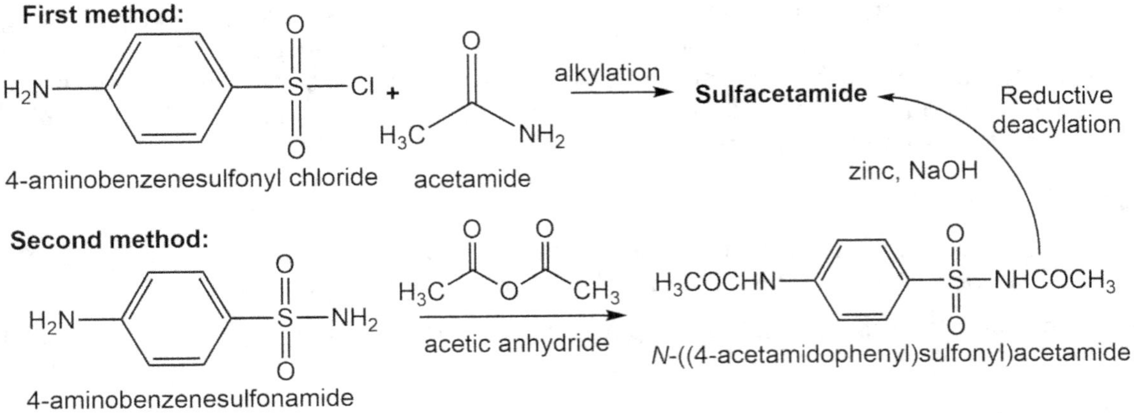

First method:

4-aminobenzenesulfonyl chloride   acetamide

alkylation → **Sulfacetamide** ← Reductive deacylation

zinc, NaOH

Second method:

4-aminobenzenesulfonamide

acetic anhydride → *N*-((4-acetamidophenyl)sulfonyl)acetamide

Fig. 4.51 Synthesis of Sulfacetamide.

Mechanism of Action

Most bacteria must produce their own folate in order to survive; they cannot obtain it from other sources. Humans, on the other hand, do not synthesise folate and must receive it through their diet. Sulphacetamides are folate synthesis inhibitors. The drug competes with p-aminobenzoic acid (PABA), which is the initial step of folate synthesis. The enzyme dihydropteroate synthase catalyses the following reaction. It causes the inhibition of tetrahydrofolate (THF) production and the prevention of DNA synthesis. This prevents bacteria from growing (a bacteriostatic effect).

Uses

1. Sulphacetamide sodium is used to treat eye infections and injuries.

2. This drug has antibacterial activity against *streptococci, pneumococci, staphylococci, meningococci,* and *gonococci.*

3. In neonates and adults, it is used to treat pneumonia, purulent (discharging pus) tracheobronchitis (cough), urinary tract infections, and gonorrheal disorders of the eyes.

4.7.5 Sulphapyridine

Historical Background

Lionel Whitby, a British scientist, of May & Baker Ltd., found it in 1937. It was used to treat bacterial pneumonia and made headlines after treating Winston Churchill, the British Prime Minister.

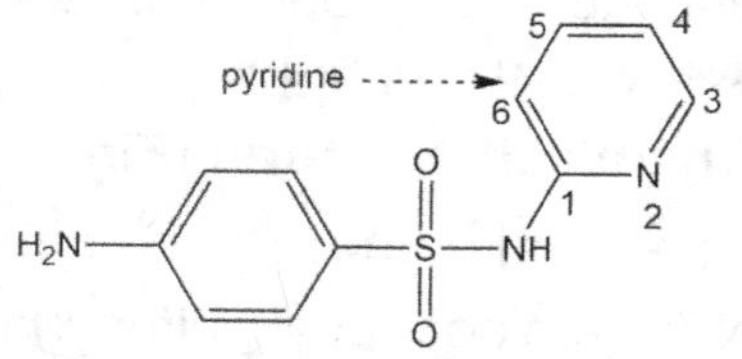

Chemical Structure: (Fig. 4.52)

Chemical Name:
4-amino-N-(pyridin-2-yl)benzenesulfonamide

Fig. 4.52 Chemical structure of Sulfapyridine.

Mechanism of Action

Sulfapyridine inhibits the bacterial enzyme dihydropteroate synthetase, which is a competitive inhibitor. In these species, it inhibits the synthesis of folic acid by blocking the substrate, para-aminobenzoic acid (PABA), in the reaction. The activity of dihydropteroate synthetase is important for the synthesis of folate, which is essential for cells to produce nucleic acids like DNA and RNA. As a result, if DNA molecules cannot be formed, the cell will not be able to divide.

Uses

1. This drug is antibacterial against *streptococci, pneumococci, staphylococci, meningococci, gonococci,* colon bacillus, and pathogenic dysentery.

2. It's used to treat dermatitis herpetiformis (Duhring's disease), which is a skin condition.

4.7.6 Sulfamethoxazole

Historical Background

In 1961, it was first introduced in the United States. It's now almost always used with trimethoprim. The sulphamethoxazole and trimethoprim combination was available in the mid-1970s. The WHO Model List of Essential Medicines lists this combination as a first-line treatment for urinary tract infections.

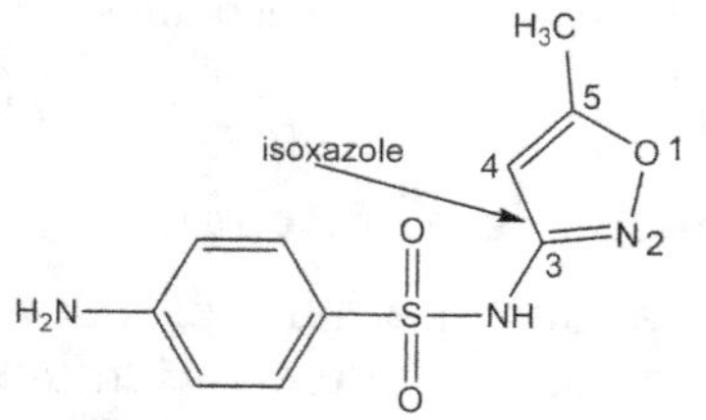

Fig. 4.53 Chemical structure of Sulfamethoxaole.

The ideal sulfamethoxazole/trimethoprim ratio is 20:1.

Chemical Structure: (Fig. 4.53)

Chemical Name:
4-amino-*N*-(5-methylisoxazol-3-yl)benzenesulfonamide;
4-amino-*N*-(5-methyl-3-isoxa- zolyl) benzenesulphanilamide

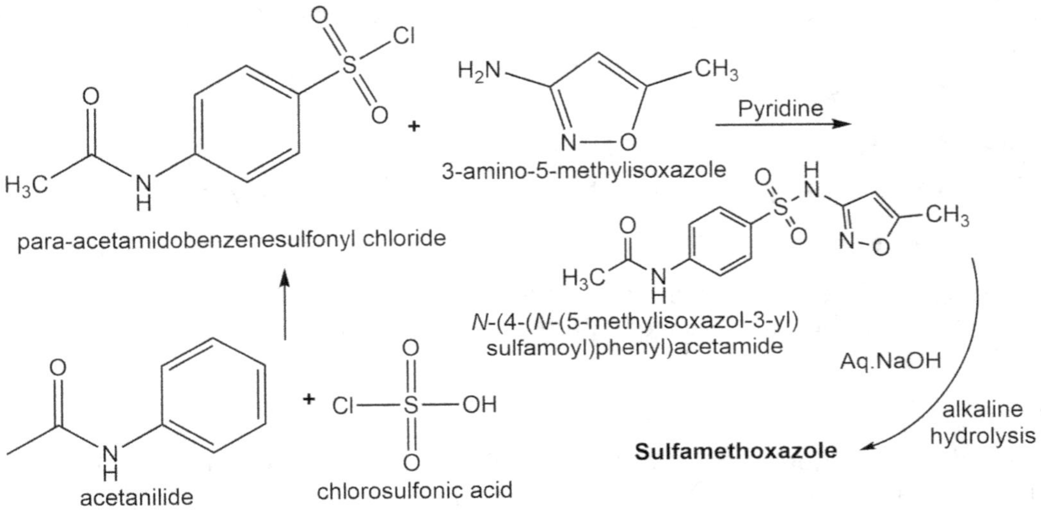

Fig. 4.54 Syntheis of Sulfamethoxazole.

Synthesis

Sulfamethoxazole is prepared by reacting 3-amino-5-methylisoxazole with para-acetamidobenzenesulfonyl chloride (treatment of acetanilide with chlorosulfonic acid yields para-acetamidobenzenesulfonyl chloride) in the presence of pyridine, and then alkaline hydrolyzing the intermediate. Sulfamethoxazole is produced by cleaving the acetyl group. (Fig. 4.54)

Mechanism of Action

Sulfamethoxazole is a structural analogue of para-aminobenzoic acid (PABA). The drug competes with PABA for binding to dihydropteroate synthetase by preventing PABA. Thus, the drug prevents dihydropteroate diphosphate from being converted to dihydrofolic acid or dihydrofolate. It causes the inhibition of normal bacterial folic acid synthesis when the formation of the dihydrofolate intermediate (folate) is inhibited. Folate involves DNA synthesis, especially thymidylate and purine biosynthesis, and amino acid synthesis, including serine, glycine, and methionine biosynthesis, making it a crucial metabolite for bacterial growth and replication. As a result, inhibiting folate production reduces bacterial growth by inhibiting folate-dependent metabolic pathways. Sulfamethoxazole belongs to the bacteriostatic since it suppresses bacterial growth.

Uses

A combination of sulfamethoxazole and trimethoprim is used to treat ear infections, urinary tract infections, bronchitis, diarrhea, shigellosis, and pneumonia.

4.7.7 Sulfadiazine

Historical Background

Sulfadiazine is an antibacterial sulfonamide that is used to treat mild to moderate infections. In 1973, the US FDA approved the use of sulfadiazine in the United States.

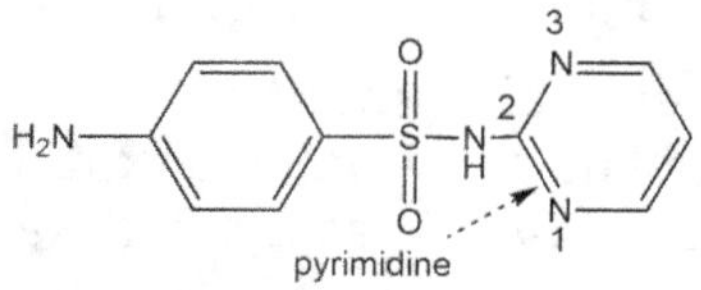

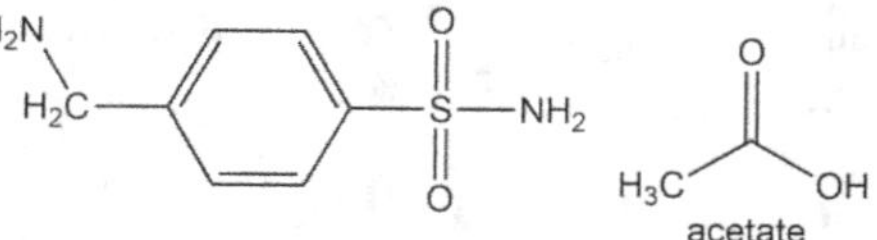

Fig. 4.55 Chemical structure of sulfadiazine.

Chemical Structure: (Fig. 4.55)

Chemical Name:

4-amino-*N*-(pyrimidin-2-yl)benzenesulfonamide; N^1-(Pyrimidin-2-yl)sulphanilamide

Mechanism of Action

Sulfadiazine has bacteriostatic effects. It prevents bacterial cells from synthesizing folic acid by inhibiting the formation of tetrahydrofolic acid from para-aminobenzoic acid (PABA).

Uses

1. Sulfadiazine is generally used to treat UTIs. The preferred regimen for *T. gondii* infection is a combination of sulfadiazine and pyrimethamine.

2. In burn victims, silver sulphadiazine and mafenide acetate are used topically for their antimicrobial properties.

3. Silver sulphadiazine cream is applied to treat skin infections, particularly in second and third-degree bums, infected leg ulcers, and pressure sores.

4.7.8 Mafenide Acetate

Historical Background

Mafenide was first used as a topical burn therapy in the mid-1960s. Mafenide acetate, a drug used by the Germans to heal open wounds during WWII, was developed for treating burns by microbiologist **Robert Lindberg** and surgeon **John Moncrieff** at the Institute of Surgical Research in San Antonio.

Fig. 4.56 Chemical structure of Mafenide acetate.

Chemical Structure: (Fig. 4.56)

Chemical Name: 4-(aminomethyl)benzenesulfonamide Mafenide acetate

Mechanism of Action

Mafenide has a distinct mode of action from sulfonamides. Mafenide is unaffected by PABA. There is no relationship between bacterial sensitivity to mafenide and sulfonamides. Changes in the acidity of the environment do not affect its activity. Mafenide acts by lowering the bacterial population in the avascular tissues of burns, allowing deep partial-thickness burns to heal on their own.

Uses

1. It's mostly used as a cream or a solution to help prevent and cure bacterial infections in second and third-degree burns.

2. Infected or contaminated wounds have been sterilized with povidone-iodine wound irrigation or wound soaking with mafenide.

3. The antibacterial properties of silver sulphadiazine and mafenide acetate applied topically to burn patients.

4.7.9 Sulfasalazine

Historical Background

Sulfasalazine was first designed to treat rheumatoid arthritis in the 1930s. However, before the previous two decades, this drug was mainly used to treat inflammatory bowel disease. Professor **Nana Svartz** developed sulphasalazine synthetically in Stockholm in the 1940s. In 1950, the US FDA approved sulfasalazine for medicinal use in the United States. It is listed as an essential medicine by the World Health Organization.

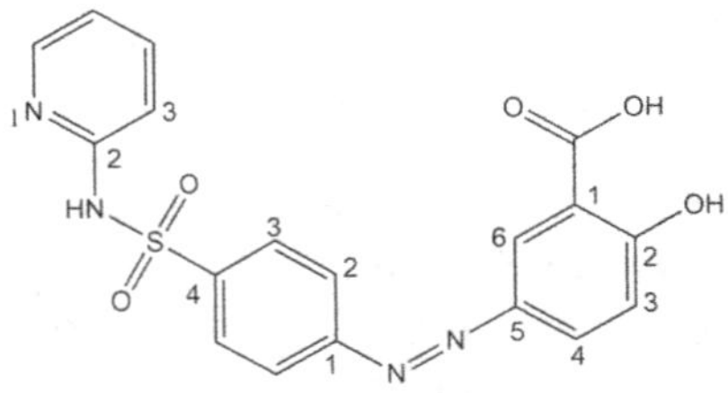

Fig. 4.57 Chemical structure of Sulphasalazine.

Sulphasalazine is an azo molecule that is a combination of sulphapyridine and 5-aminosalicylic acid. This drug's pharmacological effects are mainly due to its breakdown products, 5-aminosalicylic acid, and sulfapyridine. It has anti-inflammation, immunosuppressive, and antibacterial properties.

Chemical Structure: (Fig. 4.57)

Chemical Name:

2-hydroxy-5-((4-(*N*-(pyridin-2-yl)sulfamoyl)phenyl)diazenyl)benzoic acid

Pharmacology

It is a 5-aminosalicylic acid (5-ASA) and sulfapyridine combination (SP). In the small intestine, the drug is absorbed as intact sulfasalazine (SSZ). The drug is subsequently circulated through the enterohepatic system and delivered to the large intestine, where it is split into 5-ASA and SPs by the action of gut flora. SP is absorbed at this point, but 5-ASA is retained in the large intestine lumen. Through hydroxylation and acetylation, the SP moiety is metabolized in the liver. Individuals who are "slow acetylators" may have increased toxicity due to genetic variances in acetylation rates.

Mechanism of Action

Sulfapyridine kills bacteria by serving as a competitive antagonist for para-aminobenzoic acid. It involves blocking some folate-metabolizing enzymes.

Uses

1. It has been used as the primary treatment for ulcerative colitis and regional enteritis (Crohn's disease – GIT disorder).

2. It's suitable to treat rheumatoid arthritis and inflammatory bowel diseases.

3. It is not worthy for people who have thrombocytopenia, severe liver illness, or active viral hepatitis.

4.8 Folate Reductase Inhibitors

Several biological components can only be synthesized by prokaryotic and eukaryotic cells using reduced folic acid biomolecules. While most bacteria and plants synthesize these folic compounds from the start, some bacteria and mammalian cells employ folates and have recovery routes for decreased folates and pyrimidines. Six enzymes, including dihydrofolate reductase, are involved in the production of tetrahydrofolic acid (THF) from guanosine triphosphate, as illustrated in (Fig. 4.58). Purines, some amino acids, and thymidine are all produced by bacteria using tetrahydrofolate molecules.

DHFR (dihydrofolate reductase) is involved in the formation of cellular THF and subsequent components and aids in cell growth and proliferation. THF is produced solely by DHFR, which is rapidly incorporated into growing cells. Several key antibacterial drugs target this enzyme. There are clear differences between eukaryotic and prokaryotic DHFRs, which led to the discovery of trimethoprim as an antibacterial drug (TMP). TMP binds bacterial DHFRs 10^5 times more strongly than it binds vertebrate DHFRs. Antibacterial DHFR inhibitors work by preventing the production of DNA, RNA, and proteins, thereby stopping cell growth.

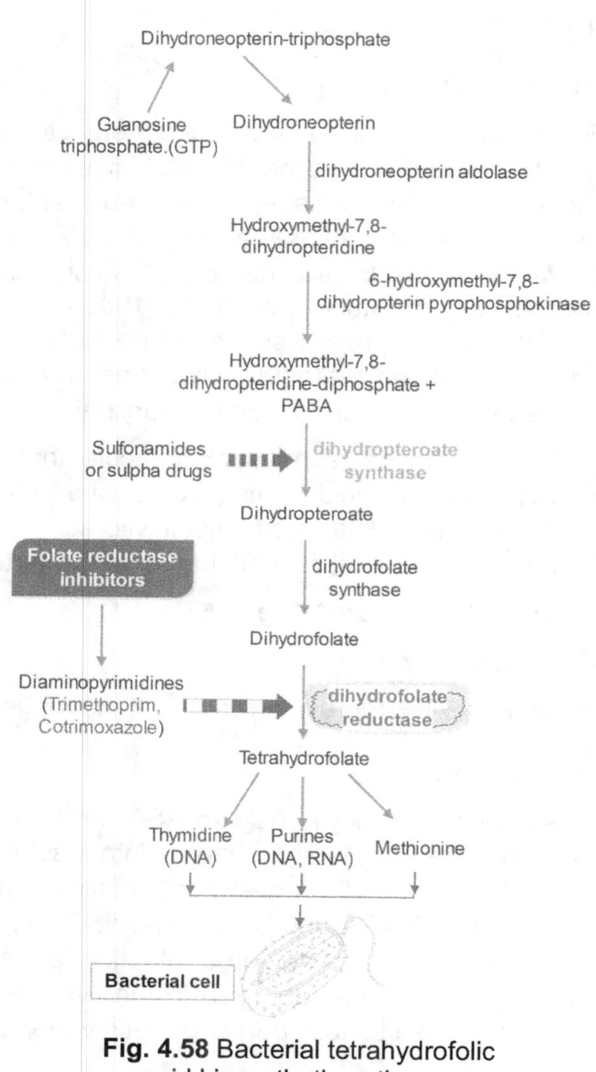

Fig. 4.58 Bacterial tetrahydrofolic acid biosynthetic pathway.

All living cells require tetrahydrofolate biomolecules for the production of purines, some amino acids, and particularly thymidine from GTP. It is one of the chemical components required for RNA synthesis during the transcription process. Furthermore, 3D structures of DHFR provide information to study inhibitor binding, enzyme: inhibitor complexes, and the distinctions between bacterial and mammalian DHFR. The abundance of data on DHFR makes it a promising therapeutic target for antimicrobial therapy. Moreover, knowledge of the mechanism of action and causes of resistance opens the way to new research and the discovery of antibacterial drugs that work by inhibiting DHFR specifically and selectively.

Indeed, diaminopyrimidines (trimethoprim, pyrimethamine) are effective dihydro-folate reductase inhibitors. The affinity of this chemical for receptive areas of dihydrofolate reductase is most likely due to the structural similarity between these drugs (as well as the structural similarity between the pteridine ring of folic acid and the diaminopyrimidine fragment of pyrimethamine).

Trimethoprim and pyrimethamine are diaminopyrimidines. These are antibacterial drugs and dihydrofolate reductase inhibitors that can be used alone or in combination with sulfanilamides, particularly with sulfamethoxazole (co-trimoxazole). When used in combination with sulfamethoxazole, it has a very significant effect on a wide range of bacteria. According to current research, the ideal sulfamethoxazole/trimethoprim ratio is 20:1. Drugs with a 5:1 ratio are suitable to get this ratio in the plasma (Fig. 4.58).

4.8.1 Trimethoprim

Historical Background

Sulfonamides and trimethoprim are antibacterial agents developed at opposite ends of the time scale. Trimethoprim, on the other hand, was first used in clinical practice in the late 1960s. Trimethoprim's antibacterial spectrum is comparable to that of sulphonamides. It can be bacteriostatic or bactericidal, depending on the microorganisms' growing circumstances.

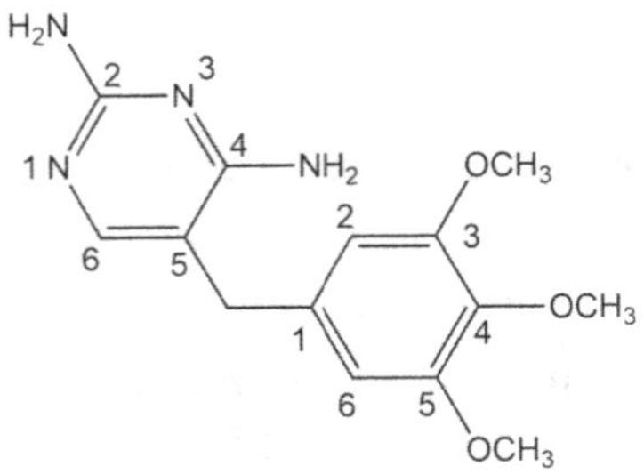

Fig. 4.59 Chemical structure of Trimethoprim.

Chemical Structure: (Fig. 4.59)

Chemical Name

5-(3,4,5-trimethoxybenzyl)pyrimidine-2,4-diamine;2,4-diamino-5-(3,4,5-trimethoxybenzyl) pyrimidine

Synthesis

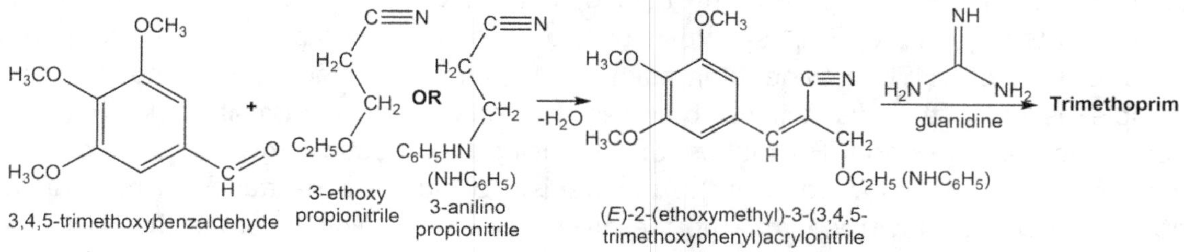

OCH_3 ; H_3CO ; H_3CO — 3,4,5-trimethoxybenzaldehyde + $C \equiv N$; H_2C ; CH_2 ; C_2H_5O — 3-ethoxy propionitrile **OR** $C \equiv N$; H_2C ; CH_2 ; C_6H_5HN (NHC_6H_5) — 3-anilino propionitrile $\xrightarrow{-H_2O}$ OCH_3 ; H_3CO ; H_3CO ; $C \equiv N$; C ; H ; CH_2 ; OC_2H_5 (NHC_6H_5) — (E)-2-(ethoxymethyl)-3-(3,4,5-trimethoxyphenyl)acrylonitrile $\xrightarrow[\text{guanidine}]{NH,\ H_2N,\ NH_2}$ Trimethoprim

Fig. 4.60 Synthesis of Trimethoprim.

Condensation of 3,4,5-trimethoxybenzaldehyde with 3-ethoxy- or 3-anilinopropionitrile yields the corresponding benzylidene derivative. The resultant derivative, which reacts directly with guanidine to provide trimethoprim. (Fig. 4.60)

Mechanism of Action

Trimethoprim's efficacy is due to its potent inhibition of bacterial dihydrofolate reductase, the enzyme that follows the sulfonamide-blocking phase in folic acid production. Trimethoprim is 50,000-100,000 times more effective than dihydrofolate reductase in bacteria than in humans. It prevents the conversion of dihydrofolate to tetrahydrofolate, which is a precursor to folinic acid and, eventually, purine and DNA synthesis. Sulfonamides and trimethoprim work together to disrupt the same metabolic pathway. Thus, resulting in a high level of synergistic action against a wide range of bacteria. Humans do not produce folic acid but need it in their food, and trimethoprim's enzyme suppression has no effect on human purine synthesis.

Uses

- ✓ It's used to treat infections of the urinary system, such as cystitis.
- ✓ It has occasionally been used to treat various infections, such as chest infections and acne.
- ✓ It is used in the treatment of urinary tract infections, prostatic infections, otitis media in children, Shigella eradication, and *Pneumocystis carinii* pneumonia in combination with sulfonamides.
- ✓ Trimethoprim is also effective for acute conjunctivitis when coupled with polymyxin B.

4.8.2 Cotrimoxazole

Historical Background

Co-trimoxazole is a wonder drug with a broad antibacterial spectrum that makes it effective for treating a wide range of illnesses and good tissue penetration that makes it useful for infections affecting numerous body systems.

In patients with AIDS, the combination of sulfamethoxazole and trimethoprim has proven to be the most effective treatment and prophylactic for pneumocystis. This combination was first reported in 1975 and became the main treatment strategy by 1980. To treat both pneumonia and extrapulmonary infections, this combination is beneficial. Co-trimoxazole inhibits both the incorporation of p-aminobenzoic acid (PABA) into folic acid and the conversion of dihydrofolic acid to tetrahydrofolic acid by dihydrofolate reductase.

Trimethoprim

Sulphamethoxazole

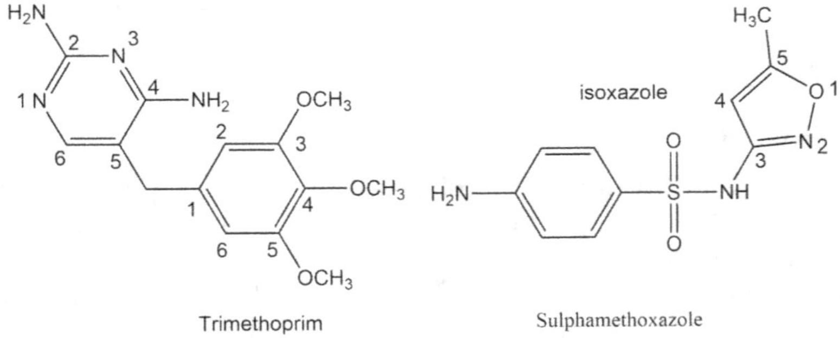

Fig. 4.61 Chemical structure of Co-trimoxazole.

Chemical Structure: (Fig. 4.61)

Chemical name:

5-(3,4,5-trimethoxybenzyl)-2,4-pyrimidinediamine (Trimethoprim)-4-Amino-*N*-(5- methyl-1,2-oxazol-3-yl)benzenesulfonamide (sulphamethoxazole) - 1:1

Mechanism of Action (Fig. 4.62)

Trimethoprim and sulfamethoxazole prevent bacteria from making tetrahydrofolic acid, which is the physiologically active form of folic acid and an essential cofactor for the production of thymidine, purines, and bacterial DNA. Sulfamethoxazole is a sulfonamide drug that suppresses the formation of the intermediate dihydrofolic acid from its precursors. It is a structural analogue of para-aminobenzoic acid. Trimethoprim is a structural counterpart of dihydrofolic acid's pteridine component that inhibits dihydrofolate reductase and, as a result, tetrahydrofolic acid formation from dihydrofolic acid. This bactericidal activity is achieved by sequentially blocking two enzymes in one pathway.

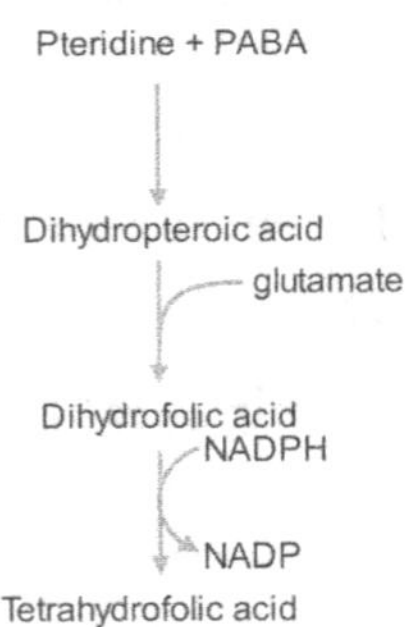

Fig. 4.62 Folate metabolism steps are hindered by sulfonamides and trimethoprim in a specific order.

Uses

Co-trimoxazole is used to treat bacterial infections such as pneumonia, bronchitis, and infections of the urinary system, ears, and intestines. It's also used for the treatment of diarrhea.

4.9 Sulfones

Diaryl sulfones are the most common type of drug used to treat leprosy. Studies looking into the SAR of sulfonamides led to the discovery of sulfones. Other active compounds have been developed through a variety of chemical changes, but none have proven to be more useful than the original lead, 4,4'-diaminodiphenylsulfone (Dapsone). In 1943, dapsone became the first drug to cure leprosy.

4.9.1 Dapsone

Historical Background

Eric Fromm., and **J. Wittmann**, chemists at the University of Freiburg, released a report on the synthesis of dapsone on June 15, 1908. The therapeutic potential of dapsone was unknown and unused for almost three decades after that until the rise of sulfa drugs turned scientific attention to the medical characteristics of sulfur-containing compounds. Dapsone was not intended as a medicinal treatment at the time, but rather as a product of pure chemical science ambitions. In the context of sulfonamide research, two organisations in England and France were the first to examine dapsone as an antibacterial agent in 1937. Researchers quickly identified chemically related compounds, such as dapsone, as prospective additions to this family of drugs. **R. G. Cochrane** and his associates studied dapsone in 1949 and discovered it to be "the most potent anti-leprosy treatment". A wide range of disorders, including tuberculosis, leprosy, and AIDS-related pneumonia, were treated with the drug dapsone between 1936 and 1996.

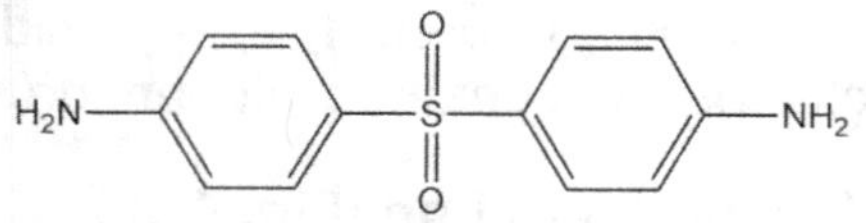

Fig. 4.63 Chemical structure of Dapsone.

Chemical Structure: (Fig. 4.63)

Chemical Name: 4,4'-sulfonyldianiline; 4,4-diaminodiphenylsulfone

Synthesis: (Fig. 4.64)

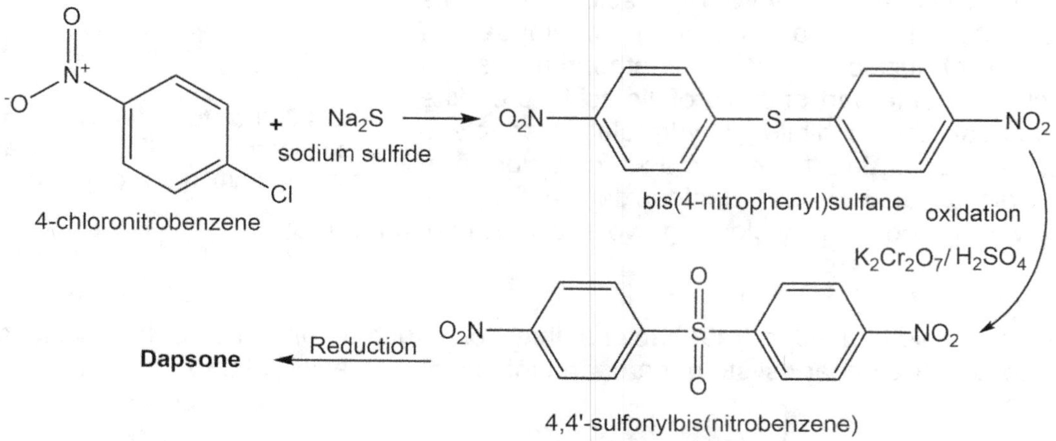

Fig. 4.64 Synthesis of Dapsone.

It is prepared either from 4-chloronitrobenzene or the sodium salt of 4-acetamido-benzenesulfonic acid. Reacting 4-chloronitrobenzene with sodium sulphide yields 4,4-dinitrodiphenylthioester and oxidising the sulphur atom in this molecule with potassium dichromate in sulfuric acid yields 4,4-dinitro-diphenyl sulfone. With hydrochloric acid tin dichloride, the nitro group is reduced to yield the desired product, namely dapsone.

Structure-Activity Relationship: (Fig. 4.65)

1. Dapsone is a synthetic sulfone compound that has similar activity to sulfonamide drugs. It targets dihydropteroate synthase, a key enzyme in bacteria.

2. In order to increase the activity of dapsone, several derivatives of dapsone have been developed. Out of which, thiazolsulfone was formed through isosteric substitution (thiazole ring) of one benzene ring. It is less effective than dapsone, even though it is still active.

3. Acetosulfone is created by substituting an acetamide group in one of the aromatic rings. The resultant product has decreased activity compared to dapsone while increasing water solubility and decreasing GI discomfort.

4. Adding a methanesulfinate group to dapsone to make sulfoxone sodium is an effective substitute. In vivo, this water-soluble form of the subsequent product is a breakdown to yield dapsone. Individuals who are unable to tolerate dapsone due to GI irritation should take sulfoxone sodium, which must be taken in a dose three times that of dapsone due to the poor metabolism of dapsone.

5. Chemical modification of dapsone derivatives is examined in the hopes of discovering additional drugs for the treatment of Mycobacterium leprae resistant strains.

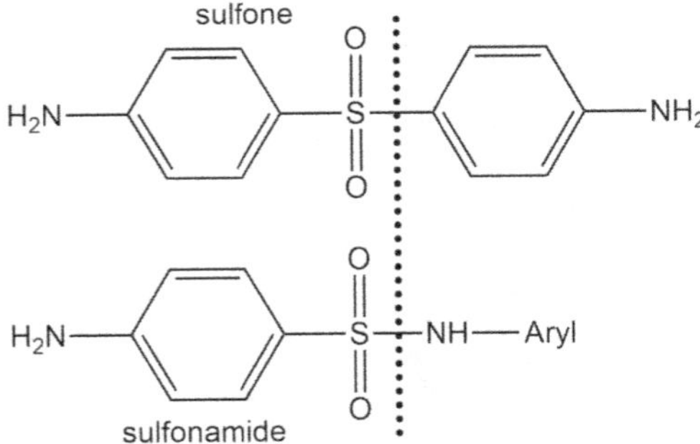

Fig. 4.65 Structural difference between sulfone and sulfonamide.

Mechanism of Action

Dapsone is not a sulfonamide. However, it functions in the same way as sulfonamide by competing for the active site of dihydropteroate synthase with para-aminobenzoic acid.

It works as a bacteriostatic antibacterial agent. It mimics the activity of sulphonamides in inhibiting the formation of dihydrofolic acid by competing with para-aminobenzoic acid for the active site of dihydropteroate synthetase. Sulfones have been shown to inhibit the growth of a wide range of pathogenic bacteria, including *streptococci*, *staphylococci*, *pneumococci*, and *mycobacteria*.

Uses

- ✓ Dapsone is a sulfone drug that is primarily used to treat leprosy. It is beneficial in specific types of refractory skin lupus, such as bullous lupus (blisters on the skin.).

- ✓ It is also in the treatment of lupus profundus (Inflammation of the skin).

- ✓ Dapsone has been used treatment of uncomplicated malaria in combination with pyrimethamine and chlorproguanil.

CHAPTER 5

INTRODUCTION TO DRUG DESIGN AND COMBINATORIAL CHEMISTRY

5.1 Introduction to Drug Design

Drug design, also known as rational drug design, is the process of developing drug candidates based on knowledge of a biological target. The drug is usually an organic small molecule that activates or inhibits the action of a biomolecule, such as a protein. This approach provides a therapeutic benefit to the patient.

The simplest term for drug design is to create molecules that are complimentary in shape and charge to the biomolecular target with which they interact and bind the active site. Computer modelling approaches are commonly used in drug development. Computer-aided drug design (CADD)(Fig. 5.1) is a term used to describe this type of modelling. Finally, structure-based drug design refers to drug development that is based on knowledge of the biomolecular target's three-dimensional structure. Biopharmaceuticals, which include peptides and, in particular, therapeutic antibodies, are becoming a more important class of drug design.

Drug design is simply the development of molecules with complementary 3D structures and charge distributions to the protein target in order to maximize molecular recognition and binding. Molecular docking opens the door to *in silico* creation and optimization of virtual compounds by predicting molecular recognition and binding affinity.

is a more correct phrase for "drug design" (i.e., the design of a molecule that will bind firmly to its target, such as a protein). Although design strategies for predicting binding affinity are quite successful, many other qualities, such as bioavailability, metabolic half-life, side effects, and so on, must first be improved before a ligand can be made into a safe and effective medicine. During the clinical phases of drug development, more emphasis is given to selecting candidate drugs with physicochemical properties. It is predicted to result in fewer development complications and, as a

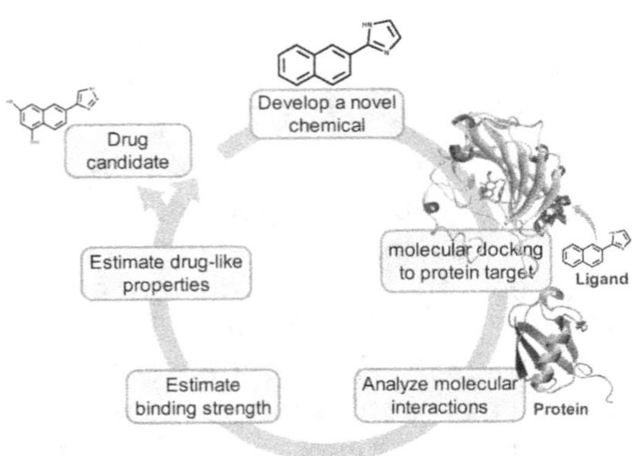

Fig. 5.1 Computer-Aided Drug Design.

197

result, is more likely to lead to a drug that is approved and marketed. *In vitro* tests, in combination with computational methods, are increasingly being utilised in early drug development to choose molecules with better ADME (absorption, distribution, metabolism, and excretion) and toxicity profiles.

To create possible drugs, such as inhibitors of viral proteins or RNA, drug designers use the information of the 3D structure of the binding site (or the structure of the complex with a ligand). A force field is required in addition to the 3D structure to analyze the interaction between the protein and the ligand (to predict binding energies). Virtual screening is putting a library of molecules through their paces on a computer to see how well they can attach to a macromolecule.

The present drug design and development process is a complex one (Fig.5.2). Drugs were initially discovered by observing the impact of numerous natural ingredients on sick and healthy people throughout history. Willow bark has been used to treat pain for thousands of years, and its effectiveness has been linked to its salicylic level. The discovery of salicylate (salicylic acid) as an active component of willow bark gave one of the earliest 'lead compounds' (salicylic acid) for therapeutic development, leading to the discovery of aspirin.

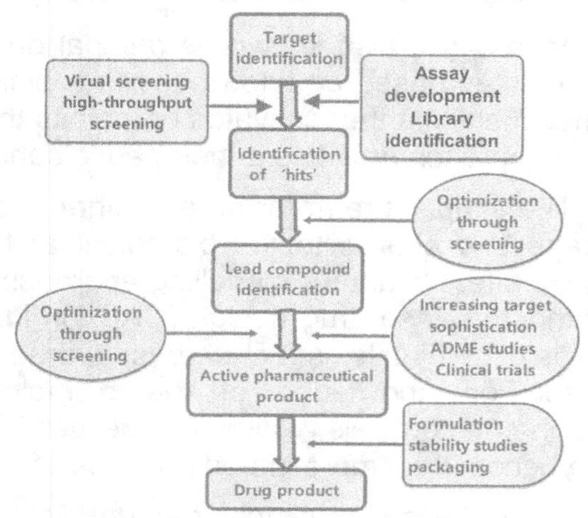

Fig. 5.2 The process for developing a new drug.

Pharmacologically active compounds are only part of a drug's design process (Fig.5.3), whereas it includes several other steps. For example, unwanted side effects must be eliminated, or pharmacokinetic behaviour improved by chemically altering a lead component.

Salicylic acid was the active ingredient in aspirin for pain relief, but it caused gastrointestinal irritation; acetylation of the o-hydroxyl group produced the therapeutic derivative used today. The transition of physostigmine from a natural substance to a drug is another example. , the

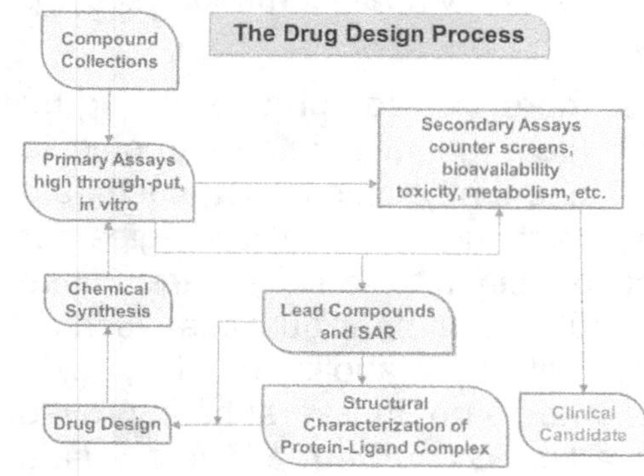

Fig. 5.3 Schematic diagram of drug discovery cycle.

active component of the Calabar bean (Physostigma venenosum) found in tropical Africa. It was suspected of containing a lethal poison. Physostigmine, a competitive inhibitor of acetylcholine esterase was identified 60 years ago. Early research identified physostigmine as a lead chemical for a class of cholinesteric drugs, leading to novel derivatives including phenserine, which is being studied for the treatment of Alzheimer's disease. It is now common practice in drug discovery to use structural biology as well as high throughput screening and computer models for virtual screening.

Various approaches used in drug design

Drug design is essentially the creation of small drug molecules with 3D shapes and charge distributions. The designed molecule is complementary to the protein target in order to maximize molecular recognition and binding. Molecular docking opens the door to in silico creation and optimization of virtual compounds by predicting molecular recognition and binding affinity.

Before the twentieth century, human beings used herbs as drugs. The efforts to extract and purify active substances (i.e., the pure chemicals responsible for the therapeutic characteristics) from various sources to cure diseases did not begin until the mid-nineteenth century. Many of the pharmaceutical businesses we know today owe their existence to the success of these initiatives. Several naturally occurring drugs have been obtained since then, and their structures have been determined. For instance, morphine from opium, cocaine from coca leaves, quinine from the bark of the cinchona tree.

These natural chemicals inspired a massive synthetic effort, with chemists creating thousands of analogues in an attempt to improve on what nature had already provided. Although much of this work depends on a trial-and-error process, the results show numerous general principles behind drug design. Researchers relied on the lead molecule, an active principle derived from nature, or a synthetic product synthesized in the laboratory.

Over the last century, chemistry has had a positive impact on life expectancy and quality in the design and production of drugs. It is common knowledge that the design and development of a new medicine costs more than a billion dollars and takes at least ten years. Despite these efforts, only a small percentage of drug discovery initiatives will result in a new drug. CADD is one of several technologies that have been created to streamline the process by reducing time, cost, and dropout rate. CADD makes use of computational resources, algorithms, and 3D visualization of the drug molecule. This technique helps in the production of noble drug molecules. It improves rational thinking about how to make or change molecules, as well as decision-making during the drug design process.

There are two types of CADD technologies: A. structure-based and B. ligand-based approaches.

A. Structure-based drug design (SBDD):

Definition: It is the process of designing and optimizing a chemical structure to identify a substance appropriate for clinical testing — a therapeutic candidate. It is based on a complete understanding of the drug's three-dimensional structure, as well as how the drug's shape and charge cause it to interact with its biological target, resulting in a therapeutic benefit.

In comparison to the traditional methods (such as random screening, trial & error method, ethnopharmacology approach, serendipity method, and classical pharmacology), SBDD is becoming an indispensable tool for faster and more cost-effective lead discovery. Numerous new targets and approaches for drug discovery have emerged as a result of genomic, proteomic, and structural studies.

Because of the large number of target proteins available, the completion of the human genome project and developments in bioinformatics have accelerated drug development. The availability of 3D structures of therapeutically significant proteins helps the discovery of binding cavities and has paved the way for SBDD. This is becoming an increasingly important component of both industrial drug development initiatives and academic research purposes. Because it works with the 3D structure of a target protein and knowledge about the disease at the molecular level, SBDD is a more specific, efficient, and quick technique for lead discovery and optimization. Structure-based virtual screening (SBVS), molecular docking, and molecular dynamics (MD) simulations are the most prevalent computational approaches employed in SBDD. These methods can be used to analyze binding energetics, ligand-protein interactions, and the conformational changes that occur during the docking process. A tremendous rise in software packages for efficient drug discovery processes has pushed recent improvements in the drug design process. In addition, the availability of supercomputers, computer groups, and cloud computing has accelerated the identification and evaluation of lead compounds.

When the three-dimensional structure of the protein target is available or reliably reconstructed, SBDD techniques could apply in this case. It is thought that molecular docking is the foundation of structure-based drug design. Anti-influenza drugs like zanamivir and oseltamivir (Tamiflu) are two of the most effective treatments.

A small molecule's ability to bind to a specific protein target is the first and most important goal in structure-based drug design. If it does, the strength of the molecular recognition will be determined by this prediction. The first goal can be fulfilled with a docking algorithm, which optimises the interactions between both chemical groups to allow for the most likely geometry shape and position of a small molecule at the surface of a protein. Many docking systems, including web-based utilities like SwissDock.ch and Autodock, and the Autodock Vina programme (free software), can be used to determine the molecular binding position. The concept of molecular docking is simple, which can be explained to any beginner.

For instance, we found favorable findings when 3D models of cyclooxygenase (COX) and ibuprofen, a well-known anti-inflammatory drug that binds to COX. It is possible to analyze the COX model, revealing the binding site that accepts ibuprofen. To automate the docking process by employing computer algorithms to treat many types of molecules.

The second objective, measuring the small molecule's affinity for the protein, can be accomplished using a binding free energy estimator. There is computer-assisted software that can be used for this purpose. They're primarily based on high-level methodologies involving physical chemistry and statistical physics principles. Theoretically complicated concepts like fitness or score might, however, be concealed by more basic concepts. A docking software usually produces a rough estimate of the binding free energy, which can be determined as a score to optimize the drug molecule.

SBDD (Fig.5.4) is a computer technique and is usually practised by scientists and pharmaceutical firms. SBDD has discovered several drugs that are currently on the market. Isoniazid (tuberculosis), norfloxacin (UTI), dorzolamide (glaucoma), amprenavir (HIV), and flurbiprofen (rheumatoid arthritis) are the most well-known success stories of the SBDD study.

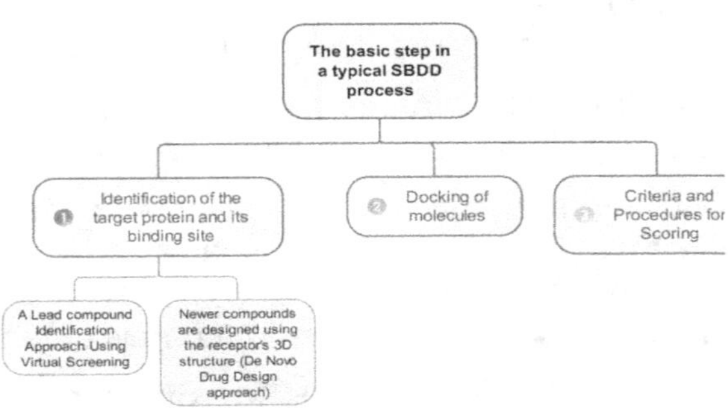

Fig. 5.4 The basic step in a typical SBDD process.

SBDD is a multi-cycle procedure that leads to the development of an optimized drug candidate for clinical trials. The identification and confirmation of the target protein is the first stage in a typical SBDD procedure. Here, the following steps are involved during the optimization of molecular structures.

1. **Identification of the target protein and its binding site:** NMR, X-ray crystallography, or cryo-electron microscopy are preferred to determine the 3D structures of proteins. But if a solution structure is not available, in silico methods are employed to model the protein's 3D structure. There are three well-known structure prediction methods, such as comparative modeling, threading, and *ab initio* modeling. Homology modelling is one of the best and most reliable ways because it predicts the 3D shape of a target protein based on the structure of homologous proteins with >40% similarity. The next step is to identify the binding pocket after the target protein's structure has been determined. The next stage is to find hits by docking chemical libraries into the target protein's binding cavity. SBDD utilizes two distinct strategies for locating hits: virtual screening and *de novo* design

I. **A Lead compound Identification Approach Using Virtual Screening:** This strategy involves computationally screening databases containing millions of drug-like or lead-like chemicals against target proteins with well-known 3D structures. Docking is a method of screening compound libraries in which ligands are screened based on their binding affinity. The computational screening's top hits are next put to the test *in vitro*. Through computer algorithms, the target protein is docked with vast libraries of drug-like chemicals that are commercially available. Afterward, experimental assays is carried out to confirm the binding's validity once a scoring function has run.

II. **Newer compounds are designed using the receptor's 3D structure (*De Novo* Drug Design approach):**

De novo drug design is a technique for creating novel chemical compounds from molecular components. The idea behind this method is to design chemical structures for small molecules that have a high affinity for binding to the target binding cavity. It is classified into two groups: (i) ligand-based and (ii) receptor-based. The latter method is more common.

2. **Docking of molecules:** Molecular docking is classified into two types: flexible-ligand search docking and flexible-protein docking.

   Docking is a virtual simulation tool for molecular interactions. Molecular docking is the most prevalent SBDD technique because it accurately predicts the shape and binding of ligands inside a target active site. A ligand-binding position and intermolecular interactions for complex stability can be studied using this method.

3. **Criteria and Procedures for Scoring:** A docking programme can use a scoring algorithm to dig further into the ligand-binding region. The scoring function calculates binding affinity once a significant binding confirmation has been identified. Scoring functions, as a result, are expected to have a significant impact on docking. Scoring functions are developed using a training dataset of chemicals from a similar class for which experimental binding affinity data is available. There are four types of scoring functions: force field, empirical, knowledge-based, and machine learning.

B. Ligand-based drug design (LBDD): Ligand-based drug design is a technique used when there is a limitation of 3D information for receptors and focuses on knowledge about molecules that bind to the biological target of interest. The most essential and extensively used techniques in ligand-based drug design are 3D quantitative structure-activity relationships (3D QSAR) and pharmacophore modeling. They can generate prediction models that can be used to identify and optimize leads (Fig. 5.5).

Application of LBDD:

I. QSAR Studies:

QSAR is defined as a technique that quantitatively links structural molecular features (descriptors) with functions (e.g., physicochemical qualities, biological activities, toxicity, and so on) for a group of related substances.

QSAR is an alternative technique and one of the most frequently applied ligand-based drug discovery approaches in the lack of good structural knowledge. The term QSAR

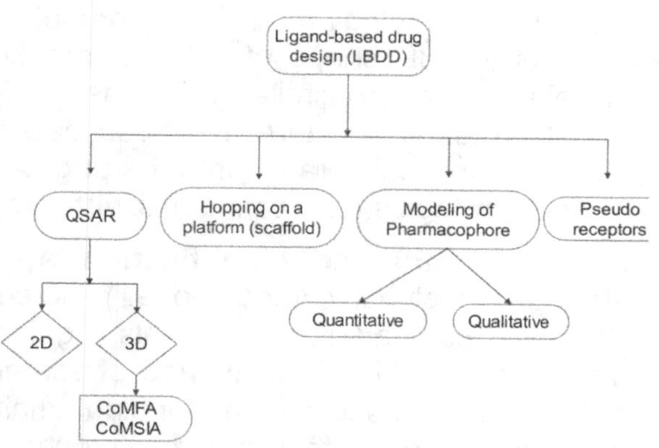

Fig. 5.5 LBDD types of drug design.

refers to approaches that connect molecular structure with qualities such as in vitro or in vivo biological activity. When QSAR relates to toxicological data, these methods are called the quantitative structure toxicity relationship (QSTR), and when modelling physicochemical attributes with QSAR, they are known as the quantitative structure-property relationship (QSPR). The idea behind QSAR is that a molecule's structure (i.e., its geometric, steric, and electronic properties) must contain the features that are responsible for its physical, chemical, and biological activities.

QSAR is defined as a technique (Fig.5.6) that quantitatively links structural molecular features (descriptors) with functions (e.g., physicochemical qualities, biological activities, toxicity, and so on) for a group of related substances.

II.   Strategies for Pharmacophore Modeling:

In the early 1900s, **Paul Ehrlich** proposed the term pharmacophore to refer to the molecular structure of the compound that carries (phoros) the properties which are important for a drug's biological activity (pharmacon). **Peter Gund** described it later in 1977 as a set of structural properties in a molecule that is recognized at the receptor site and is responsible for that molecule's biological activity.

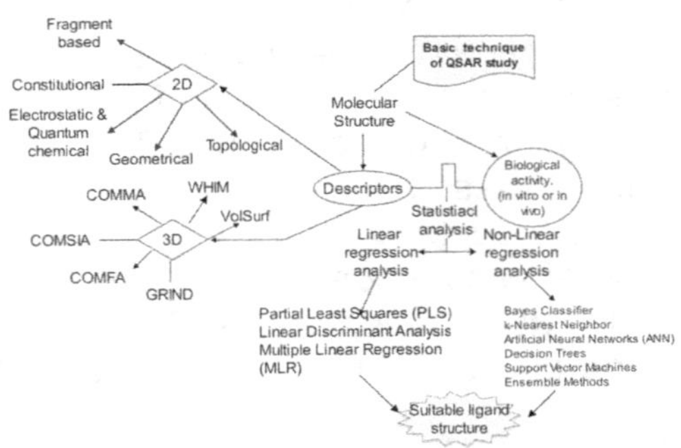

Fig. 5.6 Basic technique of QSAR study.

Virtual screening based on pharmacophores has recently become a highly valuable technique for the hit design step of drug development. It has become the most widely used method in drug design research where the target's three-dimensional (3D) structure is unknown.

The key benefit of this method is that it allows for quick screening of millions of chemicals to identify promising candidates. Three processes are involved in the pharmacophore mapping/modeling of the drug. They are First identifying the features required for a specific biological activity; second determining the confirmation of molecular structure (i.e., the bioactive conformation); and third, developing a superposition or alignment rule for the series of compounds.

Drug target selection, database preparation, pharmacophore model building, and 3D screening are all processes in the pharmacophore-based virtual screening process. Catalyst, Ligand Scout, DISCO, GASP, Phase, MOE, and other software programs now provide automated pharmacophore mapping.

Hydrogen bond acceptor (A), hydrogen bond donor (D), hydrophobic (H), negative ionic/ionizable (N), aromatic rings (R), and positive ionic/ionizable (P) are the most common types of interaction sites detected by pharmacophore software programme. All of these strategies rely on activity to create pharmacophore models that can distinguish between active and inactive compounds while eliminating the latter.

III. Scaffold Hopping:

Scaffold hopping is a technique for identifying structurally diverse compounds and preserving a specific biological function, i.e., keeping the 3D interaction capabilities of a scaffold while changing the structural skeleton. If structurally varied compounds are determined, this will aid in the discovery of new classes of chemicals that can be used to combat the target protein. There are only a few automated scaffold hopping methods available.

IV. Modeling of Pseudoreceptors:

Pseudoreceptor modelling is a new approach in computer-aided drug design that allows for the reconstruction of an unknown target's three-dimensional structure using the structures of its ligands (known bioactive compounds). It integrates existing methodologies while also greatly expanding their capabilities by creating a specific receptor model. This model can then be used to estimate affinity and perform other receptor-based modelling activities. Pseudoreceptor models connect the dots between ligand- and receptor-based drug development. In computational chemistry, Pseudoreceptor models are termed as 3D QSAR approaches.

5.2   QSAR

Medicinal chemistry is an interesting subject area that includes organic chemistry, biochemistry, computational chemistry, pharmacology, pharmacognosy, molecular biology, and physical chemistry. This field of chemistry refers to the discovery, design, synthesis, and testing of novel drugs for human and animal use. It also entails the investigation of commercially available pharmaceuticals, their biologic features, and quantitative structure-activity connections (QSAR).

The numerous approaches that can be employed in drug development. Several of these efforts entailxed reshaping the drug to better 'fit' its target receptor binding site. Changes in functional groups or substituents were used in other ways to improve the drug's pharmacokinetics or binding site interactions. Analogues with various substituents on aromatic or heteroaromatic rings or accessible functional groups were often synthesized. If we tried to create analogues with every possible substituent and combination of substituents, the number of possible analogues would be limitless. To solve this difficulty, researchers used the quantitative structure-activity relationship (QSAR) method.

The QSAR method aims to identify and measure a drug's physicochemical qualities to evaluate if any of them have an impact on the drug's biological activity. If such a relationship exists, the medicinal chemist can create an equation that quantifies the relationship and allows them to conclude with some certainty that the property of the drug plays a substantial role in the drug's pharmacokinetics or pharmacodynamics. It also gives the medicinal chemist some predictive ability. There are two benefits to doing so. First, it enables the medicinal chemist to focus on analogues with improved biological activity by reducing the number of analogues required. Second, if an analogue has not fit the equation, it indicates that another parameter may attribute significance and suggests a direction for additional research.

The QSAR approach must be applied correctly and appropriately. First, A compound's structure, target, and mechanism of action must all be similar. Second, proper testing processes must be employed. For example, *In vitro* testing on isolated enzymes is important for QSAR studies since the actions of different inhibitors are directly involved in how they bind to the active site. However, *in vivo* experiments for enzyme inhibitors are invalid due to pharmacodynamic and pharmacokinetic considerations. It prevents the construction of a QSAR equation.

It is impossible to quantify and correlate all of a drug's features with its biological activity at the same time. Simpler and more practicable is to alter one or two physicochemical aspects of the drug while keeping other properties constant. It is not always possible to change one property without impacting another. It has worked in many QSAR studies.

QSAR attempts to design drugs by creating a mathematical relationship between quantifiable physicochemical properties including lipophilicity, shape, and size of the molecule, biological activity, and electron distribution or electronic effects within the molecule.

5.2.1 Physicochemical Parameters used in QSAR

The field of medicinal chemistry investigates how chemical structure affects biological activity. Therefore, understanding the mechanism by which a drug works, as well as how the molecular and physicochemical features of the molecule influence the pharmacokinetics (absorption, distribution, metabolic processing, and excretion) and pharmacodynamics (what the drug does to the body) of the drug are vital.

The term "physicochemical properties" describes how a molecule's functional groups affect its acid-base characteristics, water-solubility, partition coefficient, crystal structure, stereochemistry, and ability to interact with biologic systems, including enzyme active sites and receptor sites. The relative contribution of each functional group (i.e., pharmacophore) to the total physicochemical properties of the molecule must be studied in order to create better medicinal agents. This form of research entails changing a molecule systematically and then determining how these changes alter biological activity. Structure-activity relationships (SARs) are studies that look at how structural properties of a molecule contribute to or subtract from the desired biologic activity.

The QSAR method has been used to investigate a variety of physical, structural, and chemical properties, but the most prevalent are hydrophobic, electronic, and steric properties. This is because these effects can be quantified. Complete compounds or individual substituents can have their hydrophobic characteristics easily measured. However, quantifying electronic and steric properties for entire molecules is more difficult, and this is only really practicable for individual substituents.

QSAR investigations are more commonly conducted on compounds with the same structure but different substituents on aromatic rings or available functional groups. The QSAR analysis then evaluates how the substituents' hydrophobic, electronic, and steric characteristics affect biological activity.

5.2.2 Hydrophobicity

The hydrophobicity of a drug affects its ability to cross cell membranes and may play a role in receptor interactions. It's possible that substituent changes to a drug's hydrophobic nature — and hence its biological activity — will have prime effects. As a result, it is essential to quantify the hydrophobicity of a drug molecule.

5.2.2.1 The Partition Coefficient: (*P*)

A molecule's hydrophobicity character could be evaluated by its log P-value, while P is known as the partition coefficient.

The partition coefficient (log P) is a physicochemical measure. It is defined as the ratio (in logarithms) between the equilibrium concentrations of a drug dissolved in a two-phase system containing polar and non-polar solvents. These two phases are frequently limited to two liquid solvents, water and n-octanol, in the life and pharmaceutical sciences.

The hydrophobicity of a drug can be determined experimentally by measuring its relative distribution in an *n*-octanol/water mixture. In this two-phase system, hydrophobic molecules prefer to dissolve in the n-octanol layer, while hydrophilic molecules prefer the aqueous layer. The partition coefficient (*P*), which stands for the relative distribution of the molecule between two phases, can be calculated using the following equation:

$$P = \frac{\text{Concentration of drug in octanol}}{\text{Concentration of drug in aqueous solution}}$$

The P-value of hydrophobic molecules is high, while the P-value of hydrophilic compounds is low.

In other words, when hydrophobicity increases, biological activity increases. The above result indicates that the drug's hydrophobicity is increased, making it easier for it to pass through cell membranes and reach its target areas. This could imply that by increasing hydrophobicity, one could continue to increase activity. In actuality, this is not the case at all. The majority of QSAR experiments are undertaken on compounds with a narrow log P value range. If compounds were produced with a considerably wider range of log P values, an optimum log P value beyond which activity would fall would be identified. The below formula would result in a parabolic curve (Fig. 5.7), where k_1 k_2 and k_3 are constants.

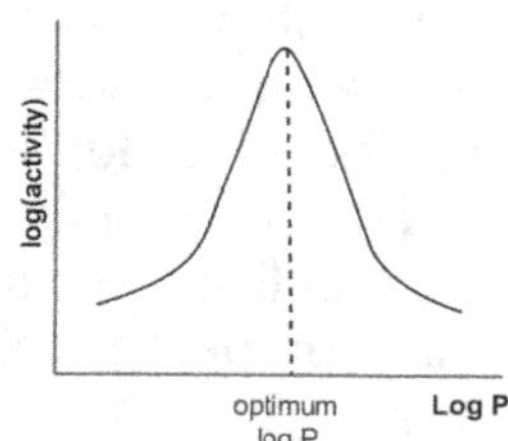

Fig. 5.7 Parabolic curve relating log(activity) vs. log P.

$$\log(\text{activity}) = -k_1(\log P)^2 + k_2 \log P + k_3$$

In this equation, the $-(\log P)^2$ input has a detrimental influence on activity, but the logP entry has a beneficial effect. Log P is more significant than $-(\log P)^2$ when P is low. As a result, log P is more significant in the first half of the curve, and activity increases as log P increases. The $-(\log P)^2$ component takes over in the second half of the curve, and activity decreases.

Since biological activity is dependent on drugs that pass-through cell membranes, log P is present in the majority of QSAR equations when considering their in vivo activity. The log P factor may be less important or perhaps negligible when activity is undertaken in an in vitro study.

A series of analogues with varied hydrophobicities and, hence, varying P values will be produced by modifying the lead compound's substituents. By graphing these P values against the biological activity of these drugs, it is possible to determine whether there is a relationship between the two characteristics. The biological activity is denoted as 1/C, where C denotes the drug concentration required to achieve a specific level of biological activity. The reciprocal of the concentration (1/C) is employed because more active drugs have a defined biological activity at a lower concentration.

A straight-line graph (Fig.5.8) is made by graphing log (1/C) against log P. The graph indicates that there is a link between hydrophobicity and biological activity. The equation for such a line is:

$$\log \left(\tfrac{1}{c}\right) = -k_1 \log P + k_2$$

Fig. 5.8 Biological activity versus log P.

5.2.2.2 Substituent Hydrophobicity Constant

The partition coefficient indicates a molecule's overall hydrophobicity, but it is also feasible to measure the hydrophobic character of individual substituents of the compound by using sets of tables that provide hydrophobicity constants (π) for each substituent. The hydrophobicity of a substituent relating to hydrogen is called the substituent hydrophobicity constant. The value could be determined empirically by comparing the logP values of a standard chemical with and without the substituent. The following equation has to get the hydrophobicity constant (π_x) for the substituent (X):

$$\pi_X = \log P_X - \log P_H$$

P_x is the partition coefficient for the analogue containing the substituent, while P_H is the partition coefficient for the standard compound. If π is greater than zero (positive value), the substituent has a higher hydrophobicity than hydrogen. The substituent is less hydrophobic than hydrogen, if π is a negative value obtained.

This calculated value would be advantageous if the hydrophobicity of the molecule as a whole had previously been determined. There are two reasons, though, why such constants might be valuable. First, hydrophobicity constants can be used to determine logP values for various compounds, hence eliminating the need to measure each logP value

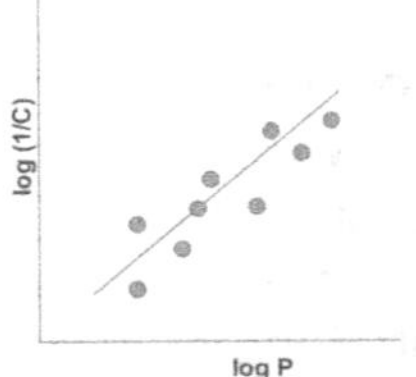

Fig. 5.9 LogP calculation for para-bromoanisole.

experimentally. For example, Para-logP bromoanisole's value can be computed as 2.97 using benzene's logP value (2.13), andπ constants for the bromine and methoxy 0.86 and -0.02 respectively could be obtained from the set of the table as substituent constant (Fig.5.9).

The π constants are only meaningful for the structures that determined them. As a result, the aromatic π constants apply to substituted benzenes but not to heteroaromatic ring complexes. Similarly, the aromatic π constants are irrelevant for aliphatic substituents. For the molecular skeletons being examined, precise π values should ideally be determined experimentally.

For the second reason, π values can be used in QSAR to see if hydrophobic substituents at specific locations on the molecular skeleton have any localized effect on activity. A QSAR equation can contain both logP and π. The former examines how the molecule's overall hydrophobicity affects activity, such as its ability to cross cell membranes, whereas the latter shows any localised hydrophobic effects. If, hydrophobic substituents in the para position of an aromatic ring are favourable to activity. Then there may be a hydrophobic binding pocket in the binding site which can induce the fit of the substituents.

5.2.3 Hammet's Electronic Parameter

The electronic characteristics of specific substituents can also have a significant impact on biological function. The **Hammett substitution constant**, σ, describes the electronic properties of aromatic substituents. These constants were given in separate tables and were determined experimentally by observing the influence of substituents on benzoic acid dissociation. Benzoic acid is a weak acid that ionizes only partially in the water (Fig. 5.10). The **equilibrium** or **dissociation constant** K_H (the subscript H indicates that there are no substituents on the aromatic ring) is established between the ionized and nonionized forms, and the relative proportions of these species are known as the equilibrium or dissociation constant:

$$K_H = \frac{C_6H_5COO^-}{C_6H_5COOH}$$

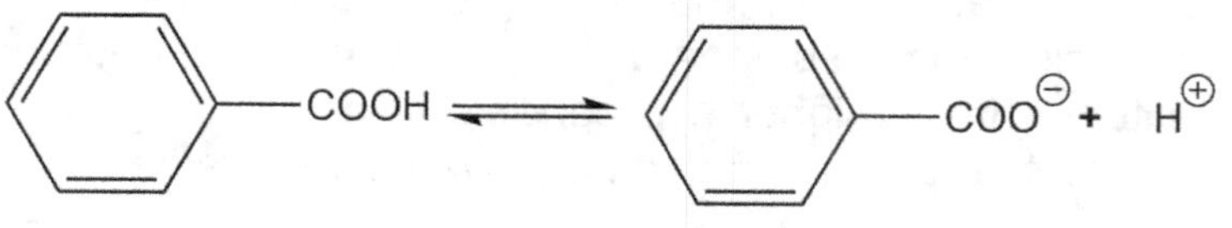

Fig. 5.10 Ionization of benzoic acid.

This equilibrium will be affected by substituents on the aromatic ring. The carboxylate anion will be stabilized by substituting electron-withdrawing groups, and the equilibrium will move to the ionized form, resulting in a greater equilibrium constant. Substitution of an electron-donating group destabilizes the carboxylate ion, causing the equilibrium to move to the left and the equilibrium constant to decrease. The following equation gives the Hammett substituent constant (σ_x) for a specific substituent (X):

$$\sigma_x = \log \frac{K_x}{K_H} = \log K_x - \log K_H$$

These constants, like hydrophobic constants, are only correct for the chemical structures from which they are derived. Electron-donating substituents (e.g., CH_3, CH_2CH_3) have a negative value while electron-withdrawing substituents (e.g., Cl, CN, CF_3) have a positive value.

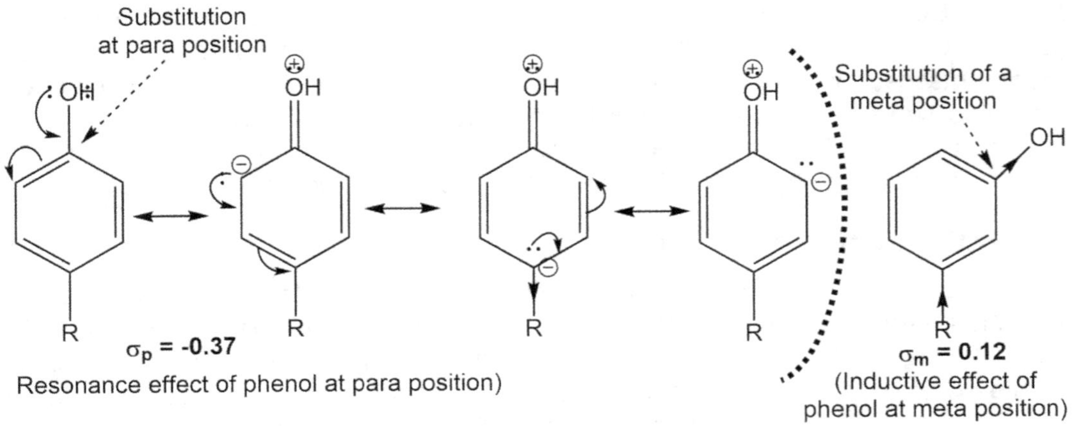

Fig. 5.11 The electronic effect of phenol in the para and meta regions.

The Hammett substituent's value to consider both inductive and resonance effects (σ_m and σ_p) and the could depend on whether the substituent is meta or para to the remainder of the molecule. For example, the electron-withdrawing influence felt at the meta position due to induction effect, σ_m value is 0.12 for a phenol group. When the phenol group is in the para position, σ_p value is -0.37, indicating that the group is now electron-donating due to resonance at that location (Fig. 5.11). Because ortho substituents can have both a steric and an electronic influence, aromatic substitution constants for ortho substitution are inaccurate.

As stated previously, the Hammett substitution constants account for both inductive and resonance effects. However, the inductive effect (F) or the resonance effect (R) of aromatic substituent constants could be quantified individually.

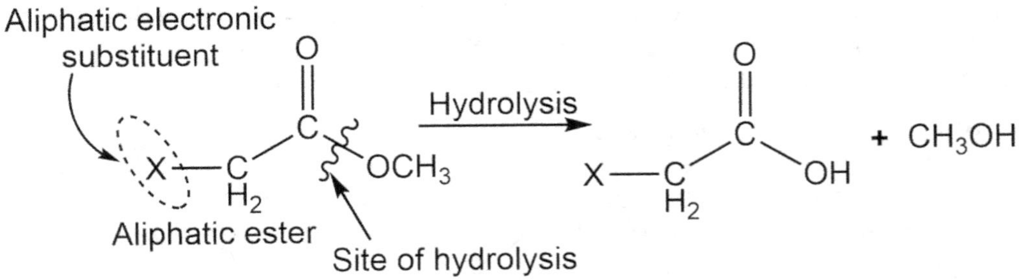

Fig. 5.12 An aliphatic ester undergoes hydrolysis.

Aliphatic electronic substituent constants are usually measured by monitoring the rates of hydrolysis of a series of aliphatic esters (Fig.5.12). Here, methyl ethanoate has been taken as the parent ester. The rate of hydrolysis of the aliphatic compound depends on the substituent's electronic effect, which is due to inductive influences. Electron donating groups have negative values because they slow down the rate of hydrolysis. Electron withdrawing groups have positive values and improve the rate of hydrolysis. Bulky substituents may have a steric effect on the hydrolysis rate by protecting the ester from hydrolysis. Hydrolysis rates under basic and acidic environments can be used to distinguish between these two (steric and electronic) effects. The two factors are essential in basic conditions, whereas only steric factors are important in acidic ones. Values for the electronic effect (σ_I) and the steric effect (E_s) can be calculated by comparing the hydrolysis rates of aliphatic compounds.

5.2.4 Taft's Steric Parameter

The chemical compound's biological activity is linked with the size of different substituents attached. Bulky groups can reduce activity by preventing drugs from binding effectively. A bulky substituent, in contrast, can boost activity by pushing a molecule into the active conformation required for binding. It's not as easy to determine a substituent's steric qualities as it is to estimate its hydrophobic or electronic nature. However, the three most common approaches to determining the steric effect of the studied compound are as follows:

To examine the size of the substituent in the chemical structure, researchers used an experimental technique known as **Taft's steric factor** (E_s). This technique involves observing how different substituents affect the rate at which a chemical reaction occurs in the parent structure. Large substituents near the reaction centre slow down the reaction more than smaller substituents; hence, reaction rate differences are used to determine the size of a substituent.

Additionally, using the substituent's molecular weight (MW), density (d), an index of refraction (n), one may compute the substituent's **molar refractivity** (MR) as a measure of the size of the substituent.

$$MR = \frac{(n^2-1)}{(n^2+2)} \times \frac{MW}{d}$$

The volume is defined by the formula MW/d, whereas the correction factor $(n^2-1)/(n^2+2)$ specifies how easily the substituent can be polarized. It is especially important if the substituent contains π or lone pairs of electrons.

Sterimol, a computer-based software application, generates steric factors known as Verloop steric parameters. It is a third technique of estimating the size of the substituents. This programme could apply to measuring the substituent's standard bond angles, van der Waals radii, bond lengths, and potential conformations of the substituents at the binding site. The advantage of this technique is being able to determine a Verloop steric parameter for any substituent without the requirement for any experimental data.

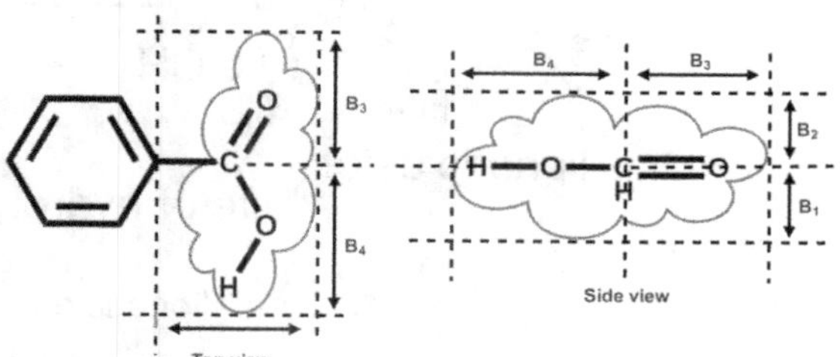

Fig. 5.13 Steric parameter determination of carboxylic acid by Verloop.

For example, the Verloop steric characteristics of a carboxylic acid group are illustrated in Fig. 5.13. The length of the substituent is L, while the radii of the group are B1-B4.

5.2.5 Hansch Analysis

The QSAR equation relating physicochemical properties to activity is known as the Hansch equation. These equations typically incorporate many parameters, the most common of which are logP, π, σ, F, R, MR, and E_s. The following is an example of a Hansch equation.

$$\log \left(\tfrac{1}{C}\right) = -k_1(\log P)^2 + k_2\log P + k_3\pi + k_4\sigma + k_5 E_s + k_6$$

Where k_1-k_6 are constants. To produce the best fitting line, these constants would be determined by a computer. A drug's biological activity is commonly measured as 1/C, where C is the drug concentration required to produce a specific biological effect (for example, the drug concentration required to produce 50% inhibition of an enzyme). If a drug is more potent, then a lower concentration of the drug is necessary, and the value of 1/C increases accordingly. The following equation is an example of a Hansch equation for the inhibitory action of a sequence of N-(phenyloxyethyl) cyclopropylamines (Fig. 5.14) against the enzyme monoamine oxidase.

$$\log \tfrac{1}{c} = 0.398\pi + 1.089\sigma - 1.03E_s(3,5) + 4.541$$

Positive values of π and σ indicates the increase activity, and shown that electron-withdrawing hydrophobic substituents are advantageous for activity. The Taft steric properties of any substituents in the meta position are represented by the E_s (3,5) factor. Bulky groups have a negative E_s value, indicating that they are unfavorable for activity.

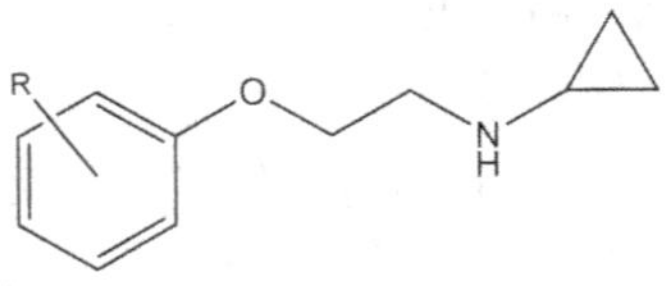

Fig. 5.14 N-(phenyloxyethyl) cyclopro-pylamines series compound.

It's important to remember that the quality of a QSAR equation is directly related to the quality of the input data. Typically, several compounds are produced to determine the impact of two or three physical characteristics (for example, π and σ) on biological activity. However, to analyze compounds, it is critical to select a correct set of compounds. It means that the substituents must provide a wide range of values for the physical parameters in interest while also distinguishing among them so that they are not correlated (i.e., follow the same trend). Let's take the substituents F, Cl, Br, and I as an example of how they differ. The electron-withdrawing effect of these substituents follows the F, Cl, Br, I pattern, with I being the most electron-withdrawing and F being the least effective. The hydrophobic property of these substituents, however, increases in the same order. Without such information, it is impossible to determine if any similar trend in biological activity is attributable to the hydrophobic or electronic properties of the substituents. Craig plots can be used to find acceptable substituents for QSAR experiments.

5.2.6 Hansch Analysis: An Update

Hansch's analysis is based on earlier attempts to link pharmacological activity to observable chemical properties by researchers such as **Richardson** (1867), **Richet** (1893), **Meyer** (1899), **Overton** (1901), **Ferguson** (1939), and **Collander** (1954). In the early 1960s, Hansch and his colleagues proposed a multiparameter solution based on the drug's lipophilicity and the electronic and steric effects of groups contained in its structure. They realized that a compound's biological activity has estimated by its capacity to reach and bind to its target position of a biological system. According to Hansch, Drug action can be separated into two stages:

A. The delivery of a drug to its actual site of action

B. The drug's affinity for the target location

He described the drug's distribution as a "random walk" from the place of administration to the region of action. The ability of a drug to reach its target depends on its lipophilicity throughout this 'walk'. In mathematical terms, this capacity is a function of the drug's partition coefficient P or the p values of relevant substituents. However, the shape, electron distribution, and polarizability of the groups implicated in the interaction determine how well the drug binds to the target site once it reaches it. The Hammett electronics and Taft E_s constants are two of the most popular parameters used to explain each of these elements of pharmacological activity.

Hansch proposed that all or some of these parameters may be linked to a drug's biological activity using simple mathematical calculations based on the following general format:

$$\log \left(\frac{1}{C}\right) = k1 \text{ (partition parameter)} + k2 \text{ (electronic parameter)}$$

$$+ \ k3 \text{ (steric parameter)} + k4$$

k1, k2, k3, and k4 are numerical constants generated by entering the data into a suitable computer statistical tool, and C is the minimal concentration required to produce a specific biological response. These parameter values are derived from the literature (for example, p, π and E_s) or determined experimentally.

The accuracy of Hansch equations, and the effectiveness of QSAR investigations, is dependent on the number of analogues used, the precision of the data, and the parameters chosen. The following factors influence the level of the Hansch equation.

a) The higher the number of analogues employed in a study, the more likely an accurate Hansch equation will be derived. A basic guideline is that the minimum number of compounds in the study should not be fewer than 5x, where x is the number of parameters utilized to obtain the relationship. When substituents are varied, it's also important to employ as many distinct substituents in as many different positions as necessary.

b) To develop a Hansch equation, biological data of the chemical compound must be accurate because the relationship's value depends partially on the subject being measured. Thus, to derive the Hansch equation, a sufficient number of measurements of any biological data, such as a compound's activity, must be taken.

Extreme parameter values should also be avoided, as they tend to dominate regression analysis and produce inaccurate Hansch equations. Their presence indicates that the parameter is either unsuitable or uncorrelated.

c) The choice of parameter is crucial since one parameter may produce an acceptable regression constant while another may not. For example, it may be able to correctly connect dipole moments of a sequence of analogues with biological activity but not with Hammett constants. Also, some parameters like p and π are connected, so using them in the same equation can be confusing.

Hansch equations are commonly used to either determine and quantify the parameters that control analogue activity or to estimate the structure with the optimum activity. In this situation, the Hansch equation is employed to find the most active analogue parameter values and relate them to substituents that either match or best fit these ideal values. Tables can be used to find these values.

Hansch analysis has a prime drawback in that its parameters ignore the three-dimensional nature of biological systems. Three-dimensional QSAR attempts to address this issue.

5.2.7 Pharmacophore Modeling

The **pharmacophore** defines the relative positioning of prime atoms or functional groups allowed to bind to a specific target. Existing compounds can be screened through computers to know the presence of the desired pharmacophore, which could lead to the discovery of new lead compounds.

The pharmacophore is a diagram that depicts the prime binding groups which are essential for biological activity and their relative positions in space. For example, the two phenol groups, the aromatic ring, and the nitrogen atom are the most important binding groups for our hypothetical drug glipine. The pharmacophore will be as illustrated in Fig. 5.15. The two-dimensional (2D) pharmacophore is shown in structure I, whereas the three-dimensional (3D) pharmacophore is shown in structure II. The latter describes the relative spatial placement of the major groups. In this scenario, the nitrogen atom is 5.063A from the phenolic ring's centre and at an angle of 18 from the ring's plane.

A bonding type of pharmacophore is a 3D pharmacophore - Structure III (Fig. 5.15). The bonding qualities of each functional group are defined in the 3D pharmacophore here. It includes the aromatic ring, which is determined by the centroid. To specify their placements, pharmacophoric triangles connect all the points. The phenol groups of the structure can act as hydrogen bond donors or acceptors, during interaction with the receptor. The aromatic ring can also take part in van der Waals interactions, and the amine, if protonated, can operate as a hydrogen bond acceptor or as an ionic center.

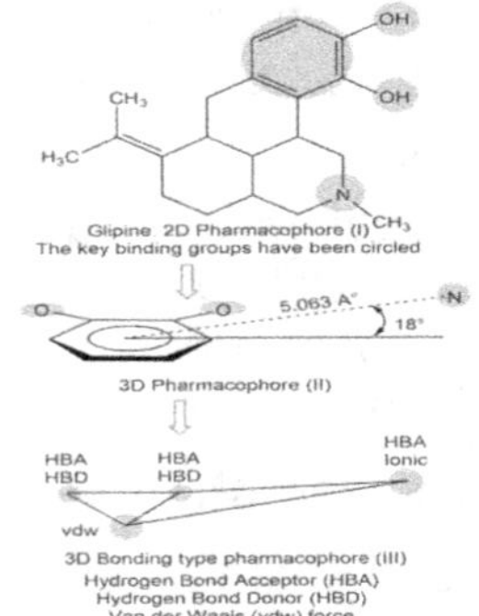

Fig. 5.15 A pharmacophore of Glipine (hypothetical drug).

After a century of research, pharmacophore methods have emerged as one of the most common techniques in drug discovery. Various ligand-based and structure-based approaches for enhanced pharmacophore modelling have been developed, and they have been effectively and widely used in virtual screening, de novo design, and lead optimization. Despite these advances, pharmacophore techniques have not reached their full potential, especially in reducing the present high overall cost of drug discovery and development.

Historical Background: In 1909, **Paul Ehrlich** defined pharmacophore as "a molecular framework that carries (phoros) the key features responsible for a drug's (pharmacon) biological activity". According to IUPAC's A pharmacophore model is a group of steric and electronic properties required to achieve optimal supramolecular interactions with a given biological target and to trigger (or block) its biological response. Günd and Wermuth have studied the evolution and history of the pharmacophore concept over the last century.

Following the breakthroughs in computational chemistry over the last 20 years, a plethora of automated tools for pharmacophore modelling and their applications have emerged regularly.

Types of pharmacophore:

A pharmacophore model has two types. They are either ligand-based or structure-based techniques. A ligand-based pharmacophore model could be constructed by superimposing a series of active molecules and identifying common chemical characteristics that are important for their bioactivity. Structure-based pharmacophores are created by probing potential contact locations between the macromolecular target and the ligands. Virtual screening, *de novo* design, lead optimization, and multitarget drug discovery have all developed from pharmacophore approaches (Fig. 5.16).

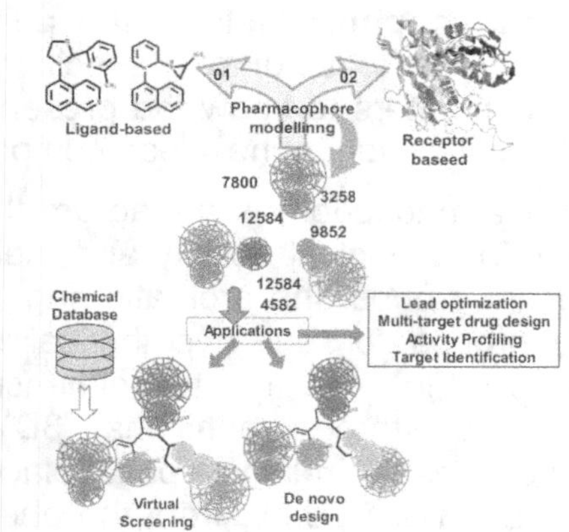

Fig. 5.16 The complete pharmacophore design framework.

Pharmacophore models are 3D representations of the chemical and steric properties required for a small molecule to interact with a target protein. These properties are related to chemical functions such as hydrogen bond acceptor (HBA), hydrogen bond donor (HBD), hydrophobic region (H), aromatic ring (AR), positively/negatively ionizable groups (PIs/NIs), and exclusion volume.

A. Ligand-based pharmacophore modeling:

Ligand-based pharmacophore (LBP) modelling has become a significant computational technique for helping drug discovery. The LBP model is developed by extracting common chemical characteristics from the 3D structures of a known set of ligands that describe fundamental interactions between the ligands and a macromolecular target.

Regarding LBP modelling, there are two major steps: first, creating a conformational space for each ligand in the training set to represent conformational flexibility and align the multiple ligands in the training set, and second, determining the essential common chemical features to build the pharmacophore model. The most challenging step in LBP modelling is the conformational study of ligands and their molecular alignment.

Numerous ligand-based modelling computational tools are available. However, nearly all of them are commercial (LigandScout, Discovery Studio, MOE, PHASE, etc.). PharmaGist is a well-known free programme for creating ligand-based pharmaco-phores. Different techniques such as genetic optimization, clique detection, and pharmacophore alignment are used in these applications to identify common pharmacophores.

B. Structure-based pharmacophore modeling:

SBP modeling is entirely dependent on the three-dimensional structures of macromolecular targets or macromolecule-ligand complexes. SBP approaches have gained popularity as the number of experimentally defined 3D target structures has expanded dramatically. The approach is contemporary with docking procedures, offering the same degree of information and requiring less computational resources. SBP modeling includes assessing the active site's complimentary chemical properties and their spatial correlations, as well as building a pharmacophore model assembly with selected features.

SBP modeling comes in two types: macromolecule-ligand complex-based and macromolecule-based (without ligand). The macromolecule-ligand complex-based technique is useful for finding the macromolecular target's ligand-binding site and determining the critical points of interaction between ligands and the target protein. LigandScout is a software tool that uses a macromolecule-ligand complex-based approach. A similar approach is used by programmes like Pocket v.2 and GBPM. The requirement for a 3D structure of the macromolecule-ligand combination is a key drawback of this method. As a result, it can't be used in circumstances when no ligands targeting the desired binding site are known. The macromolecule-based approach can help with this. A classic example of a macromolecule-based methodology is the SBP method, which is implemented in the Discovery Studio software.

Docking techniques:

Definition:

Docking: It is a molecular modeling technique for evaluating how well a ligand and its binding site (receptor) fit together.

Ligand: A ligand is a corresponding companion molecule that binds to the receptor to allow an efficient bimolecular response. It includes small drug molecules, neuro-transmitters, hormones, lymphokines, lectins, and antigens.

Concept of docking:

The study of how two or more molecular structures (for example, drug and enzyme or protein) fit together is known as molecular docking. Docking is a molecular modelling technique that predicts how a protein interacts with small molecules (ligands). The ability of a protein (enzyme) or nucleic acid to form a supramolecular complex with small molecules affects protein dynamics and can increase or decrease biological function. Molecular docking describes how small molecules behave in target protein binding sites. This approach identifies correct ligand positions in a protein's binding pocket and predicts ligand-protein affinity. Docking is classified (Fig. 5. 17) by the ligands used.

Classification:

Protein-small molecule (ligand) docking is a basic process, and numerous systems exist that facilitate predicting compounds that may inhibit the proteins. Protein-protein docking is usually significantly more difficult. The reason that proteins have a wide range of conformational options is that they are highly flexible.

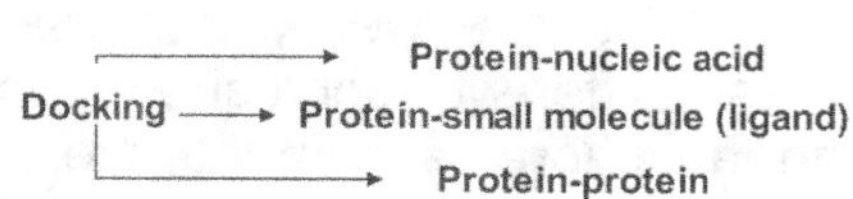

Fig. 5.17 Classification of docking.

Docking approaches for protein-nucleic acid have to predict the 3D structures of macromolecular complexes from their atomic coordinates. Theoretical models of macromolecular structures can provide enough information to establish a working hypothesis and direct subsequent experimental analysis to identify essential amino acids or nucleotide residues. However, they are less specific than experimental measurements.

Docking studies: Docking is a tool for predicting the optimal orientation of ligands at the active site of receptors when they are linked together to form a stable complex. Due to its capacity to determine the binding conformation of a small molecule (ligand) to the appropriate target binding site, it is one of the most often utilized methods in structure-based drug design. These techniques allow many compounds to be evaluated for biological activity at an early step in the drug development process.

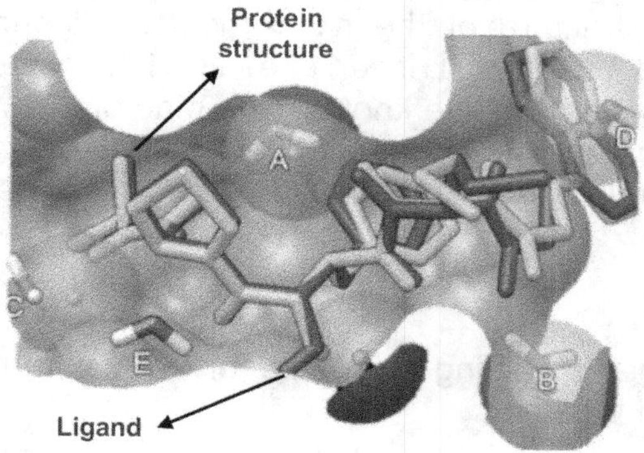

Fig. 5.18 Complexation of Drug (ligand) and Receptor (protein).

Rigid docking and flexible docking are the two types of docking. In rigid docking, the bond angles and lengths between the protein and the ligand are fixed. This technique of docking is highly rapid. But it is not applied practically because it does not consider the conformational degrees of freedom of the ligands involved. Flexible docking allows for conformational alterations and is commonly employed nowadays. However, it takes more time and depends on its computing capability.

Docking involves inserting rigid molecules or fragments into the active site of a protein (Fig.5.18) using techniques such as clique-searching, geometric hashing, or pose clustering. The search algorithm [e.g., Monte Carlo (MC) methods, genetic algorithms (GAs), fragment-based methods, Tabu searches, distance geometry methods, and scoring functions such as force field (FF) methods and empirical free energy scoring functions] determines the performance of docking. The creation of a composition of all potential conformations and orientations of the protein combined with the ligand is the first stage in docking. The scoring function then takes the data and provides a number indicating a favourable interaction.

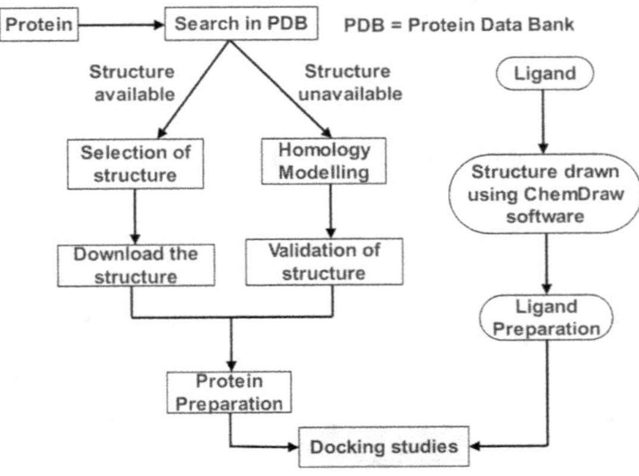

Fig. 5.19 Overview of the docking technique.

To determine the protein's active site. At first, choose the required X-ray co-crystallized structure from the protein data bank (PDB) and then extract the bound ligand to optimize the protein active site of interest. When the bound ligand is not available from the crystal structure, identifying the active position in a protein is extremely difficult. In that scenario, one must follow the steps below (Fig.5.19):

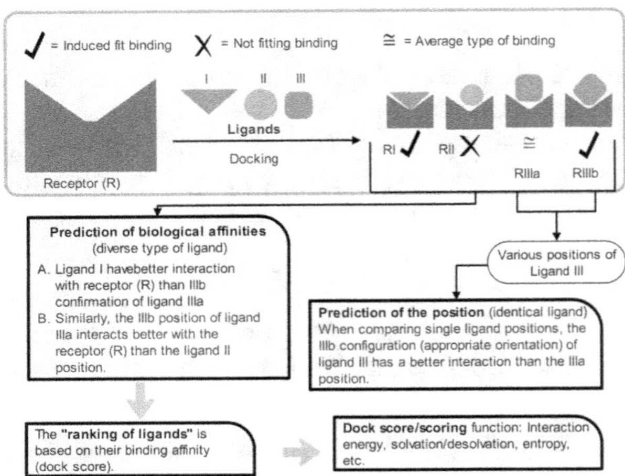

Fig. 5.20 Commonly used concepts in docking studies are displayed graphically.

1. The active site of proteins can be determined by reviewing the source literature (from which the X-ray crystal structure is included in PDB).

2. If the protein has a known drug with the same pharmacological activity, the active sites for that drug should be identified. Initially, these residues can behave as active binding sites for test ligands.

3. Each docking software tool has its algorithm for identifying the protein's active site by permitting ligand binding in different parts of the protein and examining the best probable binding position (Fig.5.20).

5.3 Combinatorial Chemistry

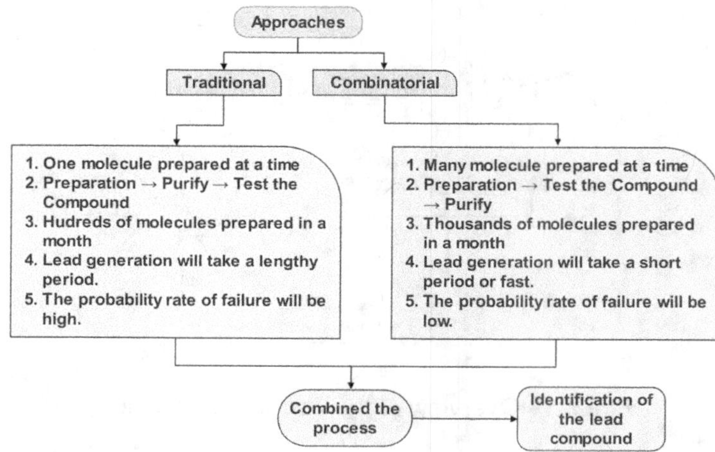

Fig. 5.21 The main differences between a traditional and a combinatorial drug discovery technique.

5.3.1 Concept of Combinatorial Chemistry

Definition

Combinatorial chemistry is the preparation of large numbers (tens of thousands or even millions) of chemical compounds in a single process. The series of chemical compounds can be generated by using computer software as a tool in the form of mixtures, sets of individual compounds, or chemical structures. Small chemical compounds and peptides can be synthesized by using combinatorial chemistry.

Chemical compounds can be manufactured in thousands and examined for biological activity using combinatorial chemistry. The development of high throughput screening techniques has mechanized the screening process, allowing for more biological experiments. The process has cut the time from discovery to market from 10-14 years to 5-8 years.

The chemist performs the usual reaction A + B $\Rightarrow$ C in a traditional organic synthesis lab. However, in combinatorial chemistry, A is a mixture of possibly

5 components and B is a mixture of 10, so the chemist now obtains 50 products instead of one. This rapidly generated collection of molecules is referred to as a library. The developed library accepts a single generic structure, such as benzodiazepine, and outputs a whole variety of benzodiazepine derivatives in a defined molecular weight range that varies in the composition of the various R groups. The result of this produces several benzodiazepine derivatives. Combinatorial chemistry is an advanced method for finding a new chemical compound from complexes due to its small changes around a general structure.

Combinatorial chemistry (Fig. 5.21) is a novel technology developed by academics and researchers in the pharmaceutical and biotechnology industries to cut the time and expense of developing effective, marketable, and competitive new drugs. Often, it is preferred by chemists to generate vast collections of compounds that can be efficiently screened via high-throughput screening. It aids in producing enormous libraries of compounds in a relatively short time.

The pharmaceutical industry has widely adopted this method for use during the drug design and screening stages of test compounds. If the drug design team discovers a "lead or promising chemical molecule," then the combinatorial technique is utilized to evaluate a large number of derivatives for the chemical compound's efficacy.

It is defined by a variety of automated high throughput synthesis strategies for producing large quantities of small organic molecules for drug discovery screening against a variety of biological targets. Synthesis, candidate screening, and purification of library products are the three basic stages in combinatorial chemistry, but chromatography is chiefly used in the final two processes.

Various analytical approaches can be used to verify library products during drug candidate screening. HPLC-MS, HPLC-DAD-MS, and HPLC-MS-MS are among these that have become key routine tools for combinatorial chemists because they offer structural information that allows them to identify the compounds that have been synthesized.

The prime goal of computer-assisted combinatorial chemistry is to create thousands of structurally varied compounds as libraries, maximizing their diversity, which is then considered in an experimental parallel automated synthesis and screening based on their properties.

The introduction of combinatorial techniques has revived random screening as a model for drug discovery and created considerable optimism about the promise of identifying new and essential drugs quickly and affordably.

5.3.2 Application of Combinatorial Chemistry

The concept of combinatorial chemistry emerged in the mid-1980s when Geysen's multi-pin technology and Houghten's tea-bag technology were implemented to simultaneously synthesize hundreds of thousands of different peptides on the solid support. Combinatorial peptide libraries with solution-phase mixtures and one-bead one-compound (OBOC) combinatorial peptide libraries were introduced in 1991. **Bunin** and **Ellman** described the first small-molecule combinatorial library in 1992. Scientists were able to generate and decode a large diversity of small molecule organic, peptide, and macrocyclic libraries in the mid-2000s.

Defination: Combinatorial synthesis is the use of automated solid phase synthetic processes to create numerous unique structures on a small scale.

Solid phase synthesis: Solid-phase processes can be carried out when the starting material is attached to a solid support like a resin bead. The linker molecule can then undergo a series of reactions. The final structure is separated from the solid support. It has various advantages by adopting the process:

1. Since the starting material, intermediates, and final product are all attached to a solid support, excess reagents or unbound by-products from each reaction can be easily removed by washing the resin.

2. A substantial surplus of reagents can be used to complete the reactions since excess reagents are easily eliminated from the process.

3. All intermediates in the reaction are bound to the bead and do not need to be purified.

4. The polymeric support can be regenerated and reused if appropriate cleavage conditions and anchor/linker groups are chosen.

5. It is possible to streamline the process.

6. In combinatorial synthesis (Fig. 5.22), different starting ingredients can be bonded to individual beads. The beads can be combined to treat all the beginning components in a single experiment. Because they are bonded to different beads, the raw components and finished products are still physically distinct. In most situations, combining the initial elements in solution chemistry leads to a sticky mess due to polymerizations and side reactions. After the experiment, the individual beads can be separated to give an individual product.

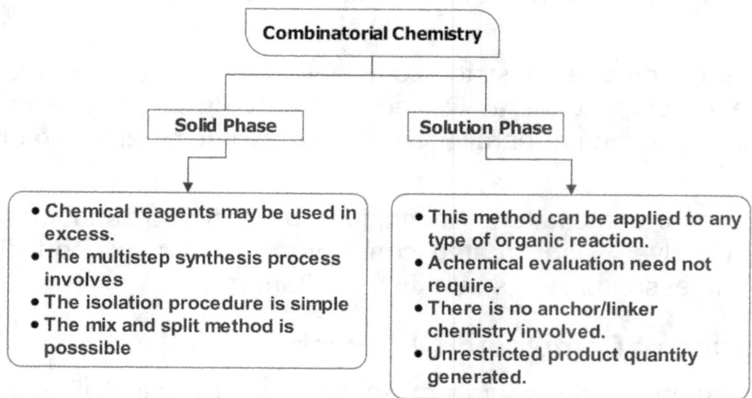

Fig. 5.22 Characteristics of combinatorial chemistry in the solid and solution phases.

The following are the prime parameters for solid-phase synthesis:

1. A synthetically inert cross-linked polymeric support (e.g., a resin bead).
2. The anchor, also known as a linker, is covalently bonded and contains a reactive functional group that can be used to attach a substrate.
3. A stable bond connects the substrate to the linker at the reaction conditions used in the synthesis.
4. A technique for separating the products or intermediates from the linker
5. Safeguarding groups for functional groups are not participating in the synthetic route.

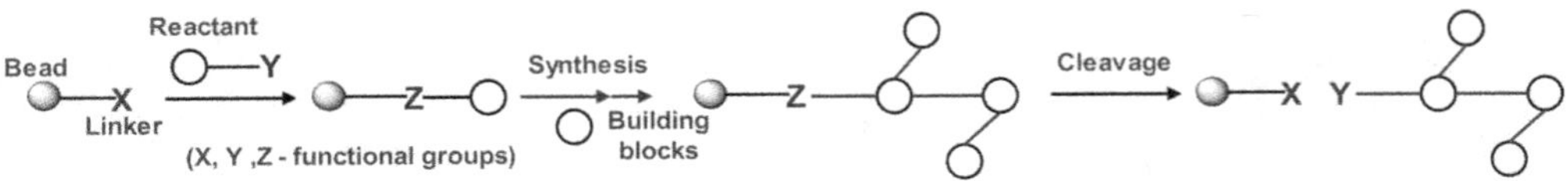

Fig. 5.23 Synthesis of solid phases.

Polymeric resins, such as beads, are used in solid-phase synthesis. Linker molecules are functionalized into each bead, allowing beginning materials to be covalently attached to the bead. After that, structures are built while still linked to the bead. Because synthetic intermediates do not need to be separated, more reagents can be used at each reaction stage, increasing overall yield.

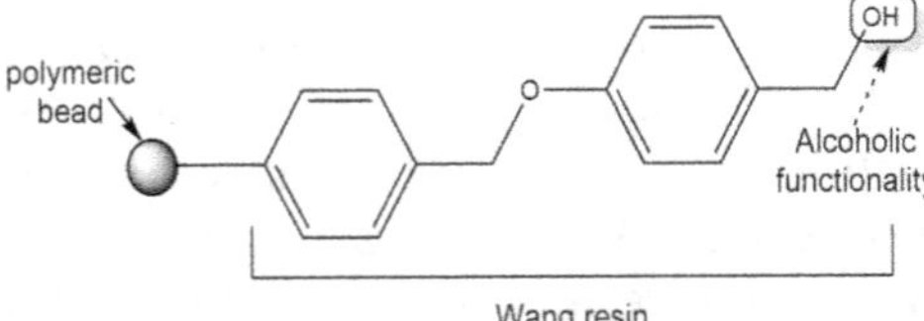

Fig. 5.24 Wang's resin.

Combinatorial synthesis makes use of solid-phase synthesis because it's well-suited to automated processes. Solid-phase synthesis requires polymeric support or resin that is inert to the reaction conditions. It is frequently in the form of tiny beads. A functional group (a linker) must also be present on the resin for molecules to be covalently attached to the solid support. The first molecule in a solid-phase synthesis is linked to the solid phase, and then the rest of the synthesis is carried out on the polymer-bound structure (Fig.5.23). The link connecting the structure to the polymer must remain stable throughout the whole reaction process. Finally, the product must be released from the polymer using appropriate reaction conditions that do not destroy the end product.

Solid-phase synthesis has various advantages, the most important of which is higher yields. There is no need to identify and purify reaction intermediates because the reaction sequence is carried out on a polymer-bound structure. Large volumes of reagents can be used to force reactions to completion, and the surplus chemicals can be easily removed by washing the resin with suitable solvents.

A variety of solid supports with diverse linkers are available, allowing molecules to be linked via various functional groups. Wang's resin, which contains an alcohol functional group as part of the linker unit, is one of the most often utilized solid supports (Fig. 5.24). As a result, carboxylic acids or carboxylic acid derivatives can be attached to this resin.

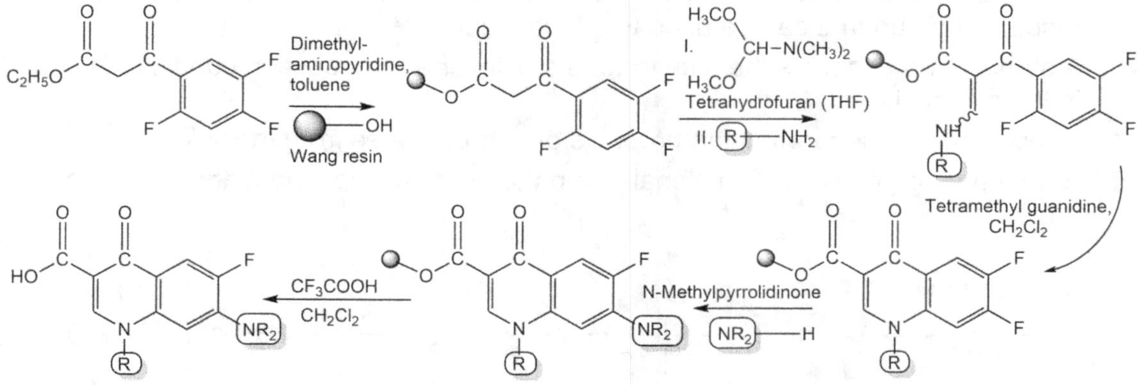

Fig. 5.25 Synthesis of fluoroquinolones by a combinatorial approach.

Fluoroquinolones are antibacterial compounds synthesized through combinatorial synthesis (see Fig.5.25). The synthesis begins with a covalent bond between the first structure and the Wang resin via an ester bond. Once the resin has been connected in the process, the remainder of the synthesis can be completed. And the final product is obtained by treating the resin with trifluoroacetic acid and drying it.

Solution phase synthesis: The initial focus of combinatorial chemistry was on solid-phase techniques because of the numerous advantages. Combinatorial chemists did not consider solution-phase synthesis suited for their work due to the time and effort required for isolation and purification. It was initially employed for compound classes [amides, sulfonamides, ureas, heterocycles (thiazole)] that were easily produced. Solution-phase combinatorial synthesis is becoming increasingly popular these days due to several advantages.

Advantages

1. In the solution phase, many reactions can be optimized.
2. There are starting materials with all reactive groups obtainable.
3. There are no restrictions on the resin's thermal or chemical stability.
4. Synthesis takes one or two stages less.
5. Reactions in solution usually require a significantly shorter time.
6. When there are insoluble components involved, the reaction is restricted to the solution phase.
7. Simple methods for monitoring reactions (TLC, NMR, UV) are available.
8. In general, reaction volumes are require less compared to end product volumes.

Parallel or solution combinatorial synthesis uses the same reaction sequence but distinct reactants and reagents for each reaction glass jar. Each vial's beads will have the same structure. However, the architecture of various vials will vary based on the reactants and reagents used. Because each reaction vial has its unique product, the structure of the molecule may be determined by the reagents used. As shown in Fig. 5.26 the amines (RNH_2 and R_2NH) introduced to each vial determine the fluoroquinolone produced.

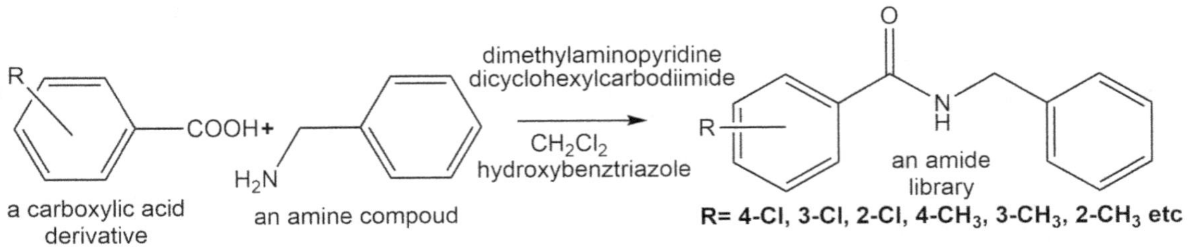

Fig. 5.26 Coupling reaction during solution-phase synthesis.

Parallel (solution phase) synthesis involves performing a reaction in a sequence of wells, each containing one product. This process is a 'quality above quantity' method that is frequently employed in lead optimization research. This process makes it efficient; the standard organic synthesis obstacles must be removed or simplified. It is possible to make one or two novel compounds per week using conventional organic synthesis methods. It allows the same researcher to synthesize dozens of pure chemicals at the same time, improving synthetic output and speeding up lead optimization.

Consider the synthesis of an amide, which is commonly accomplished by reacting a carboxylic acid with an amine in the presence of a coupling reagent such as dicyclohexylcarbodiimide (DCC) (Fig.5.26). Traditionally, once the reaction is complete, a work-up step is required. It comprises removing unreacted amine from the organic solution by washing it with aqueous acid (HCl). Subsequently, the aqueous and organic layers have been separated, the organic layer is washed with an aqueous base (NaOH, KOH, etc.) to eliminate unreacted acid. Then, the organic and basic layers are separated, and the organic layer is dried using magnesium sulfate. The drying agent is removed with filtration, followed by the removal of solvent, to produce the crude amide. Thereafter, crystallization or chromatography are required for the purification process. All of these procedures would have to be repeated to synthesize a small 12-component amide library by reacting different carboxylic acids with the same amine.

BIBLIOGRAPHY

[1] Abongwa, M., Martin, R. J., and Robertson, A. P. (2017). A brief review on the mode of action of antinematodal drugs. Acta veterinaria, 67(2):137.

[2] Adebayo, J., Tijjani, H., Adegunloye, A., Ishola, A., Balogun, E., and Malomo, S. (2020). Enhancing the antimalarial activity of artesunate. Parasitology Research, pages 1–16.

[3] Al-Badr, A. and Tariq, M. (1987). Mebendazole. In Analytical Profiles of Drug Substances, volume 16, pages 291–326. Elsevier.

[4] Alsaqabi, S. M. and Lotfy, W. M. (2014). Praziquantel: a review. Veterinary Science & Technology, 5(5):1.

[5] Anonymous (1987). Sulphamethoxazole, volume 79, page 361–378. WHO.

[6] Anonymous (2021a). Global tuberculosis reports 1997-2020. World Health organization.

[7] Anonymous (2021b). Hansch analysis. Pharmacological Sciences.

[8] Anonymous (2021c). Our history - merck.

[9] Aoki, F. Y. (2015). 45 - antivirals against herpes viruses. In Bennett, J. E., Dolin, R., and Blaser, M. J., editors, Mandell, Douglas, and Bennett's Principles and Practice of Infectious Diseases, pages 546–562.e7. W.B. Saunders, Philadelphia, eighth edition.

[10] Aparoy, P., Kumar Reddy, K., and Reddanna, P. (2012). Structure and ligand based drug design strategies in the development of novel 5-lox inhibitors. Current medicinal chemistry, 19(22):3763–3778.

[11] Araujo, O. E., Flowers, F. P., and King, M. M. (1990). Griseofulvin: a new look at an old drug. DICP, 24(9):851–854.

[12] Ball, P. (2000). Chapter 1 - the quinolones: History and overview. In Andriole, V. T., editor, The Quinolones, pages 1–31. Academic Press, San Diego, third edition.

[13] Bardal, S. K., Waechter, J. E., and Martin, D. S. (2011). Chapter 18 – infectious diseases. In Bardal, S. K., Waechter, J. E., and Martin, D. S., editors, Applied Pharmacology, pages 233–291. W.B. Saunders, Philadelphia.

[14] Barr, J. (2011). A short history of dapsone, or an alternative model of drug development. Journal of the history of medicine and allied sciences, 66(4):425–467.

[15] Batool, M., Ahmad, B., and Choi, S. (2019). A structure-based drug discovery paradigm. International journal of molecular sciences, 20(11):2783.

[16] B´egu´e, J. and Bonnet-Delpon, D. (2008). Chapter 13 - biological impacts of fluorination: Pharmaceuticals based on natural products. In Tressaud, A., editor, Fluorine and Health, pages 553–622. Elsevier, Amsterdam.

[17] Burnell, E. S. (2020). Chapter 10 - drugs targeting mitochondrial functions. In Patrick, G. L., editor, Antimalarial Agents, pages 375–402. Elsevier.

[18] Burnett, B. P. and Mitchell, C. M. (2008). Antimicrobial activity of iodoquinol 1%-hydrocortisone acetate 2% gel against ciclopirox and clotrimazole. Cutis, 82(4):273–80.

[19] Cavassin, F. B., Ba´u-Carneiro, J. L., Vilas-Boas, R. R., and Queiroz-Telles, F. (2021). Sixty years of amphotericin b: An overview of the main antifungal agent used to treat invasive fungal infections. Infectious Diseases and Therapy, pages 1–33.

[20] Chen, W., Mook Jr, R. A., Premont, R. T., and Wang, J. (2018). Niclosamide: Beyond an antihelminthic drug. Cellular signalling, 41:89–96.

[21] Corea, N. (2007). Sulfasalazine. In Enna, S. and Bylund, D. B., editors, xPharm: The Comprehensive Pharmacology Reference, pages 1–5. Elsevier, New York.

[22] da Silva, V. B. R., Campos, B. R. K. L., de Oliveira, J. F., Decout, J.-L., and de Lima, M. d. C. A. (2017). Medicinal chemistry of antischistosomal drugs: Praziquantel and oxamniquine. Bioorganic & medicinal chemistry, 25(13):3259–3277.

[23] Daina, A., Blatter, M.-C., Baillie Gerritsen, V., Palagi, P. M., Marek, D., Xenarios, I., Schwede, T., Michielin, O., and Zoete, V. (2017). Drug design workshop: A webbased educational tool to introduce computer-aided drug design to the general public. Journal of Chemical Education, 94(3):335–344.

[24] Dash, A. K. (1994). Tolnaftate. In Analytical profiles of drug substances and excipients, volume 23, pages 543–570. Elsevier.

[25] Davis, J. L. (2018). Chapter 2 - pharmacologic principles. In Reed, S. M., Bayly, W. M., and Sellon, D. C., editors, Equine Internal Medicine, pages 79–137. W.B. Saunders, fourth edition.

[26] Dax, S. L. (1997a). Peptidic antibacterial agents. In Antibacterial chemotherapeutic agents, pages 346–366. Springer.

[27] Dax, S. L. (1997b). Quinolone antibacterials. In Antibacterial chemotherapeutic agents, pages 298–345. Springer.

[28] Drouhet, E. and Dupont, B. (1987). Evolution of antifungal agents: past, present, and future. Reviews of infectious diseases, 9(Supplement 1):S4–S14.

[29] Felix, N. S. (1956). Chloramphenicol: Applied pharmacology. Pediatric Clinics of North America, 3(2):317–327. Symposium on Antimicrobial Therapy.

[30] Foye, W. O. (2000). Antibacterial agents, sulfonamides. Kirk-Othmer Encyclopedia of Chemical Technology.

[31] Goldstein, E. J. (1987). Norfloxacin, a fluoroquinolone antibacterial agent: Classification, mechanism of action, and in vitro activity. The American Journal of Medicine, 82(6, Supplement 2):3–17. Norfloxacin: A Fluoroquinolone Carboxylic Acid Antimicrobial Agent.

[32] Gonzales, M. L. M., Dans, L. F., and Sio-Aguilar, J. (2019). Antiamoebic drugs for treating amoebic colitis. Cochrane Database of Systematic Reviews, 1.

[33] Gupta, M., Sharma, R., and Kumar, A. (2018). Docking techniques in pharmacology: How much promising? Computational biology and chemistry, 76:210–217.

[34] Haller, I. (1985). Mode of action of clotrimazole: Implications for therapy. American journal of obstetrics and gynecology, 152(7):939–944.

[35] Hawser, S., Lociuro, S., and Islam, K. (2006). Dihydrofolate reductase inhibitors as antibacterial agents. Biochemical Pharmacology, 71(7):941–948. Special Issue on Antibacterials.

[36] Hooton, T. M. (2015). 304 - nosocomial urinary tract infections. In Bennett, J. E., Dolin, R., and Blaser, M. J., editors, Mandell, Douglas, and Bennett's Principles and Practice of Infectious Diseases, pages 3334–3346.e3. W.B. Saunders, Philadelphia, eighth edition.

[37] Kadavakollu, S., Stailey, C., Kunapareddy, C., and White, S. (2014). Clotrimazole as a cancer drug: a short review. Medicinal chemistry, 4(11):722.

[38] Kayukova, L. and Berikova, E. (2020). Modern anti-tuberculosis drugs and their classification. part i: First-line drugs. Pharmaceutical Chemistry Journal, pages 1–9.

[39] Kester, M., Karpa, K. D., and Vrana, K. E. (2012). 4 - treatment of infectious diseases. In Kester, M., Karpa, K. D., and Vrana, K. E., editors, Elsevier's Integrated Review Pharmacology, pages 41–78. W.B. Saunders, Philadelphia, second edition.

[40] King, D. H. (1988). History, pharmacokinetics, and pharmacology of acyclovir. Journal of the American Academy of dermatology, 18(1):176–179.

[41] Kresge, N., Simoni, R. D., and Hill, R. L. (2004). Selman waksman: the father of antibiotics. Journal of Biological Chemistry, 279(48):e7–e7.

[42] Kunze, K. L., Nelson, W. L., Kharasch, E. D., Thummel, K. E., and Isoherranen, N. (2006). Stereochemical aspects of itraconazole metabolism in vitro and in vivo. Drug metabolism and disposition, 34(4):583–590.

[43] Kutlushina, A., Khakimova, A., Madzhidov, T., and Polishchuk, P. (2018). Ligandbased pharmacophore modeling using novel 3d pharmacophore signatures. Molecules, 23(12):3094.

[44] Lemke, T., Williams, D., Roche, V., and Zito, S. (2012). Foye's principles of medicinal chemistry. Wolters Kluwer Health Adis, seventh edition.

[45] Lin, H., Dai, C., Jamison, T. F., and Jensen, K. F. (2017). A rapid total synthesis of ciprofloxacin hydrochloride in continuous flow. Angewandte Chemie International Edition, 56(30):8870–8873.

[46] Liu, R., Li, X., and Lam, K. S. (2017). Combinatorial chemistry in drug discovery. Current opinion in chemical biology, 38:117–126.

[47] Lo, T. S., Hammer, K. D., Zegarra, M., and Cho, W. C. (2014). Methenamine: a forgotten drug for preventing recurrent urinary tract infection in a multidrug resistance era. Expert Review of Anti-infective Therapy, 12(5):549–554.

[48] Lundblad, R. (2016). Drug design. In Bradshaw, R. A. and Stahl, P. D., editors, Encyclopedia of Cell Biology, pages 135–140. Academic Press, Waltham.

[49] Ma, Z., Ginsberg, A., and Spigelman, M. (2007). 7.24 - antimycobacterium agents. In Taylor, J. B. and Triggle, D. J., editors, Comprehensive Medicinal Chemistry II, pages 699 730. Elsevier, Oxford.

[50] Maertens, J. (2004). History of the development of azole derivatives. Clinical Microbiology and Infection, 10:1–10.

[51] Markovic, M., Ben-Shabat, S., and Dahan, A. (2020). Prodrugs for improved drug delivery: Lessons learned from recently developed and marketed products. Pharmaceutics, 12(11):1031.

[52] Martins, N., Barros, L., Henriques, M., Silva, S., and Ferreira, I. C. (2015). Activity of phenolic compounds from plant origin against candida species. Industrial Crops and Products, 74:648–670.

[53] Masters, P. A., O'Bryan, T. A., Zurlo, J., Miller, D. Q., and Joshi, N. (2003). Trimethoprim-Sulfamethoxazole Revisited. Archives of Internal Medicine, 163(4):402– 410.

[54] McAuley, J. B., Herwaldt, B. L., Stokes, S. L., Becher, J. A., Roberts, J. M., Michelson, M. K., and Juranek, D. D. (1992). Diloxanide furoate for treating asymptomatic entamoeba histolytica cyst passers: 14 years' experience in the united states. Clinical infectious diseases, 15(3):464–468.

[55] McCarthy, J. S. and Moore, T. A. (2015). 42 - drugs for helminths. In Bennett, J. E., Dolin, R., and Blaser, M. J., editors, Mandell, Douglas, and Bennett's Principles and Practice of Infectious Diseases, pages 519–527.e3. W.B. Saunders, Philadelphia, eighth edition.

[56] McCarthy, J. S., Wortmann, G. W., and Kirchhoff, L. V. (2015). 41 - drugs for protozoal infections other than malaria. In Bennett, J. E., Dolin, R., and Blaser, M. J., editors, Mandell, Douglas, and Bennett's Principles and Practice of Infectious Diseases, pages 510–518.e3. W.B. Saunders, Philadelphia, eighth edition.

[57] McChesney, J. D. (1981). Considerations about the structure—activity relationships of 8-aminoquinoline antimalarial drugs. Bulletin of the World Health Organization, 59(3):459.

[58] Miertus, S., Fassina, G., and Seneci, P. (2000). Concepts of combinatorial chemistry and combinatorial technologies. Chemick´e listy, 94(12).

[59] Muraleedharan, K. and Avery, M. (2007). 7.27 - advances in the discovery of new antimalarials. In Taylor, J. B. and Triggle, D. J., editors, Comprehensive Medicinal Chemistry II, pages 765–814. Elsevier, Oxford.

[60] Murray, J. F., Schraufnagel, D. E., and Hopewell, P. C. (2015). Treatment of tuberculosis. a historical perspective. Annals of the American Thoracic Society, 12(12):1749–1759.

[61] Najjar, A. and Karaman, R. (2019). The prodrug approach in the era of drug design. Expert opinion on drug delivery, 16(1):1–5.

[62] Nett, J. E. and Andes, D. R. (2016). Antifungal agents: spectrum of activity, pharmacology, and clinical indications. Infectious Disease Clinics, 30(1):51–83.

[63] Nomoto, S. and Shiba, T. (1979). Syntheses of capreomycin analogs in relation to their antibacterial activities. Bulletin of the Chemical Society of Japan, 52(6):1709–1715.

[64] Nomoto, S., Teshima, T., Wakamiya, T., and Shiba, T. (1977). The revised structure of capreomycin. The Journal of antibiotics, 30(11):955–959.

[65] Offermanns, S. and Rosenthal, W. (2008). Encyclopedia of molecular pharmacology. Springer Science & Business Media.

[66] Padda, I. S. and Reddy, K. M. (2020). Antitubercular medications. StatPearls [Internet].

[67] Page, S. W. (2008). Chapter 10 - antiparasitic drugs. In Maddison, J. E., Page, S. W., and Church, D. B., editors, Small Animal Clinical Pharmacology, pages 198–260. W.B. Saunders, Edinburgh, second edition.

[68] Pandeya, S. N. (2006). A Text book of medicinal chemistry: Synthetic and biochemical approach, volume 2. SG Publisher, third edition.

[69] Pasko, M. T., Piscitelli, S. C., and Van Slooten, A. D. (1990). Fluconazole: a new triazole antifungal agent. Dicp, 24(9):860–867.

[70] Patrick, G. L. (2001). Instant notes on Medicinal chemistry. BIOS, first edition.

[71] Patrick, G. L. (2013). An introduction to medicinal chemistry. Oxford University Press, 5th edition.

[72] Patrick, G. L. (2017). An Introduction to Medicinal Chemistry. Oxford University Press.

[73] Pollak, E. and Indinavir, P. M. (2021). Indinavir. StatPearls [Internet].

[74] Quercia, R., Perno, C.-F., Koteff, J., Moore, K., McCoig, C., Clair, M. S., and Kuritzkes, D. (2018). Twenty-five years of lamivudine: current and future use for the treatment of hiv-1 infection. Journal of acquired immune deficiency syndromes, 78(2):125.

[75] Riley, T. N. (1988). The prodrug concept and new drug design and development. Journal of Chemical Education, 65(11):947.

[76] Roy, K., Kar, S., and Das, R. N. (2015). Chapter 10 - other related techniques. In Roy, K., Kar, S., and Das, R. N., editors, Understanding the Basics of QSAR for Applications in Pharmaceutical Sciences and Risk Assessment, pages 357–425. Academic Press, Boston.

[77] Samuelson, J. (1999). Why metronidazole is active against both bacteria and parasites. Antimicrobial agents and chemotherapy, 43(7):1533–1541.

[78] Sanchez, S. and Demain, A. (2011). 1.12 - secondary metabolites. In Moo-Young, M., editor, Comprehensive Biotechnology (Second Edition), pages 155–167. Academic Press, Burlington.

[79] Sands, M., Kron, M. A., and Brown, R. B. (1985). Pentamidine: a review. Reviews of infectious diseases, 7(5):625–6344.

[80] Sarukhan, A. (2019). Ivermectin: From soil to worms, and beyond.

[81] Sch¨on, T., Jur´een, P., Giske, C. G., Chryssanthou, E., Štureg°ard, E., Werngren, J., Kahlmeter, G., Hoffner, S. E., and ¨Angeby, K. A. (2009). Evaluation of wild-type mic distributions as a tool for determination of clinical breakpoints for mycobacterium tuberculosis. Journal of antimicrobial chemotherapy, 64(4):786–793.

[82] Sensi, P. (1983). History of the development of rifampin. Reviews of infectious diseases, 5(Supplement 3):S402–S406.

[83] Shafiei, M., Peyton, L., Hashemzadeh, M., and Foroumadi, A. (2020). History of the development of antifungal azoles: A review on structures, sar, and mechanism of action. Bioorganic Chemistry, 104:104240.

[84] Sharma, S. and Anand, N. (1997a). Chapter 21 - miscellaneous antiprotozoals. In Sharma, S. and Anand, N., editors, Approaches to Design and Synthesis of Antiparasitic Drugs, volume 25 of Pharmacochemistry Library, pages 468–488. Elsevier.

[85] Sharma, S. and Anand, N. (1997b). Salicylanilides. In Pharmacochemistry Library, volume 25, pages 239–257. Elsevier.

[86] Singh, H. and Kapoor, V. K. (2005). Medicinal and pharmaceutical chemistry. Vallabh Prakashan, 2nd edition.

[87] Smadel, J. E. (1949). Chloramphenicol (chloromycetin) in the treatment of infectious diseases. The American Journal of Medicine, 7(5):671–685. Symposium on Diabetes Mellitus.

[88] Storer, R. (1996). Solution-phase synthesis in combinatorial chemistry: Applications in drug discovery. Drug Discovery Today, 1(6):248–254.

[89] Stuetz, A., Georgopoulos, A., Granitzer, W., Petranyi, G., and Berney, D. (1986). Synthesis and structure-activity relationships of naftifine-related allylamine antimycotics. Journal of medicinal chemistry, 29(1):112–125.

[90] Sweeney, T. R. (1981). The present status of malaria chemotherapy: Mefloquine, a novel antimalarial. Medicinal Research Reviews, 1(3):281–301.

[91] Thai, T., Salisbury, B. H., and Zito, P. M. (2020). Ciprofloxacin. StatPearls [Internet].

[92] Thompson, P. E. andWerbel, L. M. (1972). Quinine and related alkaloids. In Thompson, P. E. and Werbel, L. M., editors, Antimalarial Agents, volume 12 of Medicinal Chemistry, pages 62–78. Elsevier.

[93] Vardanyan, R. and Hruby, V. (2006). 37 - drugs for treating protozoan infections. In Vardanyan, R. and Hruby, V., editors, Synthesis of Essential Drugs, pages 559–582. Elsevier, Amsterdam.

[94] Waller, D. G. and Sampson, A. P. (2018). 51 - chemotherapy of infections. In Waller, D. G. and Sampson, A. P., editors, Medical Pharmacology and Therapeutics, pages 581 629. Elsevier, fifth edition.

[95] Wender, P. A. (2017). Gilbert stork (1921-2017). Nature, 551(7680):566–567.

[96] Wikipedia (2021). Alexander Fleming — Wikipedia, the free encyclopedia.

[97] Wolfe, A. D. (1975). Quinacrine and other acridines, pages 203–233. Springer, Berlin, Heidelberg.

[98] Yadav, G. and Ganguly, S. (2015). Structure activity relationship (sar) study of benzimidazole scaffold for different biological activities: A mini-review. European Journal of Medicinal Chemistry, 97:419–443.

[99] Yang, S.-Y. (2010). Pharmacophore modeling and applications in drug discovery: challenges and recent advances. Drug discovery today, 15(11-12):444–450.

[100] Zinner, S. H. and Mayer, K. H. (2015). 33 - sulfonamides and trimethoprim. In Bennett, J. E., Dolin, R., and Blaser, M. J., editors, Mandell, Douglas, and Bennett's Principles and Practice of Infectious Diseases, pages 410–418.e2. W.B. Saunders, Philadelphia, eighth edition.

INDEX